Arteriogenesis and Therapeutic Angiogenesis

Arteriogenesis and Therapeutic Angiogenesis

Editors

Paul Quax
Elisabeth Deindl

MDPI • Basel • Beijing • Wuhan • Barcelona • Belgrade • Manchester • Tokyo • Cluj • Tianjin

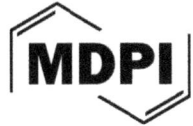

Editors
Paul Quax
Leiden University Medical
Center
The Netherlands

Elisabeth Deindl
Ludwig-Maximilians-Universität
München
Germany

Editorial Office
MDPI
St. Alban-Anlage 66
4052 Basel, Switzerland

This is a reprint of articles from the Special Issue published online in the open access journal *International Journal of Molecular Sciences* (ISSN 1422-0067) (available at: https://www.mdpi.com/journal/ijms/special_issues/Arteriogenesis_Angiogenesis).

For citation purposes, cite each article independently as indicated on the article page online and as indicated below:

LastName, A.A.; LastName, B.B.; LastName, C.C. Article Title. *Journal Name* **Year**, *Volume Number*, Page Range.

ISBN 978-3-0365-2716-1 (Hbk)
ISBN 978-3-0365-2717-8 (PDF)

Cover image courtesy of Elisabeth Deindl
Artist: Xenia Deindl: Leukocytes orchestrate vascularization

© 2021 by the authors. Articles in this book are Open Access and distributed under the Creative Commons Attribution (CC BY) license, which allows users to download, copy and build upon published articles, as long as the author and publisher are properly credited, which ensures maximum dissemination and a wider impact of our publications.

The book as a whole is distributed by MDPI under the terms and conditions of the Creative Commons license CC BY-NC-ND.

Contents

About the Editors vii

Elisabeth Deindl and Paul H. A. Quax
Arteriogenesis and Therapeutic Angiogenesis—An Update
Reprinted from: *Int. J. Mol. Sci.* **2021**, *22*, 13244, doi:10.3390/ijms222413244 1

Goren Saenz-Pipaon, Esther Martinez-Aguilar, Josune Orbe, Arantxa González Miqueo, Leopoldo Fernandez-Alonso, Jose Antonio Paramo and Carmen Roncal
The Role of Circulating Biomarkers in Peripheral Arterial Disease
Reprinted from: *Int. J. Mol. Sci.* **2021**, *22*, 3601, doi:10.3390/ijms22073601 5

Mohamed Sabra, Catherine Karbasiafshar, Ahmed Aboulgheit, Sidharth Raj, M. Ruhul Abid and Frank W. Sellke
Clinical Application of Novel Therapies for Coronary Angiogenesis: Overview, Challenges, and Prospects
Reprinted from: *Int. J. Mol. Sci.* **2021**, *22*, 3722, doi:10.3390/ijms22073722 29

Lucía Beltrán-Camacho, Marta Rojas-Torres and Mª Carmen Durán-Ruiz
Current Status of Angiogenic Cell Therapy and Related Strategies Applied in Critical Limb Ischemia
Reprinted from: *Int. J. Mol. Sci.* **2021**, *22*, 2335, doi:10.3390/ijms22052335 45

Jasni Viralippurath Ashraf and Ayman Al Haj Zen
Role of Vascular Smooth Muscle Cell Phenotype Switching in Arteriogenesis
Reprinted from: *Int. J. Mol. Sci.* **2021**, *22*, 10585, doi:10.3390/ijms221910585 73

Zeen Aref and Paul H. A. Quax
In Vivo Matrigel Plug Assay as a Potent Method to Investigate Specific Individual Contribution of Angiogenesis to Blood Flow Recovery in Mice
Reprinted from: *Int. J. Mol. Sci.* **2021**, *22*, 8909, doi:10.3390/ijms22168909 91

Matthias Kübler, Philipp Götz, Anna Braumandl, Sebastian Beck, Hellen Ishikawa-Ankerhold and Elisabeth Deindl
Impact of *C57BL/6J* and *SV-129* Mouse Strain Differences on Ischemia-Induced Postnatal Angiogenesis and the Associated Leukocyte Infiltration in a Murine Hindlimb Model of Ischemia
Reprinted from: *Int. J. Mol. Sci.* **2021**, *22*, 11795, doi:10.3390/ijms222111795 103

Matthias Kübler, Sebastian Beck, Lisa Lilian Peffenköver, Philipp Götz, Hellen Ishikawa-Ankerhold, Klaus T. Preissner, Silvia Fischer, Manuel Lasch and Elisabeth Deindl
The Absence of Extracellular Cold-Inducible RNA-Binding Protein (eCIRP) Promotes Pro-Angiogenic Microenvironmental Conditions and Angiogenesis in Muscle Tissue Ischemia
Reprinted from: *Int. J. Mol. Sci.* **2021**, *22*, 9484, doi:10.3390/ijms22179484 119

Eveline A. C. Goossens, Licheng Zhang, Margreet R. de Vries, J. Wouter Jukema, Paul H. A. Quax and A. Yaël Nossent
Cold-Inducible RNA-Binding Protein but Not Its Antisense lncRNA Is a Direct Negative Regulator of Angiogenesis In Vitro and In Vivo via Regulation of the 14q32 angiomiRs—microRNA-329-3p and microRNA-495-3p
Reprinted from: *Int. J. Mol. Sci.* **2021**, *22*, 12678, doi:10.3390/ijms222312678 141

Yasuo Yoshitomi, Takayuki Ikeda, Hidehito Saito-Takatsuji and Hideto Yonekura
Emerging Role of AP-1 Transcription Factor JunB in Angiogenesis and Vascular Development
Reprinted from: *Int. J. Mol. Sci.* **2021**, *22*, 2804, doi:10.3390/ijms22062804 . . . . **159**

Wineke Bakker, Calinda K. E. Dingenouts, Kirsten Lodder, Karien C. Wiesmeijer, Alwin de Jong, Kondababu Kurakula, Hans-Jurgen J. Mager, Anke M. Smits, Margreet R. de Vries, Paul H. A. Quax and Marie José T. H. Goumans
BMP Receptor Inhibition Enhances Tissue Repair in Endoglin Heterozygous Mice
Reprinted from: *Int. J. Mol. Sci.* **2021**, *22*, 2010, doi:10.3390/ijms22042010 . . . . **173**

Dilara Z. Gatina, Ekaterina E. Garanina, Margarita N. Zhuravleva, Gulnaz E. Synbulatova, Adelya F. Mullakhmetova, Valeriya V. Solovyeva, Andrey P. Kiyasov, Catrin S. Rutland, Albert A. Rizvanov and Ilnur I. Salafutdinov
Proangiogenic Effect of 2A-Peptide Based Multicistronic Recombinant Constructs Encoding VEGF and FGF2 Growth Factors
Reprinted from: *Int. J. Mol. Sci.* **2021**, *22*, 5922, doi:10.3390/ijms22115922 . . . . **191**

Fabiana Baganha, Laila Ritsma, Paul H. A. Quax and Margreet R. de Vries
Assessment of Microvessel Permeability in Murine Atherosclerotic Vein Grafts Using Two-Photon Intravital Microscopy
Reprinted from: *Int. J. Mol. Sci.* **2020**, *21*, 9244, doi:10.3390/ijms21239244 . . . . **207**

About the Editors

Paul Quax (PhD) obtained his PhD at the University of Leiden, the Netherlands, on the role of plasminogen activators in tissue remodeling. He kept on working on this topic in relation to vascular remodeling, first at the Gaubius Laboratory TNO and later at the Leiden University Medical Center as professor in experimental vascular medicine. His interest in arteriogenesis was driven by the lack of therapeutic options for patients with peripheral arterial disease. Therapeutic arteriogenesis and angiogenesis induced by gene therapy, growth factors, modulation of inflammatory and immune response but also by modulation of microRNAs and other noncoding RNAs in small animal model are topics of his research.

Elisabeth Deindl (Dr) graduated at the ZMBH in Heidelberg, Germany, where she worked on hepatitis B viruses. Thereafter, she joined the lab of Wolfgang Schaper at the Max-Planck-Institute in Bad Nauheim, where she started to decipher the molecular mechanisms of arteriogenesis. After a short detour on stem cells, she focused again on arteriogenesis becoming a leading expert in the field. By using a peripheral model of arteriogenesis, she demonstrated that collateral artery growth is a matter of innate immunity and presents a blueprint of sterile inflammation, which is locally triggered by extracellular RNA.

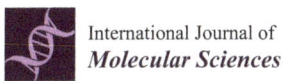

Editorial

Arteriogenesis and Therapeutic Angiogenesis—An Update

Elisabeth Deindl [1,2,*] and Paul H. A. Quax [3,*]

1. Walter-Brendel-Centre of Experimental Medicine, University Hospital, Ludwig-Maximilians-Universität, 81377 Munich, Germany
2. Biomedical Center, Institute of Cardiovascular Physiology and Pathophysiology, Ludwig-Maximilians-Universität München, Planegg-Martinsried, 82152 Munich, Germany
3. Department of Surgery, Einthoven Laboratory for Experimental Vascular Medicine, Leiden University Medical Center, 2300 RC Leiden, The Netherlands
* Correspondence: elisabeth.deindl@med.uni-muenchen.de (E.D.); p.h.a.quax@lmuc.nl (P.H.A.Q.); Tel.: +49-89-2180-76504 (E.D.); +31-71-526-1584 (P.H.A.Q.)

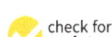

Citation: Deindl, E.; Quax, P.H.A. Arteriogenesis and Therapeutic Angiogenesis—An Update. *Int. J. Mol. Sci.* **2021**, 22, 13244. https://doi.org/10.3390/ijms222413244

Received: 3 December 2021
Accepted: 6 December 2021
Published: 9 December 2021

Publisher's Note: MDPI stays neutral with regard to jurisdictional claims in published maps and institutional affiliations.

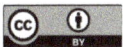

Copyright: © 2021 by the authors. Licensee MDPI, Basel, Switzerland. This article is an open access article distributed under the terms and conditions of the Creative Commons Attribution (CC BY) license (https://creativecommons.org/licenses/by/4.0/).

Vascular occlusive diseases such myocardial infarction, peripheral artery disease of the lower extremities, or stroke still represent a substantial health burden worldwide. In recent times, they have come even more into focus as thromboembolic events associated with vascular occlusive diseases are known to belong to the severe complications observed in patients with SARS-CoV-2 infection [1]. To understand the mechanisms of blood flow recovery in terms of arteriogenesis and therapeutic angiogenesis is a major goal in order to develop efficacious non-invasive treatment options for afflicted.

This Special Issue of the *International Journal of Molecular Sciences* entitled "Arteriogenesis and Therapeutic Angiogenesis" follows up with recent advances that are specific to that field of research.

One of the most important points is to identify vascular occlusive diseases already in their beginning or early progression, enabling clinicians to induce natural bypass growth—a process that is defined as arteriogenesis or that is referred to as therapeutic angiogenesis—in time [2,3]. Since patients who are at that stage are often asymptomatic, this represents a considerable challenge. In the current issue, Saenz-Pipaon et al. describe the need for reliable biomarkers for peripheral artery disease (PAD), whereby they focus on the lower limbs. PADs have a high prevalence, show a poor prognosis, and are associated with a high risk of myocardial infarction and stroke. In their article, Saenz-Pipaon et al. discuss the appropriateness of inflammatory molecules, liquid biopsies, and non-coding RNAs and even focus on the potential of machine learning methods [4].

Mohamed Sabra and colleagues describe the mechanisms of vascularization, i.e. vasculogenesis, angiogenesis, and arteriogenesis, and critically elucidate the usefulness of angiogenic therapies such as protein therapy, gene therapy, stem cell therapy, and extracellular vesical therapy. Moreover, they address the relevance of patient selection and delivery methods, and introduce bioinformatics and bioengineering as promising future tools for the treatment of patients with vascular occlusive diseases [5]. The paper by Beltrain-Camacho focusses on angiogenic cell therapy as a treatment option for critical limb ischemia, and also the use of microRNAs, exosomes, and secretomes are briefly discussed [6].

The article by Ashraf and Zen is more oriented towards basic science and deals with the function of the quiescent contractile and the proliferative synthetic phenotypes of a vascular smooth muscle cell (VSMC) as well as the molecular mechanisms and regulations of phenotype switching. Moreover, the article critically addresses the option to target phenotype switching in patients aiming to promote arteriogenesis [7].

Zeen Aref and Paul Quax highlight the difficulty of investigating the mechanisms of angiogenesis in hind limb ischemia models that are associated with arteriogenesis. They introduce an in vivo Matrigel plug assay, which is superior to current hind limb models, as it allows the analysis of ischemia-induced angiogenesis without the influence of collateral artery growth that is occurring in parallel [8]. Besides arteriogenesis also the mouse strain chosen has a major influence on the outcome of angiogenesis. Kübler et al. address this topic and explain the relevance of selecting the appropriate mouse stain depending on the scientific question that is asked. In particular, they focus on the influence of C57BL/6J and SV-129 strain-related differences in leukocyte recruitment in ischemic angiogenesis [9].

Cold-inducible RNA-binding protein (CIRP or CIRBP) is a stress inducible protein that contains RNA and protein binding domains and that has recently come into the focus of vascular research [10–12]. In the current issue of the *International Journal of Molecular Sciences*, two groups have independently shown that the absence of CIRP promotes angiogenesis in ischemic muscle tissue, and, interestingly enough, they have identified two independent mechanisms. Kübler et al. have demonstrated that the absence of extracellular CIRP results in a reduced number of M1-like polarized pro-inflammatory and an increased number of M2-like polarized regenerative macrophages associated with reduced tissue damage and an increased capillary to muscle fiber ratio [13]. Goossens et al. have identified CIRBP as a negative modulator of angiogenesis through its function to regulate the angiomiRs miR-329-3p and miR-495-3p [14], which have previously been shown to be involved in vascular regeneration [10].

Yoshitomi and colleagues present the role of the AP-1 transcription factor family Jun B in angiogenesis and highlight its function in tip cell formation and tissue-specific vascular maturation [15].

Endoglin is a co-receptor of transforming growth factor-β1 (TGF-β1), and mutations of this transmembrane protein are known to cause the vascular disorder hereditary hemorrhagic telangiectasia type 1(HHT1). By investigating *Eng+/−* mice in a myocardial infarction model, Bakker et al. were able to show that these mice display more M1-like polarized macrophages, whereas the number of M2-like polarized macrophages was reduced. These data somehow reflect data from the clinic, as patients with HHT1 also show an increased number of inflammatory macrophages. Astonishingly, the treatment of *Eng+/−* mice with a bone morphogenetic protein (BMP) receptor kinase inhibitor improved heart function and vascularization, suggesting that the BMP receptor kinase may present a promising therapeutic target for HHT1 patients in the future [16].

Gatina and co-workers investigated the serviceability of recombinant multicistronic mutagenic contructs in terms of safety and efficacy to treat ischemic disease. By using 2A-peptide-based constructs encoding vascular endothelial growth factor (VEGF) and fibroblast growth factor 2 (FGF2), they were able to demonstrate increased levels of the named recombinant proteins along with an increased number of capillary-like structures in genetically modified human umbilical vein endothelial cells (HUVECs) in vitro [17]. Last not least, Baganha et al. investigated the suitability of two-photon intravital microscopy (2P-IVM) to assess the permeability of microvessels in atherosclerotic vein grafts in mice. From their study, they concluded that 2P-IVM is a promising tool that can be used to analyze plaque angiogenesis and leakiness in preclinical atherosclerosis models in vivo [18].

In summary, we think that our new Special Issue on arteriogenesis and therapeutic angiogenesis is a rewarding collection of original and review articles in the field of vascular research that will serve as inspiration for future pioneering investigations looking into the treatment of vascular occlusive diseases.

Funding: This research received no external funding.

Conflicts of Interest: The authors declare no conflict of interest.

References

1. Preissner, K.T.; Fischer, S.; Deindl, E. Extracellular RNA as a Versatile DAMP and Alarm Signal That Influences Leukocyte Recruitment in Inflammation and Infection. *Front. Cell Dev. Biol.* **2020**, *8*, 619221. [CrossRef] [PubMed]
2. Deindl, E.; Quax, P.H.A. Arteriogenesis and Therapeutic Angiogenesis in Its Multiple Aspects. *Cells* **2020**, *9*, 1439. [CrossRef] [PubMed]
3. Faber, J.E.; Chilian, W.M.; Deindl, E.; van Royen, N.; Simons, M. A brief etymology of the collateral circulation. *Arterioscler. Thromb. Vasc. Biol.* **2014**, *34*, 1854–1859. [CrossRef] [PubMed]

4. Saenz-Pipaon, G.; Martinez-Aguilar, E.; Orbe, J.; Gonzalez Miqueo, A.; Fernandez-Alonso, L.; Paramo, J.A.; Roncal, C. The Role of Circulating Biomarkers in Peripheral Arterial Disease. *Int. J. Mol. Sci.* **2021**, *22*, 3601. [CrossRef] [PubMed]
5. Sabra, M.; Karbasiafshar, C.; Aboulgheit, A.; Raj, S.; Abid, M.R.; Sellke, F.W. Clinical Application of Novel Therapies for Coronary Angiogenesis: Overview, Challenges, and Prospects. *Int. J. Mol. Sci.* **2021**, *22*, 3722. [CrossRef] [PubMed]
6. Beltran-Camacho, L.; Rojas-Torres, M.; Duran-Ruiz, M.C. Current Status of Angiogenic Cell Therapy and Related Strategies Applied in Critical Limb Ischemia. *Int. J. Mol. Sci.* **2021**, *22*, 2335. [CrossRef] [PubMed]
7. Ashraf, J.V.; Al Haj Zen, A. Role of Vascular Smooth Muscle Cell Phenotype Switching in Arteriogenesis. *Int. J. Mol. Sci.* **2021**, *22*, 10585. [CrossRef] [PubMed]
8. Aref, Z.; Quax, P.H.A. In Vivo Matrigel Plug Assay as a Potent Method to Investigate Specific Individual Contribution of Angiogenesis to Blood Flow Recovery in Mice. *Int. J. Mol. Sci.* **2021**, *22*, 8909. [CrossRef] [PubMed]
9. Kubler, M.; Gotz, P.; Braumandl, A.; Beck, S.; Ishikawa-Ankerhold, H.; Deindl, E. Impact of C57BL/6J and SV-129 Mouse Strain Differences on Ischemia-Induced Postnatal Angiogenesis and the Associated Leukocyte Infiltration in a Murine Hindlimb Model of Ischemia. *Int. J. Mol. Sci.* **2021**, *22*, 11795. [CrossRef] [PubMed]
10. Downie Ruiz Velasco, A.; Welten, S.M.J.; Goossens, E.A.C.; Quax, P.H.A.; Rappsilber, J.; Michlewski, G.; Nossent, A.Y. Post-transcriptional Regulation of 14q32 MicroRNAs by the CIRBP and HADHB during Vascular Regeneration after Ischemia. *Mol. Ther.-Nucleic Acids* **2019**, *14*, 329–338. [CrossRef] [PubMed]
11. Kubler, M.; Beck, S.; Fischer, S.; Gotz, P.; Kumaraswami, K.; Ishikawa-Ankerhold, H.; Lasch, M.; Deindl, E. Absence of Cold-Inducible RNA-Binding Protein (CIRP) Promotes Angiogenesis and Regeneration of Ischemic Tissue by Inducing M2-Like Macrophage Polarization. *Biomedicines* **2021**, *9*, 395. [CrossRef] [PubMed]
12. Zhong, P.; Huang, H. Recent progress in the research of cold-inducible RNA-binding protein. *Future Sci. OA* **2017**, *3*, FSO246. [CrossRef] [PubMed]
13. Kubler, M.; Beck, S.; Peffenkover, L.L.; Gotz, P.; Ishikawa-Ankerhold, H.; Preissner, K.T.; Fischer, S.; Lasch, M.; Deindl, E. The Absence of Extracellular Cold-Inducible RNA-Binding Protein (eCIRP) Promotes Pro-Angiogenic Microenvironmental Conditions and Angiogenesis in Muscle Tissue Ischemia. *Int. J. Mol. Sci.* **2021**, *22*, 9484. [CrossRef] [PubMed]
14. Goossens, E.A.C.; Zhang, L.; de Vries, M.R.; Jukema, J.W.; Quax, P.H.A.; Nossent, A.Y. Cold-Inducible RNA-Binding Protein but Not Its Antisense lncRNA Is a Direct Negative Regulator of Angiogenesis In Vitro and In Vivo via Regulation of the 14q32 angiomiRs—microRNA-329-3p and microRNA-495-3p. *Int. J. Mol. Sci.* **2021**, *22*, 12678. [CrossRef]
15. Yoshitomi, Y.; Ikeda, T.; Saito-Takatsuji, H.; Yonekura, H. Emerging Role of AP-1 Transcription Factor JunB in Angiogenesis and Vascular Development. *Int. J. Mol. Sci.* **2021**, *22*, 2804. [CrossRef] [PubMed]
16. Bakker, W.; Dingenouts, C.K.E.; Lodder, K.; Wiesmeijer, K.C.; de Jong, A.; Kurakula, K.; Mager, H.J.; Smits, A.M.; de Vries, M.R.; Quax, P.H.A.; et al. BMP Receptor Inhibition Enhances Tissue Repair in Endoglin Heterozygous Mice. *Int. J. Mol. Sci.* **2021**, *22*, 2010. [CrossRef]
17. Gatina, D.Z.; Garanina, E.E.; Zhuravleva, M.N.; Synbulatova, G.E.; Mullakhmetova, A.F.; Solovyeva, V.V.; Kiyasov, A.P.; Rutland, C.S.; Rizvanov, A.A.; Salafutdinov, I.I. Proangiogenic Effect of 2A-Peptide Based Multicistronic Recombinant Constructs Encoding VEGF and FGF2 Growth Factors. *Int. J. Mol. Sci.* **2021**, *22*, 5922. [CrossRef] [PubMed]
18. Baganha, F.; Ritsma, L.; Quax, P.H.A.; de Vries, M.R. Assessment of Microvessel Permeability in Murine Atherosclerotic Vein Grafts Using Two-Photon Intravital Microscopy. *Int. J. Mol. Sci.* **2020**, *21*, 9244. [CrossRef] [PubMed]

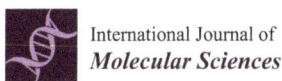

International Journal of Molecular Sciences

Review

The Role of Circulating Biomarkers in Peripheral Arterial Disease

Goren Saenz-Pipaon [1,2,†], Esther Martinez-Aguilar [2,3,†], Josune Orbe [1,2,4], Arantxa González Miqueo [2,4,5], Leopoldo Fernandez-Alonso [2,3], Jose Antonio Paramo [1,2,4,6] and Carmen Roncal [1,2,4,*]

1. Laboratory of Atherothrombosis, Program of Cardiovascular Diseases, Cima Universidad de Navarra, 31008 Pamplona, Spain; gsaenzdepip@alumni.unav.es (G.S.-P.); josuneor@unav.es (J.O.); japaramo@unav.es (J.A.P.)
2. IdiSNA, Instituto de Investigación Sanitaria de Navarra, 31008 Pamplona, Spain; esthermartinezaguilar@hotmail.com (E.M.-A.); amiqueo@unav.es (A.G.M.); leopoldofa@gmail.com (L.F.-A.)
3. Departamento de Angiología y Cirugía Vascular, Complejo Hospitalario de Navarra, 31008 Pamplona, Spain
4. CIBERCV, Instituto de Salud Carlos III, 28029 Madrid, Spain
5. Laboratory of Heart Failure, Program of Cardiovascular Diseases, Cima Universidad de Navarra, 31008 Pamplona, Spain
6. Hematology Service, Clínica Universidad de Navarra, 31008 Pamplona, Spain
* Correspondence: croncalm@unav.es; Tel.: +34-948194700
† These authors contributed equally to this work.

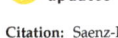

Citation: Saenz-Pipaon, G.; Martinez-Aguilar, E.; Orbe, J.; González Miqueo, A.; Fernandez-Alonso, L.; Paramo, J.A.; Roncal, C. The Role of Circulating Biomarkers in Peripheral Arterial Disease. *Int. J. Mol. Sci.* 2021, 22, 3601. https://doi.org/10.3390/ijms22073601

Academic Editors: Paul Quax and Elisabeth Deindl

Received: 26 February 2021
Accepted: 26 March 2021
Published: 30 March 2021

Publisher's Note: MDPI stays neutral with regard to jurisdictional claims in published maps and institutional affiliations.

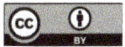

Copyright: © 2021 by the authors. Licensee MDPI, Basel, Switzerland. This article is an open access article distributed under the terms and conditions of the Creative Commons Attribution (CC BY) license (https://creativecommons.org/licenses/by/4.0/).

Abstract: Peripheral arterial disease (PAD) of the lower extremities is a chronic illness predominantly of atherosclerotic aetiology, associated to traditional cardiovascular (CV) risk factors. It is one of the most prevalent CV conditions worldwide in subjects >65 years, estimated to increase greatly with the aging of the population, becoming a severe socioeconomic problem in the future. The narrowing and thrombotic occlusion of the lower limb arteries impairs the walking function as the disease progresses, increasing the risk of CV events (myocardial infarction and stroke), amputation and death. Despite its poor prognosis, PAD patients are scarcely identified until the disease is advanced, highlighting the need for reliable biomarkers for PAD patient stratification, that might also contribute to define more personalized medical treatments. In this review, we will discuss the usefulness of inflammatory molecules, matrix metalloproteinases (MMPs), and cardiac damage markers, as well as novel components of the liquid biopsy, extracellular vesicles (EVs), and non-coding RNAs for lower limb PAD identification, stratification, and outcome assessment. We will also explore the potential of machine learning methods to build prediction models to refine PAD assessment. In this line, the usefulness of multimarker approaches to evaluate this complex multifactorial disease will be also discussed.

Keywords: peripheral arterial disease; biomarkers; inflammation; coagulation; extracellular vesicles; microRNAs; machine learning

1. Introduction

The term peripheral arterial disease (PAD) includes a range of non-coronary arterial syndromes that are caused by an alteration in the structure and function of the arteries supplying the brain, visceral organs, and extremities. Numerous pathophysiological processes can contribute to the formation of stenosis or aneurysms in the non-coronary circulation, but atherosclerosis is the most common lesion that affects the aorta and its branches [1,2]. In this review, we will focus on lower extremity PAD referring to the chronic lower limb ischemia of atherosclerotic origin.

It has been estimated that PAD affects 12–14% of the general population, approximately 202 million people across the world [2,3]. Its prevalence increases with age, affecting around 10–25% of people older than 55 years, and 40% of those older than 80 years, being associated with significant morbidity, mortality, and quality of life impairment [4,5].

PAD, frequently accompanied by atherosclerosis in other vascular beds, exhibits higher risk of ischemic events and death compared to other cardiovascular (CV) pathologies. Likewise, coronary artery disease (CAD) is present in approximately 60–80% of patients with PAD, whereas 12–25% suffer accompanying carotid artery stenosis [3,5]. In the REACH (Reduction of Atherothrombosis for Continued Health) study 4.7% of PAD patients suffered from concomitant coronary disease, 1.2% from concurrent cerebrovascular disease, and 1.6% presented both. Similarly, about one-third of men and one- quarter of women with known coronary or cerebrovascular disease are diagnosed with PAD [6]. Moreover, the severity of PAD is also associated to the prevalence of CAD. Conversely, left main coronary artery stenosis and multivessel CAD are independent predictors of PAD, and patients with PAD exhibit more advanced coronary atherosclerosis [2]. As a consequence, PAD patients present a 20–60% higher risk of myocardial infarction, and a 2–6 fold higher risk of death due to a coronary event [5,7], while the risk of stroke increases by approximately 40% [3,5]. The ARIC (Atherosclerosis Risk in Communities) study conducted among men with PAD showed 4–5 times higher risk of having a stroke or a transient ischemic attack than those without PAD, although in women, the association was not significant [8]. Indeed, it has been recently described that PAD is an equivalent risk factor to CAD for CV death [5].

Individual risk estimation of PAD is based on the Fontaine or Rutherford classification in combination with the ankle-brachial pressure index (ABI), which is the current gold standard for vascular severity categorization. The aforementioned scales divide lower extremity PAD into two major groups: namely patients with intermittent claudication (IC, Fontaine I and II), the most common clinical presentation at early stages associated to mild symptoms, and chronic limb-threatening ischemia (CLI, Fontaine III and IV) including patients at more advanced stages that can develop ischemic ulcerations or gangrene of the foot [9]. The ABI is a non-invasive test able to detect arterial occlusive disease in symptomatic patients, but more importantly, also in asymptomatic patients, presenting a sensitivity of 95% and a specificity of 100% compared with arteriography when assessing PAD vs controls. ABI values ≤ 0.90 are generally considered diagnostic of PAD although so far, no strong evidence supports its relationship with CV morbi-mortality or a reduction in thrombotic events and death by the treatment of screening-detected PAD patients [4]. Despite the high discriminative power of ABI for stenotic plaques, it is not useful to identify patients at the initial phases of the disease, when atherosclerotic lesions are not big enough to promote a hemodynamically significant stenosis. Moreover, in the subgroup of diabetic patients ABI loses sensitivity due to arterial calcification, often rendering values above 1.4, that have not been correlated clinically with increased CV morbidity and mortality [4]. In consequence, PAD is often undiagnosed and untreated, especially in the early stages of the pathology or in diabetic patients, presenting silent rates of about 50% [5], highlighting the need of early diagnosis and prognosis markers, and novel therapeutic targets for lower limb PAD.

Considering the lack of precise biomarkers for PAD assessment, and the key role of inflammation and vessel remodelling in atherosclerotic plaque progression and rupture, several authors have evaluated the levels of proteins related to those pathological processes in this regard (Figure 1). The circulating concentrations of some cytokines (C reactive protein (CRP) or Interleukin (IL)-6), coagulation factors (D-dimer or fibrinogen), proteases (Matrix metalloproteinases (MMPs) and their inhibitors, tissue inhibitors of metalloproteinases (TIMPs)) or cardiac damage markers have been reported to be increased in PAD patients according to pathological stages and CV complications [10–13], while other oxidative stress markers, and angiogenesis-related molecules rendered inconclusive results [12]. Most interestingly, extracellular vesicles (EVs) and non-coding RNAs are emerging as novel biomarkers and/or biological effectors in PAD pathophysiology [14,15]. Whether these candidates will improve the risk estimation associated to traditional CV risk factors is still unclear and will need to be further evaluated, not only by single biomarker assessment, but also and more interestingly, by combining groups of biomarkers and clinical parameters. Machine learning (ML) offers the possibility to model large datasets integrating all biological variables [16]. By doing so, these algorithms build prediction models aiming to help clinicians to better diagnose and estimate CV risk also in the context of PAD.

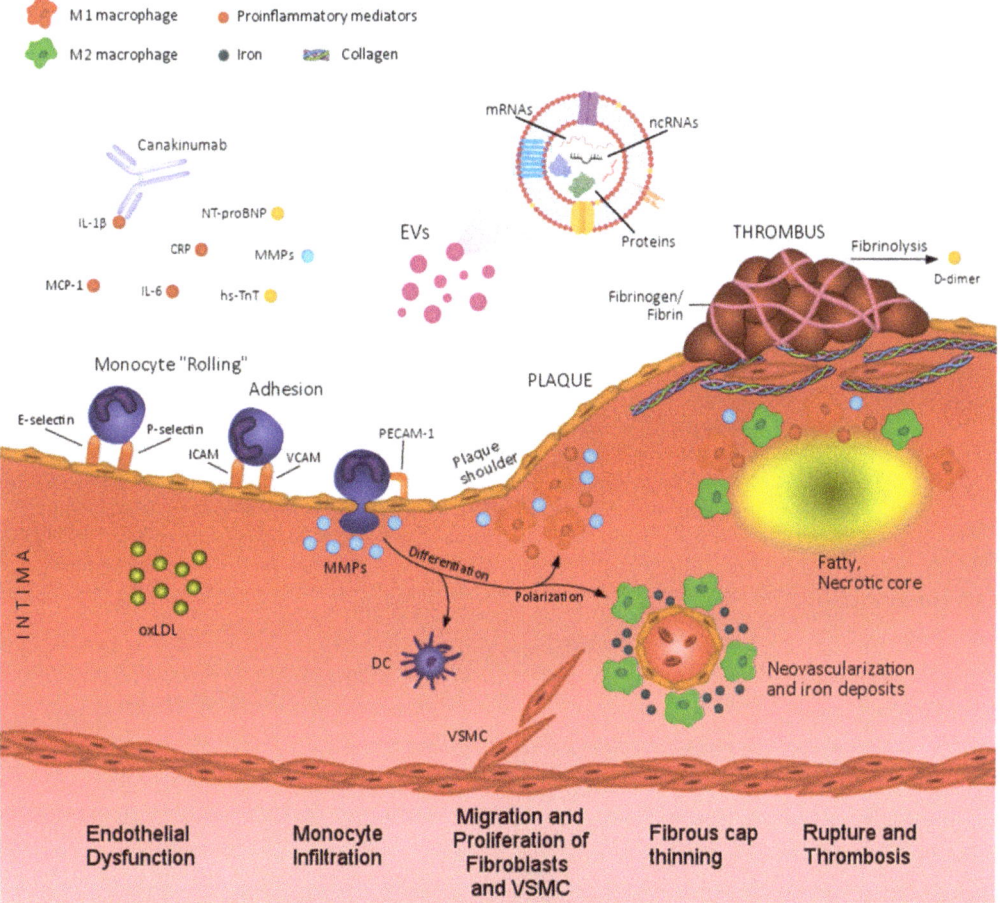

Figure 1. Circulating biomarkers in atherosclerosis and PAD pathophysiology. At early stages of atherosclerosis, endothelial dysfunction leads to increased levels of proinflammatory cytokines (IL1β, IL6, CRP, MCP-1), extracellular vesicles (EVs), proteases (MMPs), and adhesion molecules (E-selectin, P-selectin, ICAM, VCAM,) that contribute to monocyte recruitment and infiltration into the intima. Microenvironmental factors such as MMPs orchestrate plaque progression by regulating macrophage polarization towards proinflammatory (M1) or anti-inflammatory (M2) phenotypes, which are predominantly located in unstable areas (i.e.,: plaque shoulder) or neovascularization regions, respectively. In advanced lesions, inflammatory factors and MMPs exacerbate fibrous cap thinning and contribute to plaque instability, rupture, and formation of fibrin clot. Extracellular vesicles (EVs), mainly of platelet origin, also participate in thrombus formation according to the exposure of procoagulant factors (e.g.,: tissue factor and phosphatidylserine). In addition, reduced tissue perfusion due to arterial stenosis and thrombosis might cause increased levels of tissue damage-related biomarkers such as NT-proBNP or hs-TnT. CRP, C reactive protein; DC, dendritic cells; ICAM, intercellular adhesion molecule; IL, interleukin; MCP-1, monocyte chemoattractant protein; MMPs, matrix metalloproteinases; NT-proBNP, N-terminal pro-brain natriuretic peptide; oxLDL, oxidized Low Density Lipoproteins; hs-TnT, high sensitivity troponin T; VCAM, vascular cell adhesion molecule; VSMC, vascular Smooth Muscle Cells.

In this review, we will summarize the current status of different sets of circulating biomarkers, EVs, and non-coding RNAs for lower extremity PAD diagnosis and outcome assessment. Moreover, we will also discuss how the implementation of multimarker approaches and machine learning methods can produce more accurate disease classification and prediction models.

2. Inflammation and Coagulation Biomarkers in PAD

Low grade inflammation has been involved in all the phases of PAD, from atherosclerosis initiation to progression, and from plaque rupture to thrombosis. Accordingly, in the last decades several inflammatory and haemostatic molecules have been evaluated as possible biomarkers for PAD assessment, although it still remains controversial how or whether they will be able to outperform traditional CV risk factors [17,18] (Table 1). CRP, an acute phase reactant, is one of the most studied inflammatory molecules for PAD evaluation. Early in 2001, Ridker PM et al. reported the use of CRP as a potential marker of incident PAD [19], which was later confirmed by other authors [14,20]. In addition, several prospective studies have reported increased levels of CRP in PAD patients compared to controls [14,21–24] and an association with PAD severity and ABI [25–27]. CRP has also been proposed as a marker of worse outcome considering major CV events (stroke and myocardial infarction), major amputation/revascularization and mortality in high risk PAD patients [14,23,28], although it has been suggested that CRP might be more useful for short-term risk prediction rather than for long-term evaluation [29,30]. In this line, a meta-analysis by Singh TP et al. including studies with samples sizes ranging from 51 to 1157 patients reported an associated hazard ratio of 2.26 (1.65–3.09) for the categorized CRP variable and CV events and death in a follow-up ≤2 years [11]. Similarly, Kremers B et al. comprising 13 studies found that patients with increased CRP levels had a relative risk of 1.86 (1.48–2.33) for major adverse cardiovascular events (MACE), and of 3.49 (2.35–5.19) for mortality [10]. These evidences suggest the potential use of CRP for PAD diagnosis and prognosis. It is worth considering however, that some of the summarized papers were conducted with a limited number of patients (Table 1), and that in many cases risk prediction was estimated in the short term, rather than in the long term.

Table 1. Inflammatory biomarkers in lower limb PAD diagnosis and prognosis.

Assessed Biomarkers	Type of Biomarker	Studied Groups (n)	Outcome	Refs.
CRP, D-dimer, fibrinogen, NT-proBNP and cTnT	Prognosis	Systematic review and meta-analysis with 47 studies, 1990–2015. PAD patients (21,473). Minimum follow up 1 year.	Increased CRP (RR: 3.49, 95% CI: 2.35–5.19), D-dimer (RR: 2.22, 1.24–3.98), fibrinogen (RR: 2.08, 95% CI: 1.46–2.97), NT-proBNP (RR: 4.50, 95% CI: 2.98–6.81) and cTnT (RR: 3.33, 95% CI: 2.70–4.10) predicted risk of mortality in PAD patients. Association of CRP with MACE (RR: 1.86, 95% CI: 1.48–2.33).	[10]
CRP	Prognosis	Systematic review and meta-analysis with 16 studies, 2002–2017. Participants (5041). Minimum follow up 1 year.	Higher CRP levels predict MACE in PAD patients (HR: 1.38, 95% CI: 1.16–1.63, per unit increase in $\log_e$CRP).	[11]
CRP	Diagnosis Prognosis	PAD patients (317) and healthy controls (100). Mean follow up 3.6 years.	Increased CRP levels in PAD patients. Predictor of amputation (SHR: 1.76, 95% CI: 1.48–2.09) and MACE (amputation and CV mortality) (SHR: 1.53, 95% CI: 1.35–1.75).	[14]

Table 1. Cont.

Assessed Biomarkers	Type of Biomarker	Studied Groups (n)	Outcome	Refs.
CRP	Diagnosis	Prospective cohort (14916); symptomatic PAD (140) and healthy controls (140). Mean follow up 9 years.	Associated to incident PAD (RR: 2.8, 95% CI: 1.3–5.9).	[19]
CRP	Diagnosis	ARIC Study 1996–1998. Participants (9851), cases of PAD (316). Median follow up 17.4 years.	Associated to incident PAD and CLI (HR per 1 SD increase: 1.34, 95% CI: 1.18–1.52 and 1.34, 95% CI: 1.09–1.65, respectively).	[20]
CRP, IL-6 & TNF-α	Diagnosis	PAD patients (55) and healthy controls (34).	Increased CRP, IL-6 and TNF-α levels in PAD patients. IL-6 associated to PAD severity (ABI $\leq$ 0.90).	[21]
CRP, IL-6, TNF-α & ICAM-1	Diagnosis	PAD patients with intermittent claudication (75) and healthy subject (43).	Increased CRP, IL-6, TNF-α and ICAM-1 levels in PAD patients and inversely associated with maximal walking distance.	[22]
CRP, IL-6, TNF-α & VCAM-1	Diagnosis Prognosis	PAD patients (60) and healthy controls (50). Mean follow up of 2.24 years.	Increased CRP, IL-6 and TNF-α levels in PAD patients. CRP, IL-6, TNF-α and ICAM-1 associated with ABI. PAD patients with CRP > 1 mg/L had 4-fold higher risk of ischemic event or death.	[23]
CRP, IL-6, ICAM-1 & D-dimer	Diagnosis	PAD patients (62) and healthy controls (18).	Increased CRP, IL-6, ICAM-1 and D-dimer levels in PAD patients.	[24]
CRP, IL-6, TNF-α, ICAM-1 & fibrinogen	Diagnosis Prognosis	Framingham Offspring Study 1998–2001. Participants (2800), ABI < 0.9 (111).	CRP, IL-6, TNF-α and fibrinogen inversely associated to ABI. IL-6 related to ABI (OR: 1.21, 95% CI: 1.06–1.38) and intermittent claudication or lower extremity revascularization (OR: 1.36, 95% CI: 1.06–1.74).	[26]
CRP, IL-6, ICAM-1 & VCAM-1	Diagnosis	Edinburgh Artery Study 1988. Participants (2800). Follow up 5 and 12 years.	CRP, IL-6, ICAM-1 and VCAM-1 associated to PAD severity. IL-6 predicted ABI at 5 and 12 years.	[27]
CRP	Prognosis	PAD patients with (29) or without (38) adverse CV events. Follow up 5 years.	CRP levels were higher in PAD subjects with adverse CV events.	[28]
CRP	Prognosis	PAD patients (397). Average follow up 6.6 years.	CRP predicts total mortality at 2-years follow-up (HR = 1.56 per SD).	[29]
CRP & D-dimer	Prognosis	PAD patients (377). Follow up 4 years.	CRP and D-dimer predicts all-cause mortality within 1 and 2 years of follow-up (HR: 1.15, 95% CI: 1.06–1.24 and 1.14, 95% CI: 1.02–1.27, respectively).	[30]
CRP, D-dimer & fibrinogen	Diagnosis	PAD patients (45) and healthy controls (44).	CRP, D-dimer and fibrinogen were higher in PAD and associated to ABI.	[31]
CRP	Diagnosis	PAD patients (463). Mean follow up 6.1 years.	Higher CRP levels in patients with CLI compared to IC.	[25]
CRP	Prognosis	PAD patients (68). Follow up 6 months.	Pre- and post-operative (24 h) IL-6 levels and post-operative (24 h) CRP levels associated with six-month in-stent restenosis (OR: 1.11, 95% CI: 1.00–1.23, 1.04, 95% CI: 1.02–1.06 and 1.15, 95% CI: 1.04–1.26, respectively).	[32]

Table 1. *Cont.*

Assessed Biomarkers	Type of Biomarker	Studied Groups (n)	Outcome	Refs.
IL-6, TNF-α, ICAM-1 & VCAM-1	Diagnosis	PAD patients (20) and healthy controls (20).	Circulating IL-6, TNF-α, ICAM-1 and VCAM-1 levels were higher in PAD patients.	[33]
IL-6, TNF-α, ICAM-1 & VCAM-1	Diagnosis	PAD patients (80) and healthy controls (72).	All inflammatory and adhesion markers were higher in PAD patients.	[34]
CRP, IL-6, ICAM-1, VCAM-1 and D-dimer	Diagnosis	PAD patients (423).	CRP, IL-6, ICAM-1, VCAM-1 and D-dimer related to impaired lower limb functionality.	[35]
IL-6	Diagnosis	PAD patients (38). 1 year follow up.	Higher IL-6 levels were related to impaired walking distance.	[36]
VCAM-1	Diagnosis	PAD patients (51) and healthy controls (75).	VCAM-1 is increased in PAD patients.	[37]
ICAM-1, VCAM-1 & D-dimer	Diagnosis	PAD patients (60) and healthy controls (20).	ICAM-1, VCAM-1 and D-dimer increased in CLI patients.	[38]
Fibrinogen	Prognosis	FRENA registry. PAD patients (1363). Mean follow up 18 months.	High fibrinogen associated with ischemic events (HR: 1.61, 95% CI: 1.11–2.32) or major bleeding (HR: 3.42, 95% CI: 1.22–9.61).	[39]
Fibrinogen	Prognosis	LEADER trial 1992-2001. PAD patients (785). Follow up 3 years.	Fibrinogen predictor of death at 6 months (OR: 1.65, 95% CI: 0.96–2.73) and 3 years (OR: 1.44, 95% CI: 1.02–1.94).	[40]
Fibrinogen	Prognosis	PAD patients (486). Median follow up 7 years.	Fibrinogen levels predict risk of all-cause mortality (HR: 1.90, 95% CI: 1.11–3.41 for fibrinogen >12.2μmol/L) and CV death (HR: 2.68, 95% CI: 1.39–5.16 for fibrinogen >12.2 μmol/L).	[41]
D-dimer	Prognosis	BRAVO study 2009. PAD patients (595). Follow up 3 years.	D-dimer levels were increased in PAD patients 2 months before an ischemic heart event.	[42]
NLR	Diagnosis	PAD patients (733). Median follow-up 10.4 months.	Elevated NLR associated with severe PAD (OR: 1.07, 95% CI: 1.00–1.15).	[43]
NLR	Diagnosis	PAD patients (300).	NLR inversely associated with ABI.	[44]
NLR	Diagnosis	PAD patients (153) and controls (128).	NLR correlated to PAD severity.	[45]
NLR	Prognosis	CLI patients (172). Mean follow up 34.7 months.	NLR predicted amputation risk (HR: 1.14, 95% CI: 1.08–1.19).	[46]
NLR	Prognosis	PAD patients (593). Median follow-up 20 months.	High NLR (>3.0) was an independent predictor of long-term cardiovascular mortality (HR: 2.04, 95% CI: 1.26–3.30).	[47]
NLR	Prognosis	PAD patients (95). Follow up 2 years.	Postoperative high NLR (≥2.75) predicts target vessel revascularization (HR: 3.1, 95% CI: 1.3–7.7) in PAD subjects after angioplasty with stent implantation.	[48]
NLR	Prognosis	CLI patients (561). Median follow up 31 months.	Preoperative high NLR (>5) correlated with 5-year amputation-free survival (HR: 2.32, 95% CI 1.73–3.12) in PAD patients subjected to infrainguinal revascularization.	[49]

Table 1. Cont.

Assessed Biomarkers	Type of Biomarker	Studied Groups (n)	Outcome	Refs.
NLR	Prognosis	PAD patients (1228). Minimum follow up 1 year.	Preoperative NLR associated with MALE (HR: 1.09, 95% CI: 1.07–1.11) and 10-year mortality (HR: 1.09, 95% CI: 1.07–1.12) after revascularization (stenting/bypass graft).	[50]
NLR	Prognosis	PAD patients (83). Follow-up period 12 months.	PAD patients with high NLR ($\geq$5.25) had increased risk of death (HR: 1.97, 95% CI: 1.08–3.62) compared with low NLR subjects (<5.25).	[51]

CRP, C reactive protein; IL-6, interleukin-6; TNF-α, tumor necrosis factor α; ICAM-1, intercellular adhesion molecule 1; VCAM-1, vascular cell adhesion molecule 1; NLR, neutrophil-to-lymphocyte ratio; ABI, Ankle brachial index; MACE, major adverse cardiovascular events; MALE, major adverse limb events; PAD, peripheral arterial disease; IC, intermittent claudication; CLI, Critic limb ischemia; HR, Hazard ratio; SHR, Sub-Hazard ratio; RR, Relative risk; SD, standard deviation.

The impact of other inflammatory biomarkers for PAD diagnosis and prognosis has been also evaluated (Table 1). For instance, IL-6, IL-8, pentraxin-3, neutrophil gelatinase-associated lipocalin (NGAL), calprotectin or tumor necrosis factor (TNF)-α were significantly higher in PAD patients compared with healthy controls [14,21–24,33,34], and some of these candidates; IL-6, TNF-α, and pentraxin-3 were associated to PAD severity, assessed either by ABI or clinical scales [21,23,52]. Among those pro-inflammatory markers, IL-6 stands out as a prominent predictor of functional outcomes. In the Edinburgh Artery Study, IL-6 showed more consistent and stronger independent predictive value than CRP and soluble adhesion molecules for PAD progression [27]. As such, initial levels of IL-6 showed an association with ABI changes at five and 12 years of follow-up, while CRP was only associated with ABI changes at 12 years [27]. Similarly, Murabito JM et al. described that among different inflammatory molecules, namely CD40L, CRP, monocyte chemoattractant protein (MCP)-1, and myeloperoxidase, only IL-6 and TNF receptor (TNFR)-2 remained significantly associated with hemodynamic or clinical PAD after adjustment for confounding factors [26]. Levels of inflammatory biomarkers have been also explored in relation to lower limb functional impairment in PAD patients with claudication, showing an inverse correlation between high levels of IL-6 and TNF-α with the maximal walking time [22]. In line with these results, increased blood concentrations of CRP and IL-6 were significantly correlated with poorer six-minute walk performance in PAD [35]. Recently Russell KS et al. reported that reducing inflammation with an anti-IL-1β neutralizing antibody (canakinumab) improved walking performance in PAD patients and IC [36]. The canakinumab treated patients presented a reduction in blood CRP and IL-6, that was more significant and consistent for circulating IL-6 compared to CRP during the follow-up [36]. Regarding in-stent restenosis, Ueki Y et al. found no differences in the maximum change of IL-6, MCP-1, and TNF-α between patients with and without restenosis with a mean follow-up of 1 year [53], while a latest study by Guo S et al. reported an independent association between the pre- and post-operative (24 h) IL-6 levels and six-month in-stent restenosis, while for CRP the association was only found with the 24 h postintervention levels [32]. In summary, these data support a prominent role of inflammation in PAD, specially of IL-6, and suggest that its pharmacological modulation, even if indirect, might be a therapeutic alternative for PAD patients. Larger studies should be performed to corroborate the possible use of IL-6 as a biomarker for PAD and/or as pharmacological target.

The lack of reliable biomarkers in PAD has extended the study to adhesion molecules, selectins, and haemostatic candidates rendering dissimilar results. Higher circulating levels of soluble intercellular adhesion molecule (ICAM)-1, vascular cell adhesion molecule (VCAM)-1, E-Selectin, L-Selectin, P-Selectin, neopterin, serum amyloid A, and D-dimer have been reported in PAD patients compared to control groups, while for fibrinogen only a moderate increase was found [22,24,31,33,34,37]. Another study reported differences in blood levels of P-Selectin, platelet factor 4, VCAM, thrombin-antithrombin complex, prothrombin fragments 1+2, and D-dimer only when assessing CLI vs control, but not when IC was examined [38], whereas Beckman JA et al. found no differences at all in VCAM-1 and ICAM-1 levels between PAD patients and controls [23]. Similarly, blood concentrations of P-selectin, ICAM-1, and fibrinogen have been significantly related to both ABI and clinical PAD in the Framingham Offspring Study participants [26], while other authors found no such associations [23,37]. In the Edinburgh Artery Study, only ICAM-1, but not VCAM-1 or E-selectin, was independently correlated with changes in ABI at 12 years of follow-up [27]. Additionally, a slower fast-paced walking speed was associated to higher levels of VCAM-1, ICAM-1 and D-dimer in PAD patients [22,35]. Regarding other outcomes, increased fibrinogen levels were associated with subsequent ischemic events and major bleeding at the FRENA (Factores de Riesgo y Enfermedad Arterial) registry [39] and with mortality risk in other studies [40,41]. Similarly, D-dimer, the degradation product of crosslinked fibrin, was increased in PAD patients suffering ischemic heart disease compared to the non-event group [42], and was associated with all-cause mortality within 1 and 2 years of follow-up [30]. Finally, the neutrophil-to-lymphocyte ratio (NLR), obtained from the hemogram data, has been shown to be predictor of PAD diagnosis [43–45,54] and poor outcome [46,55]. Ertuk M et al. described a two-fold increase in CV mortality risk in IC and CLI patients presenting NLR>3 [47]. Moreover, in patients undergoing endovascular intervention high preoperative NLR has been independently associated to post-procedural restenosis [48], major adverse limb events (MALE) and death [49–51,54]. Despite the abundant evidences gathered in the literature, the role of adhesion and hemostatic molecules for PAD diagnosis and prognosis still remains unclear. One of the main limitations might be related to the disparity in the recruited patient numbers among different studies (Table 1). The NLR however, easier to calculate from the hemogram, seems a promising candidate in PAD assessment, although risk prediction stratification would benefit from a comparable NLR cut-off point in different scenarios.

Multimarker approach: PAD is a multifactorial disease and single biomarker determination might not be able to completely reflect the complex pathophysiological processes underlying vascular remodeling. Moreover, different inflammatory proteins might represent distinct molecular pathways operating through different mechanisms [56]. In consequence, it has been proposed that a multimarker approach might be more useful for PAD evaluation [10]. For instance, in the ARIC study the addition of galectin-3 and hs-CRP to traditional atherosclerotic predictors improved the risk prediction of PAD incidence [20]. Regarding PAD severity, Egnot NS et al. identified two biomarker groups associated to low ABI; one consisting of the inflammatory markers CRP, IL-6 and fibrinogen, and the second including the coagulation markers D-dimer and pentraxin-3 [57]. Surprisingly coagulation markers presented a stronger association with lower ABI compared to inflammatory molecules [57]. As such, the relative risk for cardiovascular mortality on IC, but not on CLI, was five times higher when considering the combination of α-defensin and CRP than when assessing either α-defensin, or CRP alone [25]. In addition, a recent report from our lab shows that the combination of calprotectin and CRP increased the risk for amputation and CV mortality when compared with each protein independently [14]. These reports suggest that single biomarker approaches might be too simplistic to predict complex multifactorial diseases such as PAD, and urge the discovery of those molecular partners that in combination might render the best outcome for PAD assessment.

3. MMPs/TIMPs in PAD

MMPs are a family of zinc-dependent enzymes that catalyse the proteolysis of extracellular matrix proteins, being negatively regulated by the TIMPs (−1 to −4) that directly bind to their catalytic domain. MMPs are produced by many inflammatory cells participating in numerous physiological and pathological processes. In atherosclerosis, MMPs dysregulation is associated with leukocyte infiltration, vascular smooth muscle cell (VSMC) migration and plaque formation. Moreover, MMPs seem to be involved in vascular remodelling, intimal thickness, and lumen narrowing during restenosis after endovascular treatment of atherosclerotic lesions.

Circulating MMPs are being increasingly recognized as biomarkers of atherosclerosis and CV risk. In PAD, MMPs have been implicated in the inflammatory process of atherosclerosis, degrading collagen and allowing VSMC migration within the vessel wall, leading to vessel occlusion and ischemia. In a large community-based study, patients with previously undetected ABI ≤ 0.9 presented higher levels of the MMP-2/MMP-9 ratio compared to non-PAD control subjects (1.4 > ABI > 0.9) [58], and high levels of both gelatinases, MMP-2 and -9, were also reported in diagnosed PAD patients compared to controls [24,34]. As for other MMPs: MMP-1, -3, -7, -10, -12, and -13 were elevated in PAD patients vs. controls, while TIMP-1 levels were lower [59,60]. Furthermore, MMP-8, -9, -10, and -13 significantly correlated with lipid levels, and MMP-10 with age and hypertension in PAD patients [59]. These data suggest that MMPs may be associated with PAD development, although to corroborate that the combined measurement of MMPs and ABI will be able to improve the diagnosis and posterior treatment of PAD, further long-term and larger studies should be performed.

Moreover, patients with CLI, the most severe form of PAD, had increased MMP-10 and TIMP-1 levels compared with IC, and those in the highest MMP-10 tertile presented an elevated incidence of mortality, either all-cause or CV [60]. In line with this results, Tayebjee MH et al. observed higher MMP-9 and TIMP-1 levels in CLI patients compared with IC, that correlated with white cell count, whereas no differences were reported in circulating TIMP-2 [61]. It has been proposed that the observed rise in circulating TIMP-1 in CLI could be related to the increased proteolytic activity of vascular patients, or reflect the enhanced fibrosis shown by these subjects [60,61]. Likewise, skeletal muscles of CLI patients presented increased mRNA and protein levels of MMP-9, -19, TIMP-1 and -2 compared to controls, whereas MMP-2 rendered inconclusive results [62]. In experimental models of hind limb ischemia, the levels and activity of MMP-2, -9, and -10 significantly increased in crural muscle after femoral artery ligation [63–65], and MMP-9 deficiency resulted in reduced tissue perfusion. The role of MMP-9 in arteriogenesis and angiogenesis still remains controversial. As such, Meisner JK et al. reported decreased necrotic and fibroadipose tissue clearance in MMP-9 knockout mice after femoral artery ligation despite normal arteriogenic and angiogenic vascular growth [66], while other authors described reduced capillary density and impaired EPC mobilization in absence of MMP-9 [67,68]. In addition, MMP-10 deficiency resulted in increased skeletal muscle necrosis and inflammatory cell infiltration early after femoral ischemia, that resulted in delayed muscle recovery at the regenerative phase [65]. These data suggest the contribution of the MMPs/TIMPs system to the pathophysiology of PAD.

Endothelial dysfunction is a key process leading to atherosclerosis and PAD, and the organism tries to counterbalance its progress by activating endothelial progenitor cell (EPC) mobilization and homing to the sites of vessel injury to induce repair. EPCs mobilization from the bone marrow is triggered by inflammation and MMPs activity. As such, Morishita T et al. investigated the pattern of EPCs mobilization and their association with inflammation and oxidative stress markers in patients with PAD [69]. They reported an increase in the number of circulating EPCs in the moderate phases of PAD, that decreased in the advanced phases of the disease, and was negatively correlated with the expression of membrane type-1 MMP (MT1-MMP) on peripheral blood mononuclear cells. MT1-MMP is an important regulator of EPC mobilization and angiogenesis [70] that cleaves CD44 adhesion molecule and reduces bone marrow stromal and progenitor cells interaction from bone marrow. These data suggest that the biphasic response of EPCs in PAD pathogenesis could be associated with changes in MT1-MMP expression [69], although its role as a potential biomarker in PAD needs to be confirmed in larger cohorts.

Vascular complications, including PAD, are more frequent among diabetics, and thus it has been hypothesized that MMPs are preferentially activated in patients with both pathologies. Increased plasma levels and zymographic activity of MMP-2 and MMP-9 has been shown in patients with type II diabetes, regardless their vascular status, in comparison with normal volunteers [71]. However, when comparing diabetic subjects with and without PAD, only plasma MMP-2 zymographic activity was higher in those presenting both pathologies vs. diabetes alone, while for MMP-9 activity no differences were observed [71]. Supporting these results, Chung AWY et al. reported an upregulation of MMP-2 and MMP-9 gene expression and gelatinolytic activity in mammary arteries of diabetic patients, that correlated positively with that of angiostatin, an antiangiogenic molecule, and negatively with VEGF, contributing likewise to impair blood vessel formation and PAD development in diabetic patients [72]. Similarly, a study with a larger sample size of type 2 diabetic patients (n = 302) reported elevated levels of MMP-2 in patients with PAD and diabetes, compared to non-PAD diabetics, which was accompanied with an increase in elastin degradation products (ELM), suggesting the regulation of MMP-2 and ELM by hyperglycemia in patients with PAD [73].

Endovascular surgery (angioplasty/stent) has become the first election therapy for most patients with PAD. However, balloon inflation and stent placement induced arterial wall damage may alter MMPs expression, contributing to constrictive remodelling, intimal thickening and re-stenosis [74,75]. In symptomatic PAD patients undergoing elective lower limb percutaneous revascularization (angioplasty/stent) the periprocedural profile of circulating MMP-2, -3, -7, and -9 and TIMP-1 and -2 has been documented. Compared to admission values, there was a significant elevation in serum MMP-3 and -7 levels 24 h after intervention, whereas no significant alterations were found in MMP-2, -9, TIMP-1 and -2 levels. The question remains on how the increased activity of specific MMPs, in this case MMP-3 and -7, after endovascular recovery affects this process and whether they might be biomarkers of post-procedure outcomes or therapeutic targets [76].

Finally, midfoot amputation, performed simultaneously to distal revascularisation, potentially leads to major amputation, and significantly increases morbidity and mortality. Despite a successful reconstruction, the failure rate of minor amputations is up to 45%, and almost 30% of patients required a major amputation [77–79]. The healing progression is closely related to extracellular matrix synthesis and degradation and is mediated by MMPs. Specifically, it has been reported that MMP-2 and MMP-9 play a major role in this process regarding their affinity for basement membrane collagen type IV and laminin [80]. Sapienza P et al. analyzed plasma MMP-2 and MMP-9 levels in three groups of patients, those that underwent an infrapopliteal vein graft and midfoot amputation, others undergoing post-traumatic midfoot primary amputation without PAD, and in healthy controls with normal LDL-cholesterol levels and without atherosclerotic lesions (excluded by ultrasonography and ABI measurements). The postoperative high levels of MMP-2 and -9 were predictive of wound healing failure at three, six, and nine months in PAD patients. Furthermore, MMP-2, and -9 were even higher and more persistent in the subgroup of patients with occlusion of the vein graft at all tested time points. These results suggest that monitoring MMP-2 and MMP-9 might help in the identification of patients at risk of healing failure of midfoot amputation after distal revascularisation, and predict the fate of the vein graft [81].

MMPs have been involved in all stages of atherosclerosis, but also in matrix remodeling in restenosis processes post angioplasty. As such, their circulating levels have been evaluated as markers of PAD incidence, diagnosis and risk stratification by different authors. However, no clear consensus has been reached on which of the studied MMPs are the most promising for PAD assessment or whether this approach will benefit from the combination of several MMPs. Studies including different MMPs in larger cohorts with longer follow-up periods will need to be performed in order to clarify their utility in this regard.

4. Cardiac Damage Biomarkers in PAD

N-terminal pro-brain natriuretic peptide (NT-proBNP) and troponin (in particular high sensitivity troponin T, hsTnT), are the most accepted specific biomarkers of cardiac damage, which are released in conditions of cardiomyocyte stress and/or injury. While the mechanisms linking PAD and the cardiac release of these biomarkers are likely multifactorial, probably related to the high coexistence of PAD and CAD, and have not been fully elucidated, several studies have reported associations between these biomarkers and the evolution and prognosis of lower extremity PAD [10].

Recent data obtained in more than 12,000 subjects from the ARIC study showed that elevated NT-proBNP and hs-TnT levels were independently associated with incident symptomatic PAD (i.e., hospitalizations with PAD diagnosis or leg revascularization), especially in the cases of CLI [82]. Similarly, NT-proBNP was associated with incident symptomatic PAD in individuals from the cardiovascular cohort of the Malmo Diet and Cancer study [83], and it was also independently associated with PAD incidence in African-Americans and with the ABI in both African-Americans and non-Hispanic whites [84]. On the other hand, detectable hsTnT in the CAVASIC study (male patients with IC) was associated with an 84% higher probability of symptomatic PAD [85]. Moreover, in patients with chronic kidney disease from the CRIC study, hsTnT was independently associated with incident PAD over a mean follow-up of 7.4 years, and its addition to the Framingham risk score improved PAD discrimination [86]. Of note, within the PAD spectrum hsTnT levels were higher in patients with CLI than in those with IC [87].

Cardiac biomarkers have also shown prognostic value in PAD patients. Indeed, NT-proBNP has been reported as an independent predictor of mortality during a 5-year follow-up in symptomatic PAD patients from the LIPAD study [88,89]. It was also associated with higher rates of CV events, including CV mortality or hospitalization for myocardial infarction, stroke or coronary revascularization in male PAD patients [90]. In addition, the combination of NT-proBNP, CRP and average day pulse pressure added on top of relevant risk factors improved risk discrimination and net reclassification index in these patients [90]. Nevertheless, there are some conflicting data on the usefulness of this biomarker; whereas male patients with peripheral arterial occlusive disease who suffered a MACE during follow-up presented higher NT-proBNP levels at baseline, this association was not maintained in multivariable regression models [91]. In a relatively small study performed with 95 PAD patients, both NT-proBNP and hsTnT were associated with a higher risk of mortality, but after adjustment by age, gender, prior cerebral artery disease and diabetes mellitus only hsTnT remained statistically significant [92]. Interestingly, in receiver operating characteristics (ROC) analyses hsTnT, NT-proBNP and their combination were superior to carotid intima-media thickness and ABI for discriminating mortality risk [92]. Reinforcing the clinical usefulness of hsTnT in this context, in the CAVASIC study detectable hsTnT was associated with a higher risk of all-cause mortality and incident CV disease during a seven-year follow-up in adjusted models [85].

Finally, cardiac biomarkers might also provide some useful information on patient evolution after endovascular revascularization. In a large retrospective study with over 1,000 patients detectable hsTnT (>0.01 ng/mL) was associated with higher rates of mortality and amputation during a 1-year follow-up and this association was maintained after adjusting for potential confounding factors [93]. Similarly, after endovascular therapy for acute limb ischemia elevated hsTnT was associated with worse in-hospital outcomes (i.e., mortality or amputation) after adjusting for clinically relevant risk factors including history of CAD [94]. Moreover, myocardial injury after revascularization in CLI, defined by a plasma hsTnT $\geq$ 14ng/L and an increase of at least 30% from the baseline value was associated with a worse outcome, including MACE and mortality [95]. Interestingly, 85% of patients with hsTnT values reflecting myocardial injury did not have ischemic clinical symptoms or electrocardiography changes [95]. Regarding the usefulness of natriuretic peptides after endovascular revascularization, elevated BNP was an independent predictor of MACE during a 2 year follow-up, but it was not related to major adverse limb events (MALE) [96].

Therefore, cumulative evidence suggests that cardiac biomarkers may be clinically useful for the diagnosis of incident PAD as well as for providing prognostic information.

5. Extracellular Vesicles as Biomarkers in PAD

Extracellular vesicles (EVs) are a heterogeneous population of small membranous particles that contain lipids, metabolites, proteins and nucleic acids from the cell of origin [97]. Their size and molecular content is determined by the type of biogenesis (i.e.,: multivesicular body exocytosis, plasma membrane budding or apoptosis) and the particular pathophysiological conditions at the time of their packaging and subsequent secretion into the extracellular space [98]. EVs in circulation contribute to the maintenance of vascular homeostasis and represent a promising component of liquid biopsy to identify novel biomarkers in CV diseases. In this review, following the last recommendations of the International Society for EVs [99], we will use the term EVs to refer to small and medium/large size vesicles also known as exosomes and microvesicles, respectively.

Circulating levels of EVs from different cellular origin are increased in response to CV risk factors (e.g., diabetes, hypertension, or hypercholesterolemia) and in patients with acute coronary syndromes, ischemic stroke or PAD [100]. Among them, platelet derived EVs (PEVs) constitute the major subtype of circulating EVs, possess high thrombogenic potential due to exposure of tissue factor and phosphatidylserine, and have been associated to atherosclerosis development and thrombosis [101]. Elevated numbers of PEVs have been found in symptomatic PAD patients compared to healthy subjects [102] and correlated to disease severity [103]. Moreover, PEVs subpopulations exposing P-selectin or CD63 were increased in PAD patients compared to age- and sex-matched controls and reflected the degree of platelet activation in vitro [104]. Endothelial EVs (EndEVs) are released into the blood flow upon endothelial injury or activation and their content could help to unravel molecular mechanisms that lead to endothelial and microcirculatory dysfunction in PAD [105]. Increased levels of circulating EndEVs have been found in several CV diseases such as stroke or CAD [106,107] being associated with endothelial dysfunction [108,109] and plaque instability [110,111]. Circulating EndEVs (CD144$^+$) were found to be significantly upregulated in PAD patients, particularly those bearing the monomeric CRP isoform, suggesting their contribution to pro-inflammatory status of this disease [112]. Moreover, EVs from different cell origins, especially those of endothelial origin, expressing the proangiogenic Sonic hedgehog morphogen correlated with the number of collateral vessels in ischemic thighs of PAD patients suggesting their possible role in neovascularization [113]. In this regard, the number of EndEVs from skeletal muscles increased 2 days after femoral artery ligation in mice, and in vitro induced a more potent bone marrow–mononuclear cell differentiation towards an endothelial phenotype when compared to EVs isolated from control muscles. As such, in vivo, the co-injection of EVs from ischemic muscles and bone marrow–mononuclear cells potentiated the proangiogenic effect of the latter [114]. Similarly, another study found upregulated expression of several microRNAs (e.g., miR-21, miR-92a and miR-126) in circulating small EVs from PAD patients and showed their capacity to modulate migration of VSMCs and ECs in vitro [115].

Advances in high-throughput technologies have contributed to depict the heterogenous content of EVs and identify novel biomarkers and therapeutic targets in CV diseases [116], however, there is still scarce EVs-related -OMICs data regarding PAD pathophysiology. Recently, by the transcriptomic study of circulating medium/large size EVs we could identify 15 protein-coding genes differentially expressed between age- and sex-matched PAD patients and healthy controls [14]. Circulating EVs from CLI subjects were enriched in pro-inflammatory genes (e.g., *Lcn2* and *S100a9*) and transcripts related to signalling pathways of platelet biology, iron homeostasis and immune response. Moreover, serum levels of calprotectin (S100A8/A9 heterodimer) were elevated in PAD and associated with an increased risk of amputation and CV mortality during the follow-up. Overall, our results suggest that the application of high-throughput technologies to EVs might be helpful to identify new molecular targets for PAD diagnosis, outcome assessment, and treatment.

Although EVs have proven a remarkable potential for the identification of new biomarkers in PAD, their study still represents a technical challenge due to their small size and heterogenicity. Moreover, biological and technical factors such as medication, co-morbidities (e.g.,: aging, tobacco smoking) or EVs isolation method can influence both the number and the content of EVs [100,117]. For instance, cilostazol induced a reduction in the number of PEVs in PAD patients [118], while atorvastatin does not modify PEVs total numbers, but specific PEVs subpopulations; those exposing P-selectin, tissue factor and glycoprotein-IIIa compared to placebo-controls [119]. Interestingly, atorvastatin displayed the opposite effect on EndEVs inducing their increase in circulation [120]. These studies demonstrate that pharmacological treatments can alter both, the number and the cargo of EVs, and might consequently modify their functional role, highlighting the importance of considering factors that can potentially influence EVs bio-dynamics.

Circulating EVs represent a potential alternative for PAD evaluation. Likewise, changes in their absolute numbers, or in the numbers of specific EVs subpopulations have been associated to PAD stages, and the study of their content, reflecting the molecular changes induced by the proatherogenic/inflammatory stimuli, may be helpful for the identification of new diagnosis, prognosis and therapeutic targets. A major drawback for EVs application into clinical practice however, is the technical challenges related to their nanometric size and scarce biological cargo, that will be overcome by current and future technological advances.

6. Role of microRNAs in PAD

MicroRNAs are small noncoding regulatory RNAs involved in the posttranscriptional modulation of gene expression. Increasing evidence suggest their involvement in the onset and progression of CV diseases, emerging as promising non-invasive biomarkers and therapeutic targets for several CV disorders [15] including PAD (Table 2).

Table 2. Circulating miRNAs as biomarkers in peripheral arterial disease (PAD).

Studied Groups (n)	Type of Biomarker	Sample Type	Candidate miRNAs	Refs.
PAD (20) and healthy controls (20)	Diagnostic	Whole blood	Among 12 miRNAs; miR-15b (AUC = 0.92), -16 (AUC = 0.93) and -363 (AUC = 0.93) had highest diagnostic value.	[121]
PAD (40) and healthy controls (19)	Diagnostic	PBMCs	29 miRNAs showed independent associations with PAD (AUC > 0.8 for all).	[122]
PAD (27) and healthy controls (27)	Diagnostic	Serum	miR-130a, -27b and -210 were upregulated in PAD. miR-210 was inversely correlated with claudication distance.	[123]
ASO (104) and healthy controls (105)	Diagnostic	Serum	mir-130a and -27b were increased in ASO and positively correlated with disease severity.	[124]
PAD (49) and healthy controls (47)	Diagnostic	Whole blood	miR-124 negatively correlated with ABI.	[125]
PAD patients with (12) and without (35) CVEs; 1 year follow up after surgery.	Prognostic	Plasma	miR-142 predicted post-femoral bypass surgery associated CVEs; (AUC = 0.861).	[126]
PAD patients with intermittent claudication (62); 2 years after surgery.	Prognostic	Serum	miR-195 independently predicted adverse ischemic events (HR per 1-SD of 0.40, 95% CI: 0.23-0.68) and target vessel revascularization (HR per 1-SD of 0.40, 95% CI: 0.22-0.75) after angioplasty with stent implantation.	[127]
PAD (146) and healthy controls (62); follow up period not specified.	Prognostic	Plasma	miR-320a (AUC = 0.766) and -572 (AUC = 0.690) predicted in-stent restenosis.	[128]
PAD patients with (74) and without (91) in-stent restenosis; follow up period not specified.	Prognostic	Serum	Serum miR-143 was lower in restenosis group and predicted in-stent restenosis; AUC = 0.866.	[129]

CVE, Cardiovascular events; PBMC, Peripheral blood mononuclear cells; ASO, Atherosclerosis obliterans; ABI, Ankle brachial index.

Stather PW et al. performed the first whole miRNA transcriptomic analysis in blood of PAD subjects and validated 12 differentially expressed transcripts in two independent sets of PAD patients and healthy controls [121] (Table 2). Three of them, miR-16, -15b, and -363, exhibited high diagnostic value when assessed by ROC curve analysis. Recently, high-throughput sequencing of miRNAs in peripheral blood mononuclear cells of patients with lower extremity PAD revealed 29 differentially expressed miRNAs predicted to target protein-coding genes involved in pathologies of atherosclerotic aetiology [122]. Those 29 miRNAs presented good performance for PAD diagnosis by ROC curves and could effectively classify PAD patients and healthy subjects using unsupervised clustering methods [122]. Besides their potential as diagnostic biomarkers, miRNAs have also been associated with PAD severity. For example, circulating miR-210 and miR-124 appeared upregulated in PAD, and inversely correlated with claudication distance and ABI respectively [123,125]. Likewise, serum miR-27b and miR-130a were also increased in atherosclerosis obliterans patients and positively correlated with Fontaine stages [124].

miRNAs have been also determined to predict worse outcome and restenosis after surgery. For instance, miR-142 was increased in plasma (1.6-fold) and femoral plaques (3.4-fold) of PAD patients subjected to femoral bypass surgery suffering coronary artery stent implantation, any other heart or vascular surgical procedures, or toe or leg amputations within 1 year of follow-up compared to those without CV events. Moreover, plasma miR-142 independently predicted the occurrence of CV events during 1-year follow up after adjustment by age and sex [126]. In addition, according to Stojkovic S et al., miR-195 was found to independently predict the adverse atherothrombotic events and the need for target vessel revascularization after stent implantation during a two-year follow up. Moreover, miR-195 improved the predictive value of clinical risk factors including age, sex, active smoking, diabetes, hypertension and hyperlipidemia [127]. Two additional studies performed in PAD subjects also identified miR-143, -320a and -572 as potential prognostic biomarkers for in-stent restenosis [128,129].

miRNAs regulate multifactorial biological processes involved in the pathogenesis of PAD and its progression to CLI, including angiogenesis, arteriogenesis, inflammation, oxidative stress, and hypoxia [130]. Angiogenesis, a key cellular mechanism for tissue reperfusion, is tightly regulated by miRNAs in response to ischemic injury. For instance, miR-26b enhanced in-vivo angiogenesis in a murine microvasculature growth model, whereas it reduced muscle fiber necrosis after femoral artery ligation [131]. miR-126 is enriched in ECs and EVs from EPCs [132,133], and its inhibition impaired angiogenesis in the gastrocnemius muscle after hindlimb ischemia in mice [134]. Conversely, miR-16 has been shown to directly target the proangiogenic molecules vascular endothelial growth factor (VEGF), VEGF receptor-2, and fibroblast growth factor receptor (FGFR)-1, and impaired angiogenesis both in-vitro and in-vivo when overexpressed [135]. Furthermore, all these three miRNAs, miR-16, -26b and -126, were found downregulated (3- to 4-fold) in peripheral blood of PAD patients compared to healthy subjects, reinforcing their biological relevance in PAD pathophysiology [121]. In contrast, miR-210 has been found upregulated in serum of PAD patients [123]. Similarly, miR-210 was elevated in murine and gastrocnemius muscles after hindlimb ischemia, and its inhibition, accentuated skeletal muscle damage due to increased mitochondrial oxidative stress [136]. Arteriogenesis is also regulated by miRNAs. For instance, inhibition of four miRNAs (miR-329, -487b, -494, and -495) by gene silencing oligonucleotides was found to individually increase perfusion and collateral artery size and density in the adductor muscles of mice subjected to femoral artery ligation [137]. Moreover, intramuscular injection of anti-miR-146a after limb ischemia in mice resulted in increased blood flow recovery and collateralization in the hypoxic thighs [138]. Macrophages, major immune cells within the skeletal muscle, orchestrate the inflammatory response upon muscle ischemia and their regulation by miRNAs is fundamental for effective muscle regeneration [139]. Intramuscular injection of miR-27b mimic reduced infiltrating macrophage content and enhanced angiogenesis post-femoral artery ligation in mice [140]. miR-93 was also found to stimulate M2-like macrophage polarization and was associated with increased neovascularization and perfusion in the ischemic muscle of the miR-106b-93-25 cluster knock-out mice [141].

The studies summarized above suggest the possible use of miRNAs as circulating biomarkers for the diagnosis and prognosis of PAD. Moreover, they provide experimental insight into the molecular mechanism underlying arterial diseases, as the basis for future therapeutic targets. Despite these promising results, additional studies are still required to verify the clinical relevance of this findings. Moreover, the technical requirements of miRNA determination in blood, including RNA isolation, several PCR steps and the need of qualified personnel, might delay their application as routine laboratory test.

7. Machine Learning and PAD

Machine learning (ML) refers to computational methods based on statistical techniques and algorithms, that can model large datasets and detect useful patterns. In medicine, those prediction models can guide clinicians into the identification of subjects that might benefit from specific pharmacological or surgical interventions or aid estimating outcomes [16]. The application of ML methods to PAD might provide a great opportunity to improve patient classification and treatment, although currently research in this area is still scarce. Baloch ZQ et al. applied ML methods to explore the relationship between PAD degree, and functional limitation and symptoms severity. They found a nonlinear relationship between symptoms and effort tolerance amongst patients with and without PAD, that with a simple linear model would have been overlooked or considered unimportant. As such, ML models might contribute to identify asymptomatic PAD patients with great functional limitations, that otherwise would be lost to PAD diagnosis by regular tests [142]. Other authors described that the combination of proteomic data and clinical information rendered algorithms able to predict angiographically significant PAD [143]. Regarding CV risk stratification, Ross EG et al. reported that state of the art ML algorithms outperformed stepwise logistic regression models for the identification of PAD and the prognostication of mortality risk in this population [144]. More recently, they have demonstrated that the application of ML to electronic health records can generate learning-based models that accurately identify PAD patients at risk of future major adverse cardiac and cerebrovascular events [145]. In addition, ML algorithms might be useful to predict not only PAD medical burden, but also its associated financial cost. Likewise, Berger JS et al. applied ML methods to a retrospective CLI cohort and identified baseline predictors of subsequent one-year all-cause hospitalizations and total annual healthcare cost in this high risk patient subgroup [146]. PAD, a multifactorial pathology with complex interactions, might considerably benefit from methods able to integrate and analyze large datasets, including multiple biomarkers, providing prediction models leading to a better understanding of PAD pathophysiology and improving its diagnosis and risk assessment.

8. Conclusions

Despite its high prevalence, the lack of awareness in PAD clinical manifestations and the limited tools for its early diagnosis, progression and prognosis evaluation in a personalized manner, has resulted in suboptimal therapeutic interventions in all its stages. Non-invasive circulating biomarkers could be of value in this setting and several candidates have been evaluated as useful for the diagnosis and risk stratification of PAD. In addition, these studies have also provided insights into the pathophysiological mechanisms involved in PAD development and evolution. Of note, some of these biomarkers have been evaluated as possible targets for pharmacological interventions. However, more conclusive evidences into the causal relationship between the studied proteins and the growth and progress of lower limb atherosclerosis will be only obtained after clinical studies involving multicentric collaborations, larger cohorts and longer follow-up periods are completed. The analysis of circulating EVs might offer a new alternative for the discovery of novel biomarkers and therapeutic targets in PAD, while non-coding RNAs might provide useful information on the regulatory pathways governing atherosclerosis initiation and progression, as well as on ischemia-induced muscle damage. It is worth considering that PAD is a complex multifactorial pathology involving diverse molecular pathways. Consequently, the evaluation of a single biomarker might not reflect those complex interactions, being a multimarker approach more suitable for this purpose. In this line, machine learning methods might be useful to obtain more accurate prediction algorithms by combining numerous biomarkers and clinical and functional parameters. This will lead to earlier diagnosis of PAD, more accurate CV risk stratification, and more personalized pharmacological or surgical treatments.

Author Contributions: Conceptualization C.R.; writing and figure designing G.S.-P.; writing and table designing E.M.-A., J.O., A.G.M. and C.R.; review and editing G.S.-P., E.M.-A., J.O., A.G.M., L.F.-A., J.A.P. and C.R. All authors have read and agreed to the published version of the manuscript.

Funding: This research was funded by "Instituto de Salud Carlos III-FEDER," Fondo de Investigaciones Sanitarias [PI18/01195] and CIBERCV (CB16/11/00371 and CB16/11/00483). G.S.-P. was funded with a Ph.D. scholarship from The Foundation for Applied Medical Research, Universidad de Navarra (Spain).

Conflicts of Interest: The authors declare no conflict of interest.

Abbreviations

ABI	Ankle brachial index
CAD	Coronary artery disease
CLI	Chronic limb ischemia
CRP	C reactive protein
CV	Cardiovascular
EML	Elastin degradation products
EPC	Endothelial progenitor cell
EVs	Extracellular vesicles
EndEVs	Endothelial Extracellular vesicles
FGFR	Fibroblast growth factor receptor
hsTnT	High sensitivity troponin T
IC	Intermittent claudication
ICAM	Intercellular Adhesion Molecule
IL	Interleukin
MACE	Major adverse cardiovascular event
MALE	Major adverse limb event
MCP	Monocyte chemoattractant protein
mi(cro)RNA	Micro ribonucleic acid
ML	Machine learning
MMP	Matrix metalloproteinase
NGAL	Neutrophil Gelatinase-Associated Lipocalin
NLR	Neutrophil-to-lymphocyte ratio
NT-proBNP	N-terminal pro-brain natriuretic peptide
PAD	Peripheral arterial disease
PEVs	Platelet extracellular vesicles
ROC	Receiver operating characteristics
TNF(R)	Tumor necrosis factor (receptor)
TIMP	Tissue inhibitor of matrix matalloproteinases
VCAM	Vascular cell adhesion molecule
VEGF(R)	Vascular endothelial growth factor (receptor)
VSMC	Vascular smooth muscle cell

References

1. Gerhard-Herman, M.D.; Gornik, H.L.; Barrett, C.; Barshes, N.R.; Corriere, M.A.; Drachman, D.E.; Fleisher, L.A.; Fowkes, F.G.R.; Hamburg, N.M.; Kinlay, S.; et al. 2016 AHA/ACC guideline on the management of patients with lower extremity peripheral artery disease: A report of the American college of cardiology/American Heart Association Task Force on Clinical Practice Guidelines. *Circulation* **2017**, *135*, e726–e779. [PubMed]
2. Frank, U.; Nikol, S.; Belch, J.; Boc, V.; Brodmann, M.; Carpentier, P.H.; Chraim, A.; Canning, C.; Dimakakos, E.; Gottsäter, A.; et al. ESVM Guideline on peripheral arterial disease. *Vasa Eur. J. Vasc. Med.* **2019**, *48*, 1–79. [CrossRef]
3. Fowkes, F.G.R.; Rudan, D.; Rudan, I.; Aboyans, V.; Denenberg, J.O.; McDermott, M.M.; Norman, P.E.; Sampson, U.K.; Williams, L.J.; Mensah, G.A.; et al. Comparison of global estimates of prevalence and risk factors for peripheral artery disease in 2000 and 2010: A systematic review and analysis. *Lancet* **2013**, *382*, 1329–1340. [CrossRef]
4. Hajibandeh, S.; Hajibandeh, S.; Shah, S.; Child, E.; Antoniou, G.A.; Torella, F. Prognostic significance of ankle brachial pressure index: A systematic review and meta-analysis. *Vascular* **2017**, *25*, 208–224. [CrossRef] [PubMed]
5. Jirak, P.; Mirna, M.; Wernly, B.; Paar, V.; Thieme, M.; Betge, S.; Franz, M.; Hoppe, U.; Lauten, A.; Kammler, J.; et al. Analysis of novel cardiovascular biomarkers in patients with peripheral artery disease. *Minerva Med.* **2018**, *109*, 443–450. [CrossRef] [PubMed]
6. Bhatt, D.L.; Steg, P.G.; Ohman, E.M.; Hirsch, A.T.; Ikeda, Y.; Mas, J.-L.; Goto, S.; Liau, C.-S.; Richard, A.J.; Röther, J.; et al. International Prevalence, Recognition, and Treatment of Cardiovascular Risk Factors in Outpatients with Atherothrombosis. *JAMA* **2006**, *295*, 180–189. [CrossRef] [PubMed]
7. Norgren, L.; Hiatt, W.; Dormandy, J.; Nehler, M.; Harris, K.; Fowkes, F. Inter-Society Consensus for the Management of Peripheral Arterial Disease (TASC II). *J. Vasc. Surg.* **2007**, *45*, S5–S67. [CrossRef] [PubMed]
8. Zheng, Z.-J.; Sharrett, A.; Chambless, L.E.; Rosamond, W.D.; Nieto, F.; Sheps, D.S.; Dobs, A.; Evans, G.W.; Heiss, G. Associations of ankle-brachial index with clinical coronary heart disease, stroke and preclinical carotid and popliteal atherosclerosis: The Atherosclerosis Risk in Communities (ARIC) Study. *Atherosclerosis* **1997**, *131*, 115–125. [CrossRef]
9. Krishna, S.M.; Moxon, J.V.; Golledge, J. A Review of the Pathophysiology and Potential Biomarkers for Peripheral Artery Disease. *Int. J. Mol. Sci.* **2015**, *16*, 11294–11322. [CrossRef]
10. Kremers, B.; Wübbeke, L.; Mees, B.; Ten Cate, H.; Spronk, H.; Ten Cate-Hoek, A. Plasma Biomarkers to Predict Cardiovascular Outcome in Patients with Peripheral Artery Disease: A Systematic Review and Meta-Analysis. *Arterioscler. Thromb. Vasc. Biol.* **2020**, *40*, 2018–2032. [CrossRef] [PubMed]
11. Singh, T.; Morris, D.; Smith, S.; Moxon, J.; Golledge, J. Systematic Review and Meta-Analysis of the Association Between C-Reactive Protein and Major Cardiovascular Events in Patients with Peripheral Artery Disease. *Eur. J. Vasc. Endovasc. Surg.* **2017**, *54*, 220–233. [CrossRef] [PubMed]
12. Hazarika, S.; Annex, B.H. Biomarkers and Genetics in Peripheral Artery Disease. *Clin. Chem.* **2017**, *63*, 236–244. [CrossRef] [PubMed]
13. Busti, C.; Falcinelli, E.; Momi, S.; Gresele, P. Matrix metalloproteinases and peripheral arterial disease. *Intern. Emerg. Med.* **2009**, *5*, 13–25. [CrossRef] [PubMed]
14. Saenz-Pipaon, G.; San Martín, P.; Planell, N.; Maillo, A.; Ravassa, S.; Vilas-Zornoza, A.; Martinez-Aguilar, E.; Rodriguez, J.A.; Alameda, D.; Lara-Astiaso, D.; et al. Functional and transcriptomic analysis of extracellular vesicles identifies calprotectin as a new prognostic marker in peripheral arterial disease (PAD). *J. Extracell. Vesicles* **2020**, *9*, 1729646. [CrossRef] [PubMed]
15. Zhou, S.-S.; Jin, J.-P.; Wang, J.-Q.; Zhang, Z.-G.; Freedman, J.H.; Zheng, Y.; Cai, L. miRNAS in cardiovascular diseases: Potential biomarkers, therapeutic targets and challenges. *Acta Pharmacol. Sin.* **2018**, *39*, 1073–1084. [CrossRef]
16. Handelman, G.S.; Kok, H.K.; Chandra, R.V.; Razavi, A.H.; Lee, M.J.; Asadi, H. eDoctor: Machine learning and the future of medicine. *J. Intern. Med.* **2018**, *284*, 603–619. [CrossRef]
17. Amrock, S.M.; Weitzman, M. Multiple biomarkers for mortality prediction in peripheral arterial disease. *Vasc. Med.* **2016**, *21*, 105–112. [CrossRef] [PubMed]
18. Tzoulaki, I.; Murray, G.D.; Lee, A.J.; Rumley, A.; Lowe, G.D.; Fowkes, F.G.R. Inflammatory, haemostatic, and rheological markers for incident peripheral arterial disease: Edinburgh Artery Study. *Eur. Hear. J.* **2007**, *28*, 354–362. [CrossRef]
19. Ridker, P.; Stampfer, M.; Rifai, N. Novel risk factors for systemic atherosclerosis. A comparison of C-reactive protein, fibrinogen, homocysteine, lipoprotein (a), and standard cholesterol screening as predictors of peripheral arterial disease. *ACC Curr. J. Rev.* **2001**, *10*, 25–26. [CrossRef]
20. Ding, N.; Yang, C.; Ballew, S.H.; Kalbaugh, C.A.; McEvoy, J.W.; Salameh, M.; Aguilar, D.; Hoogeveen, R.C.; Nambi, V.; Selvin, E.; et al. Fibrosis and Inflammatory Markers and Long-Term Risk of Peripheral Artery Disease. *Arter. Thromb. Vasc. Biol.* **2020**, *40*, 2322–2331. [CrossRef]
21. Valkova, M.; Lazurova, I.; Petrasova, D.; Frankovicova, M.; Dravecka, I. Humoral predictors of ankle-brachial index in patients with peripheral arterial disease and controls. *Bratisl. Med J.* **2018**, *119*, 646–650. [CrossRef] [PubMed]
22. Pande, R.L.; Brown, J.; Buck, S.; Redline, W.; Doyle, J.; Plutzky, J.; Creager, M.A. Association of monocyte tumor necrosis factor α expression and serum inflammatory biomarkers with walking impairment in peripheral artery disease. *J. Vasc. Surg.* **2015**, *61*, 155–161. [CrossRef] [PubMed]

23. Beckman, J.A.; Preis, O.; Ridker, P.M.; Gerhard-Herman, M. Comparison of Usefulness of Inflammatory Markers in Patients with Versus Without Peripheral Arterial Disease in Predicting Adverse Cardiovascular Outcomes (Myocardial Infarction, Stroke, and Death). *Am. J. Cardiol.* **2005**, *96*, 1374–1378. [CrossRef]
24. Engelberger, R.P.; Limacher, A.; Kucher, N.; Baumann, F.; Silbernagel, G.; Benghozi, R.; Do, D.-D.; Willenberg, T.A.; Baumgartner, I. Biological variation of established and novel biomarkers for atherosclerosis: Results from a prospective, parallel-group cohort study. *Clin. Chim. Acta* **2015**, *447*, 16–22. [CrossRef]
25. Urbonaviciene, G.; Frystyk, J.; Flyvbjerg, A.; Urbonavicius, S.; Henneberg, E.W.; Lindholt, J.S. Markers of inflammation in relation to long-term cardiovascular mortality in patients with lower-extremity peripheral arterial disease. *Int. J. Cardiol.* **2012**, *160*, 89–94. [CrossRef]
26. Murabito, J.M.; Keyes, M.J.; Guo, C.-Y.; Keaney, J.F.; Vasan, R.S.; D'Agostino, R.B.; Benjamin, E.J. Cross-sectional relations of multiple inflammatory biomarkers to peripheral arterial disease: The Framingham Offspring Study. *Atherosclerosis* **2009**, *203*, 509–514. [CrossRef] [PubMed]
27. Tzoulaki, I.; Murray, G.D.; Lee, A.J.; Rumley, A.; Lowe, G.D.; Fowkes, F.G.R. C-Reactive Protein, Interleukin-6, and Soluble Adhesion Molecules as Predictors of Progressive Peripheral Atherosclerosis in the General Population. *Circulation* **2005**, *112*, 976–983. [CrossRef]
28. Akkoca, M. The Role of Microcirculatory Function and plasma biomarkers in determining the development of cardiovascular adverse events in patients with peripheral arterial disease: A 5 year follow up. *Anatol. J. Cardiol.* **2018**, *20*, 220–228. [CrossRef] [PubMed]
29. Criqui, M.H.; Ho, L.A.; Denenberg, J.O.; Ridker, P.M.; Wassel, C.L.; McDermott, M.M. Biomarkers in peripheral arterial disease patients and near- and longer-term mortality. *J. Vasc. Surg.* **2010**, *52*, 85–90. [CrossRef] [PubMed]
30. Vidula, H.; Tian, L.; Liu, K.; Criqui, M.H.; Ferrucci, L.; Pearce, W.H.; Greenland, P.; Green, D.; Tan, J.; Garside, D.B.; et al. Biomarkers of inflammation and thrombosis as predictors of near-term mortality in patients with peripheral arterial disease: A cohort study. *Ann. Intern. Med.* **2008**, *148*, 85–93. [CrossRef]
31. Unlu, Y.; Karapolat, S.; Karaca, Y.; Kiziltunc, A.; Kızıltunç, A. Comparison of levels of inflammatory markers and hemostatic factors in the patients with and without peripheral arterial disease. *Thromb. Res.* **2006**, *117*, 357–364. [CrossRef] [PubMed]
32. Guo, S.; Zhang, Z.; Wang, L.; Yuan, L.; Bao, J.; Zhou, J.; Jing, Z. Six-month results of stenting of the femoropopliteal artery and predictive value of interleukin-6: Comparison with high-sensitivity C-reactive protein. *Vascular* **2020**, *28*, 715–721. [CrossRef]
33. Signorelli, S.S.; Mazzarino, M.C.; Di Pino, L.; Malaponte, G.; Porto, C.; Pennisi, G.; Marchese, G.; Costa, M.P.; DiGrandi, D.; Celotta, G.; et al. High circulating levels of cytokines (IL-6 and TNFα), adhesion molecules (VCAM-1 and ICAM-1) and selectins in patients with peripheral arterial disease at rest and after a treadmill test. *Vasc. Med.* **2003**, *8*, 15–19. [CrossRef] [PubMed]
34. Signorelli, S.S.; Anzaldi, M.; Libra, M.; Navolanic, P.M.; Malaponte, G.; Mangano, K.; Quattrocchi, C.; Di Marco, R.; Fiore, V.; Neri, S. Plasma Levels of Inflammatory Biomarkers in Peripheral Arterial Disease. *Angiology* **2016**, *67*, 870–874. [CrossRef] [PubMed]
35. McDermott, M.M.; Liu, K.; Ferrucci, L.; Tian, L.; Guralnik, J.M.; Green, D.; Tan, J.; Liao, Y.; Pearce, W.H.; Schneider, J.R.; et al. Circulating Blood Markers and Functional Impairment in Peripheral Arterial Disease. *J. Am. Geriatr. Soc.* **2008**, *56*, 1504–1510. [CrossRef] [PubMed]
36. Russell, K.S.; Yates, D.P.; Kramer, C.M.; Feller, A.; Mahling, P.; Colin, L.; Clough, T.; Wang, T.; LaPerna, L.; Patel, A.; et al. A randomized, placebo-controlled trial of canakinumab in patients with peripheral artery disease. *Vasc. Med.* **2019**, *24*, 414–421. [CrossRef] [PubMed]
37. Edlinger, C.; Lichtenauer, M.; Wernly, B.; Pistulli, R.; Paar, V.; Prodinger, C.; Krizanic, F.; Thieme, M.; Kammler, J.; Jung, C.; et al. Disease-specific characteristics of vascular cell adhesion molecule-1 levels in patients with peripheral artery disease. *Heart Vessel.* **2019**, *34*, 976–983. [CrossRef]
38. Zamzam, A.; Syed, M.H.; Rand, M.L.; Singh, K.; A Hussain, M.; Jain, S.; Khan, H.; Verma, S.; Al-Omran, M.; Abdin, R.; et al. Altered coagulation profile in peripheral artery disease patients. *Vascular* **2020**, *28*, 368–377. [CrossRef] [PubMed]
39. Altes, P.; Perez, P.; Esteban, C.; Muñoz-Torrero, J.F.S.; Aguilar, E.; García-Díaz, A.M.; Álvarez, L.R.; Jiménez, P.E.; Sahuquillo, J.C.; Monreal, M.; et al. Raised Fibrinogen Levels and Outcome in Outpatients with Peripheral Artery Disease. *Angiology* **2018**, *69*, 507–512. [CrossRef] [PubMed]
40. Bartlett, J.W.; De Stavola, B.L.; Meade, T.W. Assessing the contribution of fibrinogen in predicting risk of death in men with peripheral arterial disease. *J. Thromb. Haemost.* **2009**, *7*, 270–276. [CrossRef]
41. Doweik, L.; Maca, T.; Schillinger, M.; Budinsky, A.; Sabeti, S.; Minar, E. Fibrinogen Predicts Mortality in High Risk Patients with Peripheral Artery Disease. *Eur. J. Vasc. Endovasc. Surg.* **2003**, *26*, 381–386. [CrossRef]
42. McDermott, M.M.; Liu, K.; Green, D.; Greenland, P.; Tian, L.; Kibbe, M.; Tracy, R.; Shah, S.; Wilkins, J.T.; Huffman, M.; et al. Changes in D-dimer and inflammatory biomarkers before ischemic events in patients with peripheral artery disease: The BRAVO Study. *Vasc. Med.* **2015**, *21*, 12–20. [CrossRef] [PubMed]
43. Teperman, J.; Carruthers, D.; Guo, Y.; Barnett, M.P.; Harris, A.A.; Sedlis, S.P.; Pillinger, M.; Babaev, A.; Staniloae, C.; Attubato, M.; et al. Relationship between neutrophil-lymphocyte ratio and severity of lower extremity peripheral artery disease. *Int. J. Cardiol.* **2017**, *228*, 201–204. [CrossRef]
44. Selvaggio, S.; Abate, A.; Brugaletta, G.; Musso, C.; Di Guardo, M.; Di Guardo, C.; Vicari, E.S.D.; Romano, M.; Luca, S.; Signorelli, S.S. Platelet-to-lymphocyte ratio, neutrophil-to-lymphocyte ratio and monocyte-to-HDL cholesterol ratio as markers of peripheral artery disease in elderly patients. *Int. J. Mol. Med.* **2020**, *46*, 1210–1216. [CrossRef]

45. Celebi, S.; Berkalp, B.; Amasyali, B. The association between thrombotic and inflammatory biomarkers and lower-extremity peripheral artery disease. *Int. Wound J.* **2020**, *17*, 1346–1355. [CrossRef] [PubMed]
46. Luo, H.; Yuan, D.; Yang, H.; Yukui, M.; Huang, B.; Yang, Y.; Xiong, F.; Zeng, G.; Wu, Z.; Chen, X.; et al. Post-treatment neutrophil-lymphocyte ratio independently predicts amputation in critical limb ischemia without operation. *Clinics* **2015**, *70*, 273–277. [CrossRef]
47. Erturk, M.; Cakmak, H.A.; Surgit, O.; Celik, O.; Aksu, H.U.; Akgul, S.; Gurdogan, M.; Bulut, U.; Ozalp, B.; Akbay, E.; et al. The predictive value of elevated neutrophil to lymphocyte ratio for long-term cardiovascular mortality in peripheral arterial occlusive disease. *J. Cardiol.* **2014**, *64*, 371–376. [CrossRef] [PubMed]
48. Lee, S.; Hoberstorfer, T.; Wadowski, P.P.; Kopp, C.W.; Panzer, S.; Gremmel, T. Platelet-to-lymphocyte and Neutrophil-to-lymphocyte Ratios Predict Target Vessel Restenosis after Infrainguinal Angioplasty with Stent Implantation. *J. Clin. Med.* **2020**, *9*, 1729. [CrossRef]
49. González-Fajardo, J.A.; Brizuela-Sanz, J.A.; Aguirre-Gervás, B.; Merino-Díaz, B.; Del Río-Solá, L.; Martín-Pedrosa, M.; Vaquero-Puerta, C. Prognostic Significance of an Elevated Neutrophil–Lymphocyte Ratio in the Amputation-free Survival of Patients with Chronic Critical Limb Ischemia. *Ann. Vasc. Surg.* **2014**, *28*, 999–1004. [CrossRef] [PubMed]
50. Pourafkari, L.; Choi, C.; Garajehdaghi, R.; Tajlil, A.; Dosluoglu, H.H.; Nader, N.D. Neutrophil–lymphocyte ratio is a marker of survival and cardiac complications rather than patency following revascularization of lower extremities. *Vasc. Med.* **2018**, *23*, 437–444. [CrossRef]
51. Chan, C.; Puckridge, P.; Ullah, S.; Delaney, C.; Spark, J.I. Neutrophil-lymphocyte ratio as a prognostic marker of outcome in infrapopliteal percutaneous interventions for critical limb ischemia. *J. Vasc. Surg.* **2014**, *60*, 661–668. [CrossRef] [PubMed]
52. Igari, K.; Kudo, T.; Toyofuku, T.; Inoue, Y. Relationship of Inflammatory Biomarkers with Severity of Peripheral Arterial Disease. *Int. J. Vasc. Med.* **2016**, *2016*, 1–6. [CrossRef]
53. Ueki, Y.; Miura, T.; Miyashita, Y.; Ebisawa, S.; Motoki, H.; Izawa, A.; Koyama, J.; Ikeda, U. Inflammatory Cytokine Levels After Endovascular Therapy in Patients with Peripheral Artery Disease. *Angiology* **2017**, *68*, 734–740. [CrossRef] [PubMed]
54. Bath, J.; Smith, J.B.; Kruse, R.L.; Vogel, T.R. Neutrophil-lymphocyte ratio predicts disease severity and outcome after lower extremity procedures. *J. Vasc. Surg.* **2020**, *72*, 622–631. [CrossRef]
55. Paquissi, F.C. The role of inflammation in cardiovascular diseases: The predictive value of neutrophil–lymphocyte ratio as a marker in peripheral arterial disease. *Ther. Clin. Risk Manag.* **2016**, *12*, 851–860. [CrossRef] [PubMed]
56. Fowkes, F.G.R.; Aboyans, V.; McDermott, M.M.; Sampson, U.K.A.; Criqui, M.H. Peripheral artery disease: Epidemiology and global perspectives. *Nat. Rev. Cardiol.* **2017**, *14*, 156–170. [CrossRef] [PubMed]
57. Egnot, N.S.; Barinas-Mitchell, E.; Criqui, M.H.; Allison, M.A.; Ix, J.H.; Jenny, N.S.; Wassel, C.L. An exploratory factor analysis of inflammatory and coagulation markers associated with femoral artery atherosclerosis in the San Diego Population Study. *Thromb. Res.* **2018**, *164*, 9–14. [CrossRef] [PubMed]
58. Signorelli, S.S.; Anzaldi, M.; Fiore, V.; Simili, M.; Puccia, G.; Libra, M.; Malaponte, G.; Neri, S. Patients with unrecognized peripheral arterial disease (PAD) assessed by ankle-brachial index (ABI) present a defined profile of proinflammatory markers compared to healthy subjects. *Cytokine* **2012**, *59*, 294–298. [CrossRef]
59. Bayoglu, B.; Arslan, C.; Tel, C.; Ulutin, T.; Dirican, A.; Deser, S.B.; Cengiz, M. Genetic variants rs1994016 and rs3825807 in ADAMTS7 affect its mRNA expression in atherosclerotic occlusive peripheral arterial disease. *J. Clin. Lab. Anal.* **2018**, *32*, e22174. [CrossRef]
60. Martínez-Aguilar, E.; Gomez-Rodriguez, V.; Orbe, J.; Rodríguez, J.A.; Fernández-Alonso, L.; Roncal, C.; Paramo, J.A. Matrix metalloproteinase 10 is associated with disease severity and mortality in patients with peripheral arterial disease. *J. Vasc. Surg.* **2015**, *61*, 428–435. [CrossRef]
61. Tayebjee, M.H.; Tan, K.T.; MacFadyen, R.J.; Lip, G.Y.H. Abnormal circulating levels of metalloprotease 9 and its tissue inhibitor 1 in angiographically proven peripheral arterial disease: Relationship to disease severity. *J. Intern. Med.* **2004**, *257*, 110–116. [CrossRef] [PubMed]
62. Baum, O.; Ganster, M.; Baumgartner, I.; Nieselt, K.; Djonov, V. Basement Membrane Remodeling in Skeletal Muscles of Patients with Limb Ischemia Involves Regulation of Matrix Metalloproteinases and Tissue Inhibitor of Matrix Metalloproteinases. *J. Vasc. Res.* **2007**, *44*, 202–213. [CrossRef]
63. Muhs, B.; Plitas, G.; Delgado, Y.; Ianus, I.; Shaw, J.P.; Adelman, M.A.; Lamparello, P.; Shamamian, P.; Gagne, P. Temporal expression and activation of matrix metalloproteinases-2, -9, and membrane type 1-matrix metalloproteinase following acute hindlimb ischemia. *J. Surg. Res.* **2003**, *111*, 8–15. [CrossRef]
64. Muhs, B.E.; Gagne, P.; Plitas, G.; Shaw, J.P.; Shamamian, P. Experimental hindlimb ischemia leads to neutrophil-mediated increases in gastrocnemius MMP-2 and -9 activity: A potential mechanism for ischemia induced MMP activation. *J. Surg. Res.* **2004**, *117*, 249–254. [CrossRef]
65. Gomez-Rodriguez, V.; Orbe, J.; Martinez-Aguilar, E.; Rodriguez, J.A.; Fernandez-Alonso, L.; Serneels, J.; Bobadilla, M.; Perez-Ruiz, A.; Collantes, M.; Mazzone, M.; et al. Functional MMP-10 is required for efficient tissue repair after experimental hind limb ischemia. *FASEB J.* **2014**, *29*, 960–972. [CrossRef]
66. Meisner, J.K.; Annex, B.H.; Price, R.J. Despite normal arteriogenic and angiogenic responses, hind limb perfusion recovery and necrotic and fibroadipose tissue clearance are impaired in matrix metalloproteinase 9-deficient mice. *J. Vasc. Surg.* **2015**, *61*, 1583–1594. [CrossRef] [PubMed]

67. Johnson, C.; Sung, H.J.; Lessner, S.M.; Fini, M.E.; Galis, Z.S. Matrix metalloproteinase-9 is required for adequate angiogenic revascularization of ischemic tissues: Potential role in capillary branching. *Circ. Res.* **2004**, *94*, 262–268. [CrossRef] [PubMed]
68. Huang, P.-H.; Chen, Y.-H.; Wang, C.-H.; Chen, J.-S.; Tsai, H.-Y.; Lin, F.-Y.; Lo, W.-Y.; Wu, T.-C.; Sata, M.; Chen, J.-W.; et al. Matrix Metalloproteinase-9 Is Essential for Ischemia-Induced Neovascularization by Modulating Bone Marrow–Derived Endothelial Progenitor Cells. *Arter. Thromb. Vasc. Biol.* **2009**, *29*, 1179–1184. [CrossRef] [PubMed]
69. Morishita, T.; Uzui, H.; Nakano, A.; Mitsuke, Y.; Geshi, T.; Ueda, T.; Lee, J.-D. Number of Endothelial Progenitor Cells in Peripheral Artery Disease as a Marker of Severity and Association with Pentraxin-3, Malondialdehyde-Modified Low-Density Lipoprotein and Membrane Type-1 Matrix Metalloproteinase. *J. Atheroscler. Thromb.* **2012**, *19*, 149–158. [CrossRef]
70. Vagima, Y.; Avigdor, A.; Goichberg, P.; Shivtiel, S.; Tesio, M.; Kalinkovich, A.; Golan, K.; Dar, A.; Kollet, O.; Petit, I.; et al. MT1-MMP and RECK are involved in human CD34+ progenitor cell retention, egress, and mobilization. *J. Clin. Investig.* **2009**, *119*, 492–503. [CrossRef]
71. Signorelli, S.S.; Malaponte, G.; Libra, M.; Di Pino, L.; Celotta, G.; Bevelacqua, V.; Petrina, M.; Nicotra, G.S.; Indelicato, M.; Navolanic, P.M.; et al. Plasma levels and zymographic activities of matrix metalloproteinases 2 and 9 in type II diabetics with peripheral arterial disease. *Vasc. Med.* **2005**, *10*, 1–6. [CrossRef]
72. Chung, A.W.Y.; Hsiang, Y.N.; Matzke, L.A.; McManus, B.M.; Van Breemen, C.; Okon, E.B. Reduced Expression of Vascular Endothelial Growth Factor Paralleled with the Increased Angiostatin Expression Resulting from the Upregulated Activities of Matrix Metalloproteinase-2 and -9 in Human Type 2 Diabetic Arterial Vasculature. *Circ. Res.* **2006**, *99*, 140–148. [CrossRef] [PubMed]
73. Preil, S.A.R.; Thorsen, A.-S.F.; Christiansen, A.L.; Poulsen, M.K.; Karsdal, M.A.; Leeming, D.J.; Rasmussen, L.M. Is cardiovascular disease in patients with diabetes associated with serum levels of MMP-2, LOX, and the elastin degradation products ELM and ELM-2? *Scand. J. Clin. Lab. Investig.* **2017**, *77*, 493–497. [CrossRef]
74. Ward, M.R.; Pasterkamp, G.; Yeung, A.C.; Borst, C. Arterial remodeling: Mechanisms and clinical implications. *Circulation* **2000**, *102*, 1186–1191. [CrossRef]
75. Yahagi, K.; Otsuka, F.; Sakakura, K.; Sanchez, O.D.; Kutys, R.; Ladich, E.; Kolodgie, F.D.; Virmani, R.; Joner, M. Pathophysiology of superficial femoral artery in-stent restenosis. *J. Cardiovasc. Surg.* **2014**, *55*, 307–323.
76. Giagtzidis, I.T.; Kadoglou, N.P.; Mantas, G.; Spathis, A.; Papazoglou, K.O.; Karakitsos, P.; Liapis, C.D.; Karkos, C.D. The Profile of Circulating Matrix Metalloproteinases in Patients Undergoing Lower Limb Endovascular Interventions for Peripheral Arterial Disease. *Ann. Vasc. Surg.* **2017**, *43*, 188–196. [CrossRef]
77. Caruana, L.; Formosa, C.; Cassar, K. Prediction of wound healing after minor amputations of the diabetic foot. *J. Diabetes Complicat.* **2015**, *29*, 834–837. [CrossRef] [PubMed]
78. Becker, F.; Robert-Ebadi, H.; Ricco, J.-B.; Setacci, C.; Cao, P.; de Donato, G.; Eckstein, H.; De Rango, P.; Diehm, N.; Schmidli, J.; et al. Chapter I: Definitions, Epidemiology, Clinical Presentation and Prognosis. *Eur. J. Vasc. Endovasc. Surg.* **2011**, *42*, S4–S12. [CrossRef]
79. Criqui, M.H.; Aboyans, V. Epidemiology of Peripheral Artery Disease. *Circ. Res.* **2015**, *116*, 1509–1526. [CrossRef] [PubMed]
80. Sapienza, P.; Di Marzo, L.; Borrelli, V.; Sterpetti, A.; Mingoli, A.; Piagnerelli, R.; Cavallaro, A. Basic Fibroblast Growth Factor Mediates Carotid Plaque Instability Through Metalloproteinase-2 and -9 Expression. *Eur. J. Vasc. Endovasc. Surg.* **2004**, *28*, 89–97. [CrossRef]
81. Sapienza, P.; Mingoli, A.; Borrelli, V.; Brachini, G.; Biacchi, D.; Sterpetti, A.V.; Grande, R.; Serra, R.; Tartaglia, E. Inflammatory biomarkers, vascular procedures of lower limbs, and wound healing. *Int. Wound J.* **2019**, *16*, 716–723. [CrossRef]
82. Matsushita, K.; Kwak, L.; Yang, C.; Pang, Y.; Ballew, S.H.; Sang, Y.; Hoogeveen, R.C.; Jaar, B.G.; Selvin, E.; Ballantyne, C.M.; et al. High-sensitivity cardiac troponin and natriuretic peptide with risk of lower-extremity peripheral artery disease: The Atherosclerosis Risk in Communities (ARIC) Study. *Eur. Hear. J.* **2018**, *39*, 2412–2419. [CrossRef]
83. Fatemi, S.; Acosta, S.; Gottsäter, A.; Melander, O.; Engström, G.; Dakhel, A.; Zarrouk, M. Copeptin, B-type natriuretic peptide and cystatin C are associated with incident symptomatic PAD. *Biomarkers* **2019**, *24*, 615–621. [CrossRef]
84. Ye, Z.; Ali, Z.; Klee, G.G.; Mosley, T.H.; Kullo, I.J. Associations of Candidate Biomarkers of Vascular Disease with the Ankle-Brachial Index and Peripheral Arterial Disease. *Am. J. Hypertens.* **2013**, *26*, 495–502. [CrossRef] [PubMed]
85. Pohlhammer, J.; Kronenberg, F.; Rantner, B.; Stadler, M.; Peric, S.; Hammerer-Lercher, A.; Klein-Weigel, P.; Fraedrich, G.; Kollerits, B. High-sensitivity cardiac troponin T in patients with intermittent claudication and its relation to cardiovascular events and all-cause mortality—The CAVASIC Study. *Atherosclerosis* **2014**, *237*, 711–717. [CrossRef] [PubMed]
86. Janus, S.E.; Hajjari, J.; Al-Kindi, S.G. High Sensitivity Troponin and Risk of Incident Peripheral Arterial Disease in Chronic Kidney Disease (from the Chronic Renal Insufficiency Cohort [CRIC] Study). *Am. J. Cardiol.* **2020**, *125*, 630–635. [CrossRef] [PubMed]
87. Shigeta, T.; Kimura, S.; Takahashi, A.; Isobe, M.; Hikita, H. Coronary Artery Disease Severity and Cardiovascular Biomarkers in Patients with Peripheral Artery Disease. *Int. J. Angiol.* **2015**, *24*, 278–282. [CrossRef]
88. Mueller, T.; Dieplinger, B.; Poelz, W.; Endler, G.; Wagner, O.F.; Haltmayer, M. Amino-Terminal Pro–B-Type Natriuretic Peptide as Predictor of Mortality in Patients with Symptomatic Peripheral Arterial Disease: 5-Year Follow-Up Data from the Linz Peripheral Arterial Disease Study. *Clin. Chem.* **2009**, *55*, 68–77. [CrossRef]
89. Mueller, T.; Hinterreiter, F.; Luft, C.; Poelz, W.; Haltmayer, M.; Dieplinger, B. Mortality rates and mortality predictors in patients with symptomatic peripheral artery disease stratified according to age and diabetes. *J. Vasc. Surg.* **2014**, *59*, 1291–1299. [CrossRef] [PubMed]

90. Skoglund, P.H.; Arpegård, J.; Östergren, J.; Svensson, P. Amino-Terminal Pro-B-Type Natriuretic Peptide and High-Sensitivity C-Reactive Protein but Not Cystatin C Predict Cardiovascular Events in Male Patients with Peripheral Artery Disease Independently of Ambulatory Pulse Pressure. *Am. J. Hypertens.* **2014**, *27*, 363–371. [CrossRef]
91. Falkensammer, J.; Frech, A.; Duschek, N.; Gasteiger, S.; Stojakovic, T.; Scharnagl, H.; Huber, K.; Fraedrich, G.; Greiner, A. Prognostic relevance of ischemia-modified albumin and NT-proBNP in patients with peripheral arterial occlusive disease. *Clin. Chim. Acta* **2015**, *438*, 255–260. [CrossRef]
92. Clemens, R.K.; Annema, W.; Baumann, F.; Roth-Zetzsche, S.; Seifert, B.; Von Eckardstein, A.; Amann-Vesti, B.R.; Roth-Zetsche, S. Cardiac biomarkers but not measures of vascular atherosclerosis predict mortality in patients with peripheral artery disease. *Clin. Chim. Acta* **2019**, *495*, 215–220. [CrossRef] [PubMed]
93. Linnemann, B.; Sutter, T.; Herrmann, E.; Sixt, S.; Rastan, A.; Schwarzwaelder, U.; Noory, E.; Buergelin, K.; Beschorner, U.; Zeller, T. Elevated Cardiac Troponin T Is Associated with Higher Mortality and Amputation Rates in Patients with Peripheral Arterial Disease. *J. Am. Coll. Cardiol.* **2014**, *63*, 1529–1538. [CrossRef]
94. Linnemann, B.; Sutter, T.; Sixt, S.; Rastan, A.; Schwarzwaelder, U.; Noory, E.; Buergelin, K.; Beschorner, U.; Zeller, T. Elevated cardiac troponin T contributes to prediction of worse in-hospital outcomes after endovascular therapy for acute limb ischemia. *J. Vasc. Surg.* **2012**, *55*, 721–729. [CrossRef]
95. Szczeklik, W.; Krzanowski, M.; Maga, P.; Partyka, Ł.; Kościelniak, J.; Kaczmarczyk, P.; Maga, M.; Pieczka, P.; Suska, A.; Wachsmann, A.; et al. Myocardial injury after endovascular revascularization in critical limb ischemia predicts 1-year mortality: A prospective observational cohort study. *Clin. Res. Cardiol.* **2017**, *107*, 319–328. [CrossRef]
96. Stone, P.A.; Schlarb, H.; Campbell, J.E.; Williams, D.; Thompson, S.N.; John, M.; Campbell, J.R.; AbuRahma, A.F. C-reactive protein and brain natriuretic peptide as predictors of adverse events after lower extremity endovascular revascularization. *J. Vasc. Surg.* **2014**, *60*, 652–660. [CrossRef] [PubMed]
97. Dickhout, A.; Koenen, R.R. Extracellular Vesicles as Biomarkers in Cardiovascular Disease; Chances and Risks. *Front. Cardiovasc. Med.* **2018**, *5*, 113. [CrossRef]
98. Riancho, J.; Sánchez-Juan, P. Circulating Extracellular Vesicles in Human Disease. *N. Engl. J. Med.* **2018**, *379*, 2179–2181. [CrossRef]
99. Théry, C.; Witwer, K.W.; Aikawa, E.; Alcaraz, M.J.; Anderson, J.D.; Andriantsitohaina, R.; Antoniou, A.; Arab, T.; Archer, F.; Atkin-Smith, G.K.; et al. Minimal information for studies of extracellular vesicles 2018 (MISEV2018): A position statement of the International Society for Extracellular Vesicles and update of the MISEV2014 guidelines. *J. Extracell. Vesicles* **2018**, *7*, 1535750. [CrossRef] [PubMed]
100. Jansen, F.; Nickenig, G.; Werner, N. Extracellular Vesicles in Cardiovascular Disease. *Circ. Res.* **2017**, *120*, 1649–1657. [CrossRef] [PubMed]
101. Zarà, M.; Guidetti, G.F.; Camera, M.; Canobbio, I.; Amadio, P.; Torti, M.; Tremoli, E.; Barbieri, S.S. Biology and Role of Extracellular Vesicles (EVs) in the Pathogenesis of Thrombosis. *Int. J. Mol. Sci.* **2019**, *20*, 2840. [CrossRef] [PubMed]
102. Zeiger, F.; Stephan, S.; Hoheisel, G.; Pfeiffer, D.; Ruehlmann, C.; Koksch, M. P-Selectin expression, platelet aggregates, and platelet-derived microparticle formation are increased in peripheral arterial disease. *Blood Coagul. Fibrinolysis* **2000**, *11*, 723–728. [CrossRef]
103. Tan, K.T.; Tayebjee, M.H.; Lynd, C.; Blann, A.D.; Lip, G.Y.H. Platelet microparticles and soluble P selectin in peripheral artery disease: Relationship to extent of disease and platelet activation markers. *Ann. Med.* **2005**, *37*, 61–66. [CrossRef]
104. Van Der Zee, P.M.; Biró, É.; Ko, Y.; De Winter, R.J.; Hack, C.E.; Sturk, A.; Nieuwland, R. P-Selectin- and CD63-Exposing Platelet Microparticles Reflect Platelet Activation in Peripheral Arterial Disease and Myocardial Infarction. *Clin. Chem.* **2006**, *52*, 657–664. [CrossRef]
105. Hiatt, W.R.; Armstrong, E.J.; Larson, C.J.; Brass, E.P. Pathogenesis of the Limb Manifestations and Exercise Limitations in Peripheral Artery Disease. *Circ. Res.* **2015**, *116*, 1527–1539. [CrossRef]
106. Li, P.; Qin, C. Elevated Circulating VE-Cadherin+CD144+Endothelial Microparticles in Ischemic Cerebrovascular Disease. *Thromb. Res.* **2015**, *135*, 375–381. [CrossRef]
107. Koga, H.; Sugiyama, S.; Kugiyama, K.; Watanabe, K.; Fukushima, H.; Tanaka, T.; Sakamoto, T.; Yoshimura, M.; Jinnouchi, H.; Ogawa, H. Elevated Levels of VE-Cadherin-Positive Endothelial Microparticles in Patients with Type 2 Diabetes Mellitus and Coronary Artery Disease. *J. Am. Coll. Cardiol.* **2005**, *45*, 1622–1630. [CrossRef]
108. Amabile, N.; Guérin, A.P.; Leroyer, A.; Mallat, Z.; Nguyen, C.; Boddaert, J.; London, G.M.; Tedgui, A.; Boulanger, C.M. Circulating Endothelial Microparticles Are Associated with Vascular Dysfunction in Patients with End-Stage Renal Failure. *J. Am. Soc. Nephrol.* **2005**, *16*, 3381–3388. [CrossRef] [PubMed]
109. Werner, N.; Wassmann, S.; Ahlers, P.; Kosiol, S.; Nickenig, G. Circulating CD31+/Annexin V+Apoptotic Microparticles Correlate with Coronary Endothelial Function in Patients with Coronary Artery Disease. *Arter. Thromb. Vasc. Biol.* **2006**, *26*, 112–116. [CrossRef] [PubMed]
110. Schiro, A.; Wilkinson, F.L.; Weston, R.; Smyth, J.V.; Serracino-Inglott, F.; Alexander, M.Y. Elevated levels of endothelial-derived microparticles and serum CXCL9 and SCGF-β are associated with unstable asymptomatic carotid plaques. *Sci. Rep.* **2015**, *5*, 16658. [CrossRef]
111. Wekesa, A.; Cross, K.; O'Donovan, O.; Dowdall, J.; O'Brien, O.; Doyle, M.; Byrne, L.; Phelan, J.; Ross, M.; Landers, R.; et al. Predicting Carotid Artery Disease and Plaque Instability from Cell-derived Microparticles. *Eur. J. Vasc. Endovasc. Surg.* **2014**, *48*, 489–495. [CrossRef]

112. Crawford, J.R.; Trial, J.; Nambi, V.; Hoogeveen, R.C.; Taffet, G.E.; Entman, M.L. Plasma Levels of Endothelial Microparticles Bearing Monomeric C-reactive Protein are Increased in Peripheral Artery Disease. *J. Cardiovasc. Transl. Res.* **2016**, *9*, 184–193. [CrossRef]
113. Giarretta, I.; Gatto, I.; Marcantoni, M.; Lupi, G.; Tonello, D.; Gaetani, E.; Pitocco, D.; Iezzi, R.; Truma, A.; Porfidia, A.; et al. Microparticles Carrying Sonic Hedgehog Are Increased in Humans with Peripheral Artery Disease. *Int. J. Mol. Sci.* **2018**, *19*, 3954. [CrossRef]
114. Leroyer, A.S.; Ebrahimian, T.G.; Cochain, C.; Récalde, A.; Blanc-Brude, O.; Mees, B.; Vilar, J.; Tedgui, A.; Levy, B.I.; Chimini, G.; et al. Microparticles from ischemic muscle promotes postnatal vasculogenesis. *Circulation* **2009**, *119*, 2808–2817. [CrossRef] [PubMed]
115. Sorrentino, T.A.; Duong, P.; Bouchareychas, L.; Chen, M.; Chung, A.; Schaller, M.S.; Oskowitz, A.; Raffai, R.L.; Conte, M.S. Circulating exosomes from patients with peripheral artery disease influence vascular cell migration and contain distinct microRNA cargo. *JVS Vasc. Sci.* **2020**, *1*, 28–41. [CrossRef]
116. Chitoiu, L.; Dobranici, A.; Gherghiceanu, M.; Dinescu, S.; Costache, M. Multi-Omics Data Integration in Extracellular Vesicle Biology—Utopia or Future Reality? *Int. J. Mol. Sci.* **2020**, *21*, 8550. [CrossRef] [PubMed]
117. Rosińska, J.; Łukasik, M.; Kozubski, W. The Impact of Vascular Disease Treatment on Platelet-Derived Microvesicles. *Cardiovasc. Drugs Ther.* **2017**, *31*, 627–644. [CrossRef]
118. Nomura, S.; Inami, N.; Iwasaka, T.; Liu, Y. Platelet activation markers, microparticles and soluble adhesion molecules are elevated in patients with arteriosclerosis obliterans: Therapeutic effects by cilostazol and potentiation by dipyridamole. *Platelets* **2004**, *15*, 167–172. [CrossRef]
119. Mobarrez, F.; He, S.; Bröijersen, A.; Wiklund, B.; Antovic, A.; Antovic, J.; Egberg, N.; Jörneskog, G.; Wallén, H. Atorvastatin reduces thrombin generation and expression of tissue factor, P-selectin and GPIIIa on platelet-derived microparticles in patients with peripheral arterial occlusive disease. *Thromb. Haemost.* **2011**, *106*, 344–352. [CrossRef] [PubMed]
120. Mobarrez, F.; Egberg, N.; Antovic, J.; Bröijersen, A.; Jörneskog, G.; Wallén, H. Release of endothelial microparticles in vivo during atorvastatin treatment; a randomized double-blind placebo-controlled study. *Thromb. Res.* **2012**, *129*, 95–97. [CrossRef]
121. Stather, P.W.; Sylvius, N.; Wild, J.B.; Choke, E.; Sayers, R.D.; Bown, M.J. Differential MicroRNA Expression Profiles in Peripheral Arterial Disease. *Circ. Cardiovasc. Genet.* **2013**, *6*, 490–497. [CrossRef]
122. Bogucka-Kocka, A.; Zalewski, D.P.; Ruszel, K.P.; Stępniewski, A.; Gałkowski, D.; Bogucki, J.; Komsta, Ł.; Kołodziej, P.; Zubilewicz, T.; Feldo, M.; et al. Dysregulation of MicroRNA Regulatory Network in Lower Extremities Arterial Disease. *Front. Genet.* **2019**, *10*, 1200. [CrossRef] [PubMed]
123. Signorelli, S.S.; Volsi, G.L.; Pitruzzella, A.; Fiore, V.; Mangiafico, M.; Vanella, L.; Parenti, R.; Rizzo, M.; Volti, G.L. Circulating miR-130a, miR-27b, and miR-210 in Patients with Peripheral Artery Disease and Their Potential Relationship with Oxidative Stress. *Angiology* **2016**, *67*, 945–950. [CrossRef] [PubMed]
124. Li, T.; Cao, H.; Zhuang, J.; Wan, J.; Guan, M.; Yu, B.; Li, X.; Zhang, W. Identification of miR-130a, miR-27b and miR-210 as serum biomarkers for atherosclerosis obliterans. *Clin. Chim. Acta* **2011**, *412*, 66–70. [CrossRef] [PubMed]
125. Shi, Y.; Xu, X.; Luan, P.; Kou, W.; Li, M.; Yu, Q.; Zhuang, J.; Xu, Y.; Peng, W.; Jian, W. miR-124-3p regulates angiogenesis in peripheral arterial disease by targeting STAT3. *Mol. Med. Rep.* **2020**, *22*, 4890–4898. [CrossRef]
126. Barbalata, T.; Moraru, O.E.; Stancu, C.S.; Devaux, Y.; Simionescu, M.; Sima, A.V.; Niculescu, L.S. Increased miR-142 Levels in Plasma and Atherosclerotic Plaques from Peripheral Artery Disease Patients with Post-Surgery Cardiovascular Events. *Int. J. Mol. Sci.* **2020**, *21*, 9600. [CrossRef]
127. Stojkovic, S.; Jurisic, M.; Kopp, C.W.; Koppensteiner, R.; Huber, K.; Wojta, J.; Gremmel, T. Circulating microRNAs identify patients at increased risk of in-stent restenosis after peripheral angioplasty with stent implantation. *Atherosclerosis* **2018**, *269*, 197–203. [CrossRef]
128. Yuan, L.; Dong, J.; Zhu, G.; Bao, J.; Lu, Q.; Zhou, J.; Jing, Z. Diagnostic Value of Circulating microRNAs for In-Stent Restenosis in Patients with Lower Extremity Arterial Occlusive Disease. *Sci. Rep.* **2019**, *9*, 1–7. [CrossRef] [PubMed]
129. Yu, Z.-H.; Wang, H.-T.; Tu, C. Diagnostic value of microRNA-143 in predicting in-stent restenosis for patients with lower extremity arterial occlusive disease. *Eur. J. Med Res.* **2017**, *22*, 1–7. [CrossRef]
130. Pérez-Cremades, D.; Cheng, H.S.; Feinberg, M.W. Noncoding RNAs in Critical Limb Ischemia. *Arter. Thromb. Vasc. Biol.* **2020**, *40*, 523–533. [CrossRef] [PubMed]
131. Martello, A.; Mellis, D.; Meloni, M.; Howarth, A.; Ebner, D.; Caporali, A.; Zen, A.A.H. Phenotypic miRNA Screen Identifies miR-26b to Promote the Growth and Survival of Endothelial Cells. *Mol. Ther. Nucleic Acids* **2018**, *13*, 29–43. [CrossRef] [PubMed]
132. Fish, J.E.; Santoro, M.M.; Morton, S.U.; Yu, S.; Yeh, R.-F.; Wythe, J.D.; Ivey, K.N.; Bruneau, B.G.; Stainier, D.Y.; Srivastava, D. miR-126 Regulates Angiogenic Signaling and Vascular Integrity. *Dev. Cell* **2008**, *15*, 272–284. [CrossRef] [PubMed]
133. Ranghino, A.; Cantaluppi, V.; Grange, C.; Vitillo, L.; Fop, F.; Biancone, L.; Deregibus, M.; Tetta, C.; Segoloni, G.; Camussi, G. Endothelial Progenitor Cell-Derived Microvesicles Improve Neovascularization in a Murine Model of Hindlimb Ischemia. *Int. J. Immunopathol. Pharmacol.* **2012**, *25*, 75–85. [CrossRef]
134. Van Solingen, C.; Seghers, L.; Bijkerk, R.; Duijs, J.M.; Roeten, M.K.; Van Oeveren-Rietdijk, A.M.; Baelde, H.J.; Monge, M.; Vos, J.B.; De Boer, H.C.; et al. Antagomir-mediated silencing of endothelial cell specific microRNA-126 impairs ischemia-induced angiogenesis. *J. Cell. Mol. Med.* **2008**, *13*, 1577–1585. [CrossRef]

135. Chamorro-Jorganes, A.; Araldi, E.; Penalva, L.O.F.; Sandhu, D.; Fernández-Hernando, C.; Suárez, Y. MicroRNA-16 and MicroRNA-424 Regulate Cell-Autonomous Angiogenic Functions in Endothelial Cells via Targeting Vascular Endothelial Growth Factor Receptor-2 and Fibroblast Growth Factor Receptor-1. *Arter. Thromb. Vasc. Biol.* **2011**, *31*, 2595–2606. [CrossRef]
136. Zaccagnini, G.; Maimone, B.; Di Stefano, V.; Fasanaro, P.; Greco, S.; Perfetti, A.; Capogrossi, M.C.; Gaetano, C.; Martelli, F. Hypoxia-Induced miR-210 Modulates Tissue Response to Acute Peripheral Ischemia. *Antioxid. Redox Signal.* **2014**, *21*, 1177–1188. [CrossRef] [PubMed]
137. Welten, S.M.; Bastiaansen, A.J.; De Jong, R.C.; De Vries, M.R.; Peters, E.A.; Boonstra, M.C.; Sheikh, S.P.; La Monica, N.; Kandimalla, E.R.; Quax, P.H.; et al. Inhibition of 14q32 MicroRNAs miR-329, miR-487b, miR-494, and miR-495 Increases Neovascularization and Blood Flow Recovery After Ischemia. *Circ. Res.* **2014**, *115*, 696–708. [CrossRef]
138. Heuslein, J.L.; McDonnell, S.P.; Song, J.; Annex, B.H.; Price, R.J. MicroRNA-146a Regulates Perfusion Recovery in Response to Arterial Occlusion via Arteriogenesis. *Front. Bioeng. Biotechnol.* **2018**, *6*, 1. [CrossRef] [PubMed]
139. Bentzinger, C.F.; Wang, Y.X.; Dumont, N.A.; Rudnicki, M.A. Cellular dynamics in the muscle satellite cell niche. *EMBO Rep.* **2013**, *14*, 1062–1072. [CrossRef]
140. Veliceasa, D.; Biyashev, D.; Qin, G.; Misener, S.; Mackie, A.R.; Kishore, R.; Volpert, O.V. Therapeutic manipulation of angiogenesis with miR-27b. *Vasc. Cell* **2015**, *7*, 6. [CrossRef]
141. Ganta, V.C.; Choi, M.H.; Kutateladze, A.; Fox, T.E.; Farber, C.R.; Annex, B.H. A MicroRNA93–Interferon Regulatory Factor-9–Immunoresponsive Gene-1–Itaconic Acid Pathway Modulates M2-Like Macrophage Polarization to Revascularize Ischemic Muscle. *Circulation* **2017**, *135*, 2403–2425. [CrossRef] [PubMed]
142. Baloch, Z.Q.; Raza, S.A.; Pathak, R.; Marone, L.; Ali, A. Machine Learning Confirms Nonlinear Relationship between Severity of Peripheral Arterial Disease, Functional Limitation and Symptom Severity. *Diagnostics* **2020**, *10*, 515. [CrossRef]
143. McCarthy, C.P.; Ibrahim, N.E.; Van Kimmenade, R.R.; Gaggin, H.K.; Simon, M.L.; Gandhi, P.; Kelly, N.; Motiwala, S.R.; Mukai, R.; Ms, C.A.M.; et al. A clinical and proteomics approach to predict the presence of obstructive peripheral arterial disease: From the Catheter Sampled Blood Archive in Cardiovascular Diseases (CASABLANCA) Study. *Clin. Cardiol.* **2018**, *41*, 903–909. [CrossRef]
144. Ross, E.G.; Shah, N.H.; Dalman, R.L.; Nead, K.T.; Cooke, J.P.; Leeper, N.J. The use of machine learning for the identification of peripheral artery disease and future mortality risk. *J. Vasc. Surg.* **2016**, *64*, 1515–1522. [CrossRef] [PubMed]
145. Ross, E.G.; Jung, K.; Dudley, J.T.; Li, L.; Leeper, N.J.; Shah, N.H. Predicting Future Cardiovascular Events in Patients With Peripheral Artery Disease Using Electronic Health Record Data. *Circ. Cardiovasc. Qual. Outcomes* **2019**, *12*, e004741. [CrossRef] [PubMed]
146. Berger, J.S.; Haskell, L.; Ting, W.; Lurie, F.; Chang, S.-C.; Mueller, L.A.; Elder, K.; Rich, K.; Crivera, C.; Schein, J.R.; et al. Evaluation of machine learning methodology for the prediction of healthcare resource utilization and healthcare costs in patients with critical limb ischemia—Is preventive and personalized approach on the horizon? *EPMA J.* **2020**, *11*, 53–64. [CrossRef] [PubMed]

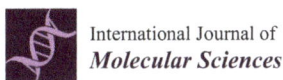

Review

Clinical Application of Novel Therapies for Coronary Angiogenesis: Overview, Challenges, and Prospects

Mohamed Sabra [1,†], Catherine Karbasiafshar [1,†], Ahmed Aboulgheit [1,2], Sidharth Raj [2], M. Ruhul Abid [1,2] and Frank W. Sellke [1,2,*,‡]

1. Cardiovascular Research Center, Rhode Island Hospital, Providence, RI 02903, USA; msabra1@lifespan.org (M.S.); ckarbasiafshar1@lifespan.org (C.K.); ahmad_aboul_gheit@brown.edu (A.A.); ruhul_abid@brown.edu (M.R.A.)
2. Division of Cardiothoracic Surgery, Alpert Medical School of Brown University, Providence, RI 02903, USA; sidharth_raj@brown.edu
* Correspondence: fsellke@lifespan.org
† These authors are equal contributing authors.
‡ Current address: MOC 530, 2 Dudley Street, Providence, RI 02905, USA.

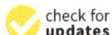

Citation: Sabra, M.; Karbasiafshar, C.; Aboulgheit, A.; Raj, S.; Abid, M.R.; Sellke, F.W. Clinical Application of Novel Therapies for Coronary Angiogenesis: Overview, Challenges, and Prospects. *Int. J. Mol. Sci.* **2021**, 22, 3722. https://doi.org/10.3390/ijms22073722

Academic Editors: Paul Quax and Elisabeth Deindl

Received: 7 March 2021
Accepted: 31 March 2021
Published: 2 April 2021

Publisher's Note: MDPI stays neutral with regard to jurisdictional claims in published maps and institutional affiliations.

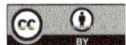

Copyright: © 2021 by the authors. Licensee MDPI, Basel, Switzerland. This article is an open access article distributed under the terms and conditions of the Creative Commons Attribution (CC BY) license (https:// creativecommons.org/licenses/by/ 4.0/).

Abstract: Cardiovascular diseases continue to be the leading cause of death worldwide, with ischemic heart disease as the most significant contributor. Pharmacological and surgical interventions have improved clinical outcomes, but are unable to ameliorate advanced stages of end-heart failure. Successful preclinical studies of new therapeutic modalities aimed at revascularization have shown short lasting to no effects in the clinical practice. This lack of success may be attributed to current challenges in patient selection, endpoint measurements, comorbidities, and delivery systems. Although challenges remain, the field of therapeutic angiogenesis is evolving, as novel strategies and bioengineering approaches emerge to optimize delivery and efficacy. Here, we describe the structure, vascularization, and regulation of the vascular system with particular attention to the endothelium. We proceed to discuss preclinical and clinical findings and present challenges and future prospects in the field.

Keywords: angiogenesis; gene therapy; stem cells; extracellular vesicles; clinical trials; bioengineering

1. Introduction

Despite substantial efforts aimed at evidence-based optimization of standards for prevention and early management, ischemic heart disease (IHD) accounts for nearly 9 million of the 18 million cardiovascular disease (CVD) deaths worldwide in 2015 [1]. The advent of therapeutic interventions and diagnostic methods have undoubtedly improved outcomes and lowered overall mortality associated with IHD. Current management of this disease comprises revascularization by means of percutaneous coronary intervention or surgical bypass grafting, in addition to pharmacological interventions aimed at mitigating risk factors, such as hypertension and dyslipidemia, in concert with correcting myocardial oxygen supply/demand mismatch. However, a common challenge encountered by clinicians is the management of advanced and diffuse multivessel disease state resistant to conventional treatment modalities, therefore, requiring the study of novel therapeutic strategies.

The term angiogenesis was first used in 1935 by Arthur Hertig to describe the formation of new blood vessels in the placenta. It was not until 1971, however, when Folkman showed that solid tumors were able to extensively vascularize their core by inducing growth of new blood vessels from contiguous vasculature of normal tissue [2]. This observation initially prompted the idea that inhibition of tumor angiogenesis could be a potential anti-neoplastic therapeutic strategy. Soon thereafter, it became evident that induction of this mechanism of autonomous blood vessel growth in tissue subject to chronic ischemia, such as the myocardium or extremities, may provide collateral blood supply and preserve viability. This notion prompted interest in the molecular mechanisms of blood vessel growth to guide future therapeutic targeting.

By the early nineties, many key angiogenic factors were characterized including various isoforms of vascular endothelial growth factor (VEGF) and fibroblast growth factor (FGF). The data from studies evaluating intramyocardial administration of recombinant growth factors in animal models of myocardial ischemia were promising, providing impetus for many clinical trials evaluating the safety and efficacy of administration of these growth factors in patients with ischemic heart disease (IHD) [3,4]. However, with increased sample sizes and extended follow-up times post-therapy, it became evident that the positive effects of new vessel growth and functional improvement were short-lived and did not culminate in sustainable long-term benefit [5]. Additionally, the incidence of adverse effects such as tissue edema with local administration of these growth factors raised concern. Since the early trials, much effort has focused on identifying issues that hinder the efficacy of novel angiogenic therapies in the clinical setting. This review will shed light on recent advances in therapeutic angiogenesis in animal models and the challenges of clinical applications of these strategies. We further review the biology of angiogenesis, summarize preclinical and clinical findings, and describe a number of translational challenges and novel angiogenic strategies.

2. Structure of the Vasculature

The adult vasculature spans a surface area of approximately 1000 m^2 and encompasses an arterial and a venous system connected by capillaries (Figure 1) [6]. Importantly, all vessels share a similar basic structure composed of four distinct layers. The innermost layer is known as the tunica intima, consisting of a single layer of endothelial cells that forms the interface with blood. Ensheathing the intima is a smooth muscle layer known as the tunica media, which is innervated by the autonomic nervous system and a major regulator of blood vessel diameter. Large elastic arteries are characterized by a prominent tunica media, whereas capillaries are solely composed of an endothelial monolayer to maximize permeation of oxygen and nutrients into the interstitial space. An adventitial connective tissue forms the tunica externa and communicates with visceral and muscular structures as blood vessels course through various anatomical regions [6].

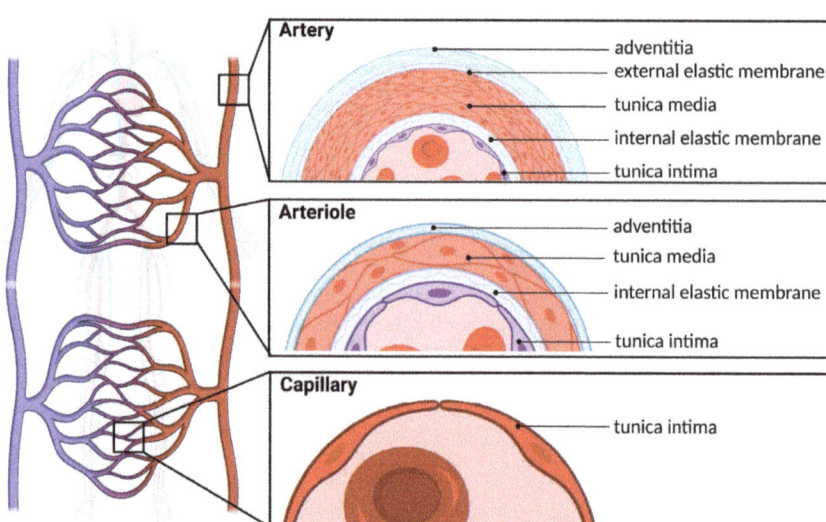

Figure 1. Structure of the arterial system. The circulatory system is a network of arteries and veins connected by capillaries where oxygen and nutrient exchange occurs. The inner lining of arteries, arterioles, and capillaries is known as the tunica intima, which is composed exclusively of endothelial cells. Arterioles and arteries additionally have a series of elastic and muscular layers.

3. Mechanisms of Vascularization

3.1. Vasculogenesis

By the third week after fertilization, blood vessels begin to form in the yolk sac and then in the growing embryo [7]. Vasculogenesis refers to the initial embryological development of nascent vascular structures, known as blood islands from endothelial progenitor cells (EPCs) (Figure 2A). Morphogenic cues, such as VEGF, trigger differentiation of these precursors and promote formation of blood islands, which then merge into primitive capillary plexuses [8]. Their subsequent growth and expansion to penetrate organs and form an interconnected network is associated with angiogenesis, which we describe next. It is important to first note that while vasculogenesis is most prominently associated with early embryonic development, recent evidence suggests that it is involved in the recruitment of circulating CD34/VEGFR2-positive and bone-marrow-derived angioblasts for in situ growth of blood vessels in post-natal life as well [9]. However, the precise mechanisms by which these angioblasts are stimulated in pathological states and the degree of contribution of this process to the formation of sustainable vasculature remain obscure.

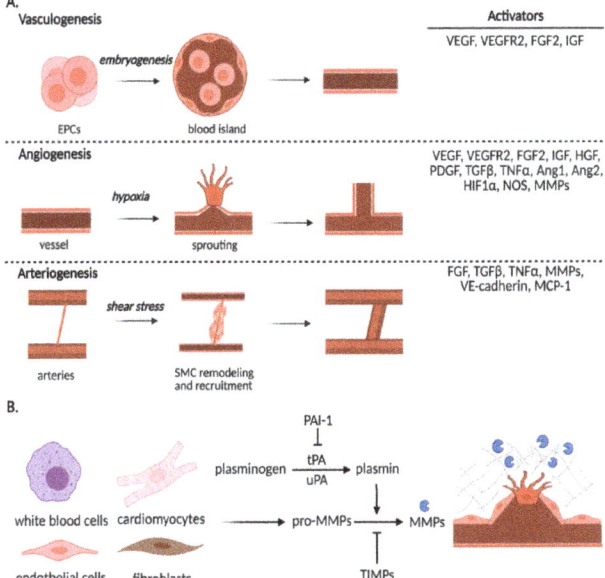

Figure 2. Mechanisms of vascularization and extracellular matrix remodeling. (**A**) Vasculogenesis describes the synthesis of de novo vessels and vasculature that occurs during embryonic development and begins with the differentiation and organization of endothelial progenitor cells. Sprouting angiogenesis is stimulated under hypoxic conditions and is characterized by phalanx, stalk, tip cell migration, proliferation, and tube formation. Arteriogenesis is the process by which shear stress signals for smooth muscle cell recruitment to support an existing vessel between arteries; this vessel then muscularizes to become an established artery. (**B**) An essential process in angiogenesis is extracellular matrix (ECM) remodeling to release growth factor stores from ECM components and promote migration of endothelial cells. A number of cell types contribute to this process in the heart by production of MMPs; their activation is tightly regulated by the plasminogen system and their inhibitors known as tissue inhibitors of metalloproteinases (TIMPs). VEGF, vascular endothelial growth factor; VEGFR2, VEGF receptor 2; FGF2, fibroblast growth factor 2; IGF, insulin growth factor; HGF, hepatocyte growth factor; PDGF, platelet-derived growth factor; TGFβ, transforming growth factor β; TNFα, tumor necrosis factor α; Ang1, angiopoietin 1; Ang2, angiopoietin 2; HIF1α, hypoxia inducible factor 1α; NOS, nitric oxide synthase; MMPs, matrix metalloproteinases; VE-cadherin; vascular endothelial cadherin; MCP1, monocyte chemoattractant protein 1.

3.2. Angiogenesis

Angiogenesis is generally considered the mainstay of neovascularization, where new vessels form from existing vessels, and occurs in many physiological processes such as wound healing, ovulation, and pregnancy. In these contexts, angiogenesis is tightly regulated by an intricate balance between pro- and anti-angiogenic factors. Disturbance of this balance results in uncontrolled blood vessel growth, which is a hallmark pathological feature seen in malignancy, retinopathy, and other disease states.

Activation of the vascular endothelium to switch from a quiescent state to a proliferative state is initiated by an increased local production of nitric oxide (NO) levels, which increases vascular permeability and upregulates expression of VEGF [10]. A series of alterations to intercellular adhesion molecules and cell membrane structure facilitate the extravasation of plasma proteins into the interstitial space. Next, proteases degrade the basement membrane and extracellular matrix (ECM), thereby clearing the path for migrating endothelial cells and, importantly, liberating cryptic adhesion sites and sequestered growth factors. Degradation of the ECM is a complex, highly regulated process. Over twenty identifiable matrix metalloproteinases (MMPs) take part in this step, which are most commonly activated by plasmin and inhibited by tissue inhibitors of metalloproteinases (TIMPs) (Figure 2B) [11,12]. This balance between proteases and their inhibitors is critical, as excessive proteolytic activity is a characteristic of pathological vessel formation in cancer and inflammatory disease.

Following migration and proliferation, tube formation or lumenogenesis occurs. At the cellular level, this process has been shown to occur via budding or cell hollowing. Molecularly, lumen formation is initiated by integrins, while lumen diameter is regulated by contractile status [13]. To this point, the endothelium acquires highly specialized characteristics according to the local tissue needs. For instance, endothelial junctions in capillaries forming the blood–brain barrier are narrow, allowing for controlled permeation of fluid as opposed to those of the glomerular capillaries, which are redundant to allow for filtration. The factors that determine such differentiation of the endothelium are largely unknown; however, the host tissue environment and VEGF signaling likely play a major role. The nascent vessels then undergo three-dimensional organization to form mature vascular networks, which is primarily directed by VEGF, and otherwise known as remodeling or branching [13]. This step occurs either by sprouting towards an angiogenic stimulus, splitting into individual daughter vessels by the formation of trans-endothelial bridges, or intussusceptive insertion of interstitial tissue columns into the lumen of pre-existing vessels. Meanwhile, the structural configuration of the newly shaped vessels composed of an endothelial mono- or double-layer is consolidated by the formation of an ECM and recruitment of peri-endothelial cells. In addition to providing structural support, vascular smooth muscle cells (VSMCs) also inhibit endothelial cell migration and proliferation, thus preventing regression of the nascent vessels.

Interestingly, differentiation of evolving vessels, i.e., artery, vein, or capillary, seems to be influenced by an interplay between external hemodynamic forces and intrinsic molecular signals. Areas of reduced blood flow favor the persistence of capillaries and may even result in complete regression of the primitive vessel if limitation of flow is significant. On the other hand, increased perfusion, pressure, and shear stress induce local recruitment of VSMCs, which lead to arterialization. Basic helix-loop-helix (bHLH) transcription factors appear to play a key role in directing angioblasts to pre-arterial or pre-venous specifications [14]. Additionally, Notch signaling and members of the large ephrin family, along with other tyrosine kinases appear to modulate differentiation of vesicular structures. Longevity of the newly formed vessels is maintained by an ongoing interaction of VEGF with the VEGFR2, P13 kinase, and β-catenin, which induces anti-apoptotic genes and promotes survival [13]. Surprisingly, hemodynamic shear forces favor inhibition of endothelial turnover and, thus, prevent tumor necrosis factor α (TNFα)-mediated apoptosis and vessel regression.

3.3. Arteriogenesis

Arteriogenesis is an adaptive phenomenon, which occurs with stenotic vascular lesions and features primary remodeling of existing collateral arteries rather than growth of new vascular structures. As opposed to angiogenesis, which is hypoxia-driven and initiated by the endothelium, arteriogenesis is predominantly stimulated by shear forces. Thus, turbulent blood flow is sensed by the endothelium, which induces the transcription of several genes including FGF2, PDGF-B, and TGFβ [15]. As a result, chloride channels open and adhesion molecules on the endothelium are upregulated, including monocyte chemoattractant protein 1 (MCP1) [16]. Circulating monocytes adhere to and invade arteriolar collaterals, initiating a myriad of inflammatory signals that recruit fibroblasts, platelets, and basophils. The local inflammatory response induces apoptosis in neighboring cells, which facilitates expansion of the collateral vessel diameter up to twenty times [17]. Importantly, the local production of growth factors such as FGF2 induces mitosis of the endothelial and smooth muscle cell layers, again forming a preliminary vascular structure that is remodeled into a final configuration [18]. To underscore that arteriogenesis occurs independent of hypoxia, it has been shown that the distance between ischemic regions and site of collateral vessel formation can be up to 70 cm. [6]. Unlike angiogenesis, arteriogenesis invariably results in competent vasculature capable of sustaining tissue viability; therefore, therapeutic targeting of arteriogenesis may prove to be a rewarding endeavor.

4. Preclinical Studies and Clinical Trials

4.1. Protein Therapy

Expanding insight into the molecular basis of neovascular formation underscored the critical role of growth factors and provided impetus for early studies, which focused on delivery of recombinant angiopeptides to target ischemic tissue. Table 1 summarizes the outcomes of clinical trials with protein therapy, in addition to gene- and stem-cell-based therapies.

Both VEGF and FGF have a central role in multiple steps of vessel development and differentiation and, therefore, are the most widely studied proteins in the search for novel angiogenic therapies. VEGF isoforms bind to and phosphorylate VEGFR1 and VEGFR2, whereas FGF binds selectively to four major receptors (FGFR1b/c, FGFR2b/c, FGFR3b/c, and FGFR4) on the vascular endothelium [19,20]. The binding of VEGF and FGF to their cognate tyrosine kinase receptor induces diverse downstream signaling pathways including MAPK, P13K, and PLC-γ. Data from preclinical studies showed increased blood vessel growth and collateral-dependent perfusion in animal models of chronic myocardial ischemia with VEGF and FGF therapy [5]. Among other growth factors that have been investigated in animal models of chronic myocardial ischemia are platelet-derived growth factor (PDGF), which positively regulates maturation of vasculature [21]. Additionally, angiopoietin-1 interaction with the Tie-2 receptor has been shown to promote stability of newly formed vessels in preclinical studies [22]. Hepatocyte growth factor (HGF) has well-documented pro-angiogenic roles in post-ischemic and post-infarcted heart failure models as well [23,24]. Although morphogens such as sonic hedgehog, Notch, and Wnt are involved in an array of pathways, taking advantage of their role in blood vessel growth has attracted attention.

Table 1. Clinical outcomes with angiogenic therapies.

Agent	Study Design (Disease; Delivery; Dose; Number of Patients)	Outcome	Ref.
Protein Therapy			
VEGF	CAD; IC day 0 and IV day 3,6,9; 17 ng/kg/min or 50 ng/kg/min; $n = 178$)	No improvement in exercise time 60 days post treatment	[25]
FGF	CAD; IC; single injection of 0, 0.3, 3, or 30 µg/kg; $n = 337$	Exercise tolerance and angina symptoms improved at 90 days; no difference at 180 days	[26]
	CAD; IC via heparin-alginate slow-release device; 1 or 10 µg; $n = 8$	Exercise tolerance and myocardial perfusion showed a trend toward improvement at 90 days, but not at 180 days	[4]
Gene Therapy			
VEGF	CAD; IM 10×; 200 µg supplemented with 6 g L-arginine per day for 3 months; $n = 19$	Improved anterior wall perfusion and anterior wall contractility at 3 months	[27]
	CAD, IM; 125 or 250 µg; $n = 15$	Angina was significantly reduced and myocardial perfusion was improved	[28]
	Angina, IM, 200 µL at 10 sites; $n = 30$	Myocardial perfusion reserve significantly increased at 3 months and 12 months compared to baseline, although no significance between 3 and 12 months.	[29]
	IHD, IM, 4×10^{10} pfu, $n = 67$	Total exercise duration and time were improved at 12 and 26 weeks	[30]
	IHD, IC, 2×10^{10} pfu, $n = 103$	Myocardial perfusion was significantly improved at 6 months; no changes in minimal lumen diameter nor % of diameter stenosis were also reported	[31]
FGF	Angina, IC, 5 different dose groups, $n = 79$	Increased exercise time at 4 weeks	[32]
	CLI; intramuscular; 4 mg at day 1, 15, 30, and 45; $n = 125$	Complete healing of at least one ulcer in the treated limb at week 25; treatment also significantly reduced the risk of all amputations by two-fold	[33]
Stem-Cell Therapy			
BM-MSC	MI; IC; day 6 post-MI on average; 7×10^5 cells; $n = 101$	LVEF was increased at 6 months; no change in LV EDV nor infarct size was observed.	[34]
	CAD; transendocardial injection; 1×10^8; $n = 92$	LV ESV nor maximal oxygen consumption were improved at 6 months	[35]
	(MI; IC; 24.6 ± 9.4 × 10^8 nucleated cells, 9.5 ± 6.3 × 10^6 CD34+ cells, and 3.6 ± 3.4 × 10^6 hematopoietic cells ~4.8 days post-MI; $n = 60$)	LVEF was improved at 6 months, but was not significant at 18 months	[36]
CPC	IHD; IM; injections at 17 sites; $n = 315$	No significant improvements in primary endpoints of MLHFQ score, 6 min walk distance; LV ESV and LV EF at 39 weeks	[37]
	IHD; IM; 600 × 106 to 1200 × 106 cells; $n = 319$	LVEF was improved with reduction in LV ESV, and improved 6-min walk distance	[38]
BMC or CPC	MI, IC, mean of 22 × 10^6 CPC or 205 × 10^6 BMC, $n = 75$	BMC treatment significantly increased LVEF compared to CPC and control groups at 3 months.	[39]

VEGF, vascular endothelial growth factor; FGF, fibroblast growth factor; BM-MSC, bone-marrow-derived mesenchymal stem cells; CPC, cardiopoietic stem cells; CAD, coronary artery disease; CLI, chronic limb ischemia; IHD, ischemic heart disease; MI, myocardial infarction; IC, intracoronary; IV, intravenous; IM, intramyocardial; LVEF, left ventricular ejection fraction; EDV, end diastolic volume; ESV, end systolic volume; EF, ejection fraction.

A plethora of data from the early clinical trials has largely demonstrated the safety and practicality of administering these growth factors to patients with refractory coronary artery disease such as the phase II VIVA trial and FIRST trial using recombinant VEGF and FGF2, respectively [25,26]. However, it was eventually recognized that the administration of these angioproteins in a clinical setting has resulted in short-lived improvements in collateral dependent perfusion that do not contribute to sustainable clinical benefit. Thus, significant limitations of these recombinant angioproteins were identified; the peptides had a short half-life and required administration of relatively large doses in order to elicit an effect, carrying the risk of significant adverse effects.

4.2. Gene Therapy

The delivery of a recombinant gene overtook protein therapy approaches, allowing for persistent expression of the encoded target protein in tissue. Indeed, the myocardium was found to be a suitable substrate for gene transfer, expressing target proteins encoded by viral vectors and non-viral vectors such as naked plasmids and liposome vehicles. Viral vectors tend to employ adenoviridae or retroviridae and are characterized by a high transfection efficiency although potentially immunogenic. The REVASC study was a large phase II randomized clinical trial that reported improved angina symptoms and exercise tolerance following intramyocardial injection of adenoviral-encoded VEGF when compared to optimal medical therapy [30]. However, the possibility of a placebo effect due to lack of blinding and occurrence of complications associated with thoracotomy procedure in four patients were limitations of this study.

Recombinant DNA delivered by means of non-viral vectors are generally more liable to destruction by circulating nucleases, which may shorten the half-life of these genes in target tissue. Nonetheless, many studies have reported meaningful therapeutic benefits with non-viral gene transfer and the lack of an immune reaction permits repeated administration. The Kuopio angiogenesis trial showed that intramyocardial injection of the recombinant VEGF gene on an adenoviral vector during percutaneous coronary angioplasty significantly increased myocardial perfusion when compared to delivery of the VEGF gene using a naked plasmid vector [31]. Moreover, phase I studies evaluating intramyocardial injection of plasmid-encoded VEGF DNA via thoracotomy in patients with end-stage coronary artery disease were associated with improvement of symptoms and blood flow to ischemic territories [27–29].

The transfer of human FGF4 bound to an adenovirus (Ad5-FGF4) vector by intracoronary infusion resulted in increased FGF mRNA production at twelve weeks, enhanced collateral dependent perfusion, and lessened the severity of symptomatic angina in patients in the AGENT trial [32]. These promising findings led to initiation of the AGENT-2, -3, and -4 trials, which were designed to assess the ultimate efficacy of Ad5-FGF4 in inducing ischemic myocardial neovascular formation in patients with stable exertional angina controlled with medical therapy (capable of exercising on a treadmill for at least three minutes) and anatomy suitable for, but not in need of, immediate revascularization. Agent-3 and Agent-4 trials, respectively, enrolled 450 and 532 patients and randomly assigned them to receive either placebo or Ad5-FGF4 as an intracoronary injection, the primary endpoint being change in exercise tolerance twelve weeks post treatment [40]. However, it was eventually found that the treatment offered no significant benefit over placebo, which led to discontinuation of these studies.

Adenoviral transfer and recombinant DNA have, therefore, faced challenges in the clinical setting likely due to breakdown in the circulation, but also includes limitations of cell turnover and risk of immune responses. CRISPR/Cas9 may hold the key to effective gene therapy approaches by offering increased precision and efficiency in comparison to conventional gene targeting approaches. In fact, Huang and colleagues designed a CRISPR/Cas9 system to deplete VEGFR2 in vascular endothelial cells, which was found to block angiogenesis in a mouse model of retinopathy [41]. While these results are recent, they provide the groundwork for future genome editing studies in the field to insert proangiogenic genes or delete inhibitory genes.

4.3. Stem Cell Therapy

Certain populations of stem and progenitor cells have the capacity to proliferate and differentiate into vascular components. Upon stimulation, angioblast-derived EPCs mobilize from the bone marrow and localize to sites of endothelial injury, differentiating into mature endothelial cells. Mesenchymal stem cells (MSCs) are another major source of adult stem cells that have been extensively studied for potential applications in cardiac regeneration, due to their reduced risk of immunogenicity and tumorigenicity. Indeed, data from animal studies showed that both bone-marrow-derived EPCs or those isolated from peripheral blood promoted vessel growth in ischemic tissue [42,43]. Subsequently, many clinical trials evaluated various methods of EPC or MSC administration to ischemic tissue.

Numerous early-phase trials of myocardial ischemia provided proof of concept that EPCs or MSCs improved vascularity in ischemic myocardial territories and overall cardiac function [34–36,38,39]. They also substantiated that intramyocardial transplantation of autologous bone-marrow-derived cells was a safe, feasible intervention that enhanced myocardial contractility and perfusion while reducing infarct size and cause-related mortality in patients with ischemic heart disease (IHD). Cytotherapy quickly gained popularity as a novel treatment for IHD and was adopted by many centers, thus generating much positive data showing improvement in various functional and symptomatic parameters following innovative methods of administration of MSCs such as NOGA guided delivery. Again, longevity of these therapeutic effects and reproducibility in larger, diverse patient populations was challenging [37–44]. Further investigation revealed that a considerable portion of the injected cells do not survive beyond the first three days and that restoration and replacement of the dying cells was lacking. Moreover, the remaining cells did not appear to conform into functional tissue that integrated into the injured myocardium. Contrarily, a trophic effect was often observable in the tissue at sites of cell transplantation.

Another caveat that impedes this cell-based therapy approach is the lack of uniform measures for characterization of cells and determination of their secretory properties. The general consensus is the use of flow cytometry to identify cells by specific markers. Such classifications may only be useful for the theoretical study of the functional behavior of cells with similar structural characteristics. In reality, however, stem and progenitor cells exhibit tremendous plasticity and may rapidly alternate phenotypes in different environments [45]. Exposure of pre-transplanted stem cells to hypoxic conditions stimulates ischemic tissue and induces the expression of many angiogenic factors and survival proteins that improve therapeutic efficacy. Growth factors such as VEGF, placental growth factor, and stem cell factor can mobilize endogenous bone-marrow-derived cells and direct their differentiation into specialized cell types with the capacity to express angiogenic factors. Another exciting approach involves engineering tissue using pluripotent stem cells and vascular progenitor cells induced to differentiate into contractile and vascular elements, respectively. Among other creative strategies that have been employed to promote survival of autologous stem cells are localized ultrasound-targeted microbubble destruction of tissue at the transplantation site to create a void that facilitates growth of the nascent cells and the use of grafts composed of cells and an ECM [46].

4.4. Extracellular Vesicle Therapy

The field of stem-cell-derived extracellular vesicles (EVs) advanced following findings that the therapeutic effects of cell-based therapies were mediated by paracrine actions [47,48]. The cardioprotective effects of EVs have since been well characterized in small and large animal models [49,50]. While EVs carry a diverse cargo of proteins, RNAs, and lipids that may mediate many pathways related to cardiac remodeling, their pro-angiogenic effects have been corroborated in vivo and in vitro. Proteomic characterization further supports the enrichment of pro-angiogenic pathways in EVs, which was shown to be regulated by NFκB signaling in an elegant study by Anderson and collaborators [51,52].

Although the field of stem-cell-derived EVs has gained much popularity amongst the research community, the translation of this therapeutic modality to the clinic has only just begun in the setting of cardiovascular diseases. Phase II and phase I studies with MSC-EV treatment for acute ischemic stroke and multiple organ dysfunction syndrome (MODS), respectively, are currently in progress (NCT03384433, NCT04356300). Challenges

5. Future of Therapeutic Angiogenesis

5.1. Patient Selection

Clinical trial eligibility criteria are essential in mitigating potential variables such as age, gender, disease state, and so forth to ensure safety, mitigate confounding factors, and isolate the effects of the treatment. Early clinical trials aiming at revascularization often targeted patients with significant severity of disease, who had previously undergone multiple failed interventions. This limited patient cohort suggests an inherent deficiency in the mechanisms needed for blood vessel growth, conferring a lack of responsiveness to growth factors and other therapies [53,54]. Additionally, many medications widely used in practice have well-documented anti-angiogenic properties including atorvastatin, spironolactone, captopril, and aspirin [55–60]. Experimental animal models may, therefore, be necessary to evaluate pro-angiogenic treatments at various time points of the disease, in addition to studying preventative measures prior to induction of the disease model. Such studies will shed light on the effectiveness of the treatment in relation to the time it was administered and the severity of the disease. Bioinformatics analysis to examine the database of clinical trial data may also be useful in evaluating the relationships between disease state, dose and delivery, and outcomes.

Additionally, lack of standardized endpoints to assess outcomes in patients enrolled in therapeutic angiogenesis trials makes interpretation difficult. Indeed, the gold standard remains the demonstration of new vessels or improved blood flow using imaging techniques or perfusion studies, respectively. However, the longevity of this vasculature and clinical significance with respect to improving quality of life and survival has been subject to controversy. Sun et al. employed simulations and statistical analysis to evaluate multiple endpoints in phase II acute heart failure clinical trials. They found that the average Z score, which considers the average among all endpoints, is most powerful [61]. Of course, the authors importantly note that sample size may require the application of different statistical methods and criteria.

5.2. Comorbidities

Preclinical studies evaluating the efficacy of therapeutics in the setting of CVDs often show promise but have little to no success when translated to the clinical setting. This discrepancy may be in part attributed to underlying comorbidities in humans that are unaccounted for in laboratory animal models. This issue is further highlighted by the high prevalence of obesity and diabetes in the U.S. population, which is, respectively, 40 and 10% as reported by the Centers for Disease Control and Prevention [62,63].

Indeed, four weeks of a high-fat diet or glucose intolerance has been associated with markedly increased expression of anti-angiogenic factors endostatin and angiostatin, increased oxidative stress and additional signaling abnormalities, which likely have a major effect in diminishing the angiogenic response to growth factors or cell therapy, or the angiogenic process in general in both animal models and in patients [64–66]. A recent study by our lab indeed found disparate gene expression and paradoxical angiogenic signaling between a chronic ischemia swine model with and without metabolic stress, when treated with EVs [67]. Therefore, future preclinical work must compare functional, cellular, and molecular effects of therapeutic treatments targeting angiogenesis in disease states with additional risk factors [68]. The widespread maladaptations that occur during cardiac remodeling, combined with underlying risk factors, also highlight the growing need for a more comprehensive or versatile treatment approach, such as combination therapies (Figure 3). In fact, therapeutic interventions such as glucose control seem to improve the potential of angiogenesis and collateral vessel growth in animal models [69].

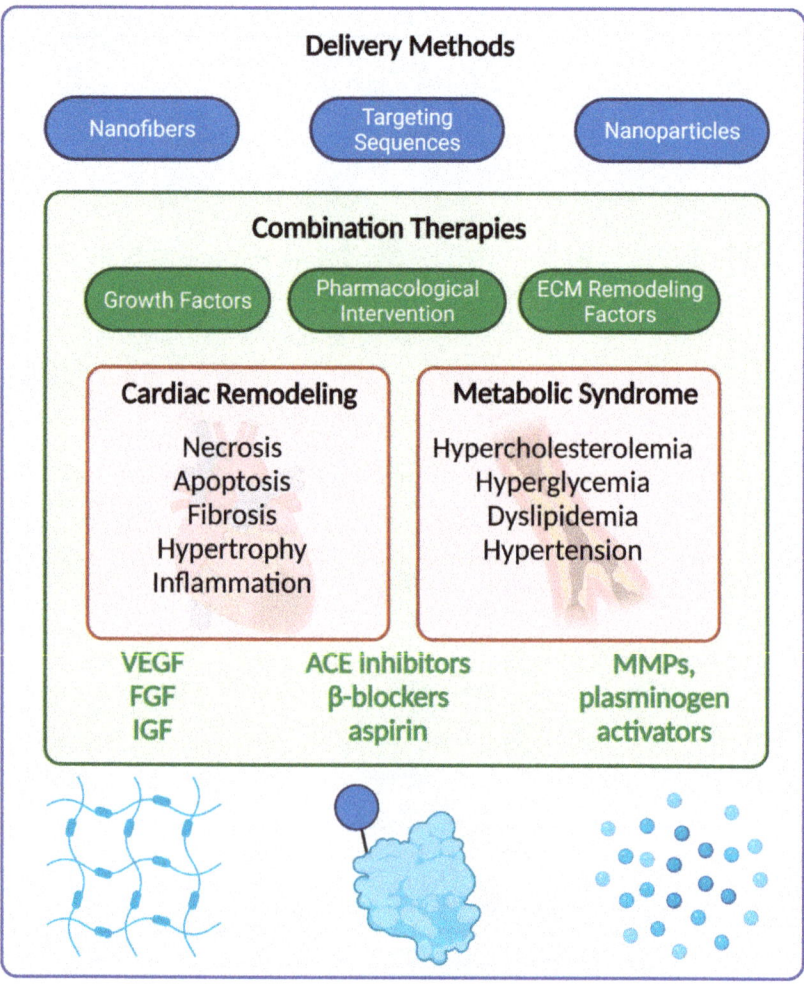

Figure 3. Future challenges and prospects in therapeutic angiogenesis. Cardiac remodeling is characterized by widespread maladaptive changes that adversely affect the structure and function of the heart; these events are further exacerbated by underlying comorbidities such as metabolic syndrome. Combination therapies have the potential to mediate the widespread changes and enhancing revascularization. Furthermore, bioengineering methods may play a valuable role in controlling the release of signaling factors, improving myocardial targeting, and encapsulating many factors.

5.3. Combination Therapies

The combination of proteins, genes, and/or cells is sound rationale to overcome the shortcomings of monotherapies. Indeed, co-administration of VEGF and PDGF, FGF2 and PDGF, or VEGF and FGF2 were found to improve revascularization compared to controls in ischemic tissues in vivo [70]. Bai and collaborators investigated single, binary, and ternary combination of growth factors with VEGF, FGF2, and bone morphogenic proteins 2 (BMP2). Together, these factors significantly improved endothelial cell angiogenesis in vitro and chorioallantoic membrane angiogenesis in vivo, with reduced concentrations of each factor [71]. Methods of modifying gene expression in BM-MSCS have had similar success; BM-MSCs overexpressing HGF or ANG1 were shown to increase vascularity in the ischemic myocardial territory [72]. The transfer of endothelial nitric oxide synthase (eNOS) to BM-MSCs using minicircle plasmid DNA also enhanced angiogenic capacity of these cells [73].

Preconditioning or priming cells with a given stimuli has also emerged to manipulate cellular cargo in place of single-gene transfections. This approach has the ability to tune the cell's contents at a much larger scale. The review by de Cássia Noronha et al. describes potential stimuli such as hypoxia, cytokine exposure, and nutrient or drug administration applied while culturing cells, and their therapeutic effects in animal models [45]. As the field of stem-cell-based therapies has been impeded by clinical findings with short-lasting improvements that are not sustained in the long-term, the field of stem-cell-derived EVs has conversely risen. Certainly, preconditioning or transfecting cells and isolating their EVs has potential in future clinical trials. A recent study by Sun and collaborators found that exosomes derived from hypoxia inducible factor 1 α (HIF1α)-overexpressing MSCs resulted in cardioprotection of a rat myocardial infarction model by inducing angiogenesis [74]. Omics studies will play a major role in characterizing EV cargo and ensure standardization for potential large-scale application. Certainly, laboratory animal models may not perfectly replicate the conditions inevitably associated with the clinical setting such as interfering comorbidities, medications, and refractory disease; however, creative and comprehensive preclinical study designs that considers comorbidities, combination therapies, and delivery systems are increasingly imperative.

5.4. Delivery

Ongoing studies aim to provide an optimal mode of delivery that does not necessitate repeated invasive procedures and ensure sustained tissue expression of the therapeutic substance. Indeed, thoracotomies and other surgical methods of delivery carry significant risks and prohibit effective control groups for clinical trials. These limitations prompted interest in employing cutting edge imaging modalities in the development of less invasive methods of administration of the gene-vectors to ischemic myocardial territories. Data from clinical trials showed that NOGA guided delivery of plasma encoded VEGF in patients with chronic symptomatic angina who are not candidates for conventional means of revascularization effectively improved Canadian Cardiovascular Society (CCS) angina class, while being well tolerated [75].

Novel delivery methods via nanofibers, nanoparticles, and targeting sequences may also be critical in overcoming these challenges. Among the nanofiber materials available, hydrogels are particularly intriguing due to their water content that is compatible with bodily tissues and support slow diffusion of bioengineered contents. An alginate-based gel containing VEGF found a stable release of the growth factor over one month in vitro and improved angiogenesis in a hindlimb ischemic model in vivo [76,77]. Of course, many polymer options can and should be explored in the development of a delivery system that maximizes and extends the angiogenic signal, such as collagens, gelatins, fibrins, peptides, and matrigels.

Nanoparticles may be sourced synthetically or from bioparticles, such as extracellular vesicles themselves; natural bioparticles may be a safer mode that avoids the risk of immunogenicity. Nonetheless, these particles—whether synthetic or natural in nature—are capable of being carriers of genes, proteins, drugs, and other molecules. The advantage to this method is protecting the molecule from potential degradation until fusion with recipient cells; furthermore, size and membrane content can be adjusted to improve delivery towards target tissue. In fact, in vivo biopanning approaches have identified cardiac-specific targeting peptides. Separate studies identified such targeting peptides, which were referred to as cardiac homing peptide (CHP) or ischemic myocardium-targeting peptide (IMTP), and conjugated them to exosomal membrane proteins [78,79]. They then proceeded to study the actions in vivo into animal models of MI and found improved delivery, biodistribution, and cardioprotection in the myocardium compared to controls [80,81].

A novel delivery platform was recently developed by Wang, designed to optimize delivery of growth factors and known as coacervate [82,83]. The coacervate forms due to electrostatic interactions that essentially polymerize into tiny oil droplets and mimic the structure of heparin along with its capability to bind many factors at once. Therefore, the coacervate has potential to deliver multiple growth factors, which may be of particular value in stimulating angiogenesis. In vitro examination supported the loading ability and controlled release of this platform; meanwhile, an in vivo study with FGF2 significantly improved angiogenesis compared to free FGF2 [82,83]. A recent study by Xiao and collaborators supported previous findings, where FGF2-loaded coacervate significantly enhanced wound healing via cell proliferation, VEGF secretion, and increased CD31 and αSMA density [84].

6. Conclusions

Ischemic heart disease is the most prevalent and deadly disease worldwide. While current standards of care have undoubtedly improved outcomes, there is consensus that novel therapies employing inherent mechanisms of revascularization are the next frontier in the management of this disease. Elucidation of angiogenic processes and their underlying mechanisms has provided key insights into activators and targets to stimulate angiogenesis. Protein, gene, and cell-based therapies have been developed; however, their translation from animal models to clinical trials have largely been disappointing. Challenges in patient selection, endpoint measures, and the prevalence of comorbidities have confounded results and interpretation. However, bioinformatic approaches and bioengineering strategies may overcome such challenges by determining optimal statistical methods that account for multiple endpoints, and improving delivery and biodistribution of factors to the damaged tissue. Combination therapies, furthermore, hold promise in mediating multiple pathways and maximizing therapeutic effects.

Author Contributions: Conceptualization, M.S., C.K., A.A., S.R., M.R.A. and F.W.S.; writing, M.S., C.K., A.A. and S.R.; reviewing and editing, M.R.A. and F.W.S.; visualization, C.K.; funding acquisition, M.R.A. and F.W.S. Figures were created with BioRender.com. All authors have read and agreed to the published version of the manuscript.

Funding: This work was supported by the NHLBI of the National Institutes of Health under award number [1R01HL133624] to M.R.A., and [R01HL128831] and [R01HL46716] to F.W.S.

Conflicts of Interest: The authors declare no conflict of interest.

References

1. Roth, G.A.; Johnson, C.; Abajobir, A.; Abd-Allah, F.; Abera, S.F.; Abyu, G.; Ahmed, M.; Aksut, B.; Alam, T.; Alam, K.; et al. Global, Regional, and National Burden of Cardiovascular Diseases for 10 Causes, 1990 to 2015. *J. Am. Coll. Cardiol.* **2017**, *70*, 1–25. [CrossRef] [PubMed]
2. Folkman, J. Tumor angiogenesis: Therapeutic implications. *N. Engl. J. Med.* **1971**, *285*, 1182–1186. [CrossRef] [PubMed]
3. Harada, K.; Friedman, M.; Lopez, J.J.; Wang, S.Y.; Li, J.; Prasad, P.V.; Pearlman, J.D.; Edelman, E.R.; Sellke, F.W.; Simons, M. Vascular endothelial growth factor administration in chronic myocardial ischemia. *Am. J. Physiol. Circ. Physiol.* **1996**, *270*, H1791–H1802. [CrossRef]
4. Sellke, F.W.; Laham, R.J.; Edelman, E.R.; Pearlman, J.D.; Simons, M. Therapeutic angiogenesis with basic fibroblast growth factor: Technique and early results. *Ann. Thorac. Surg.* **1998**, *65*, 1540–1544. [CrossRef]
5. Taimeh, Z.; Loughran, J.; Birks, E.J.; Bolli, R. Vascular endothelial growth factor in heart failure. *Nat. Rev. Cardiol.* **2013**, *10*, 519–530. [CrossRef]
6. Buschmann, I.; Schaper, W. Arteriogenesis Versus Angiogenesis: Two Mechanisms of Vessel Growth. *Physiology* **1999**, *14*, 121–125. [CrossRef] [PubMed]
7. Conway, E.M.; Collen, D.; Carmeliet, P. Molecular mechanisms of blood vessel growth. *Cardiovasc. Res.* **2001**, *49*, 507–521. [CrossRef]
8. Patan, S. Vasculogenesis and Angiogenesis. In *BT—Angiogenesis in Brain Tumors*; Kirsch, M., Black, P.M., Eds.; Springer: Boston, MA, USA, 2004; pp. 3–32. ISBN 978-1-4419-8871-3.
9. Ribatti, D.; Vacca, A.; Nico, B.; Roncali, L.; Dammacco, F. Postnatal vasculogenesis. *Mech. Dev.* **2001**, *100*, 157–163. [CrossRef]

10. Kimura, H.; Weisz, A.; Kurashima, Y.; Hashimoto, K.; Ogura, T.; D'Acquisto, F.; Addeo, R.; Makuuchi, M.; Esumi, H. Hypoxia response element of the human vascular endothelial growth factor gene mediates transcriptional regulation by nitric oxide: Control of hypoxia-inducible factor-1 activity by nitric oxide. *Blood* **2000**, *95*, 189–197. [CrossRef]
11. Nelson, A.R.; Fingleton, B.; Rothenberg, M.L.; Matrisian, L.M. Matrix metalloproteinases: Biologic activity and clinical implications. *J. Clin. Oncol. Off. J. Am. Soc. Clin. Oncol.* **2000**, *18*, 1135–1149. [CrossRef] [PubMed]
12. Brew, K.; Dinakarpandian, D.; Nagase, H. Tissue inhibitors of metalloproteinases: Evolution, structure and function. *Biochim. Biophys. Acta* **2000**, *1477*, 267–283. [CrossRef]
13. Iruela-Arispe, M.L.; Davis, G.E. Cellular and Molecular Mechanisms of Vascular Lumen Formation. *Dev. Cell* **2009**, *16*, 222–231. [CrossRef] [PubMed]
14. Carmeliet, P. Developmental biology. Controlling the cellular brakes. *Nature* **1999**, *401*, 657–658. [CrossRef]
15. Cook, D.R.; Doumit, M.E.; Merkel, R.A. Transforming growth factor-beta, basic fibroblast growth factor, and platelet-derived growth factor-BB interact to affect proliferation of clonally derived porcine satellite cells. *J. Cell. Physiol.* **1993**, *157*, 307–312. [CrossRef]
16. Cai, W.; Schaper, W. Mechanisms of arteriogenesis. *Acta Biochim. Biophys. Sin.* **2008**, *40*, 681–692. [CrossRef] [PubMed]
17. Meier, P.; Seiler, C. The coronary collateral circulation–past, present and future. *Curr. Cardiol. Rev.* **2014**, *10*, 1. [CrossRef]
18. Lin, Q.; Lu, J.; Yanagisawa, H.; Webb, R.; Lyons, G.E.; Richardson, J.A.; Olson, E.N. Requirement of the MADS-box transcription factor MEF2C for vascular development. *Development* **1998**, *125*, 4565–4574.
19. Olsson, A.-K.; Dimberg, A.; Kreuger, J.; Claesson-Welsh, L. VEGF receptor signalling—In control of vascular function. *Nat. Rev. Mol. Cell Biol.* **2006**, *7*, 359–371. [CrossRef] [PubMed]
20. Zhang, X.; Ibrahimi, O.A.; Olsen, S.K.; Umemori, H.; Mohammadi, M.; Ornitz, D.M. Receptor specificity of the fibroblast growth factor family. The complete mammalian FGF family. *J. Biol. Chem.* **2006**, *281*, 15694–15700. [CrossRef]
21. Zymek, P.; Bujak, M.; Chatila, K.; Cieslak, A.; Thakker, G.; Entman, M.L.; Frangogiannis, N.G. The role of platelet-derived growth factor signaling in healing myocardial infarcts. *J. Am. Coll. Cardiol.* **2006**, *48*, 2315–2323. [CrossRef]
22. Shyu, K.G.; Manor, O.; Magner, M.; Yancopoulos, G.D.; Isner, J.M. Direct intramuscular injection of plasmid DNA encoding angiopoietin-1 but not angiopoietin-2 augments revascularization in the rabbit ischemic hindlimb. *Circulation* **1998**, *98*, 2081–2087. [CrossRef]
23. Yang, Z.; Chen, B.; Sheng, Z.; Zhang, D.; Jia, E.; Wang, W.; Ma, D.; Zhu, T.; Wang, L.; Li, C.; et al. Improvement of heart function in postinfarct heart failure swine models after hepatocyte growth factor gene transfer: Comparison of low-, medium- and high-dose groups. *Mol. Biol. Rep.* **2010**, *37*, 2075–2081. [CrossRef]
24. Rong, S.; Wang, X.; Wang, Y.; Wu, H.; Zhou, X.; Wang, Z.; Wang, Y.; Xue, C.; Li, B.; Gao, D. Anti-inflammatory activities of hepatocyte growth factor in post-ischemic heart failure. *Acta Pharmacol. Sin.* **2018**, *39*, 1613–1621. [CrossRef]
25. Henry, T.D.; Annex, B.H.; McKendall, G.R.; Azrin, M.A.; Lopez, J.J.; Giordano, F.J.; Shah, P.K.; Willerson, J.T.; Benza, R.L.; Berman, D.S.; et al. The VIVA trial: Vascular endothelial growth factor in Ischemia for Vascular Angiogenesis. *Circulation* **2003**, *107*, 1359–1365. [CrossRef]
26. Simons, M.; Annex, B.H.; Laham, R.J.; Kleiman, N.; Henry, T.; Dauerman, H.; Udelson, J.E.; Gervino, E.V.; Pike, M.; Whitehouse, M.J.; et al. Pharmacological treatment of coronary artery disease with recombinant fibroblast growth factor-2: Double-blind, randomized, controlled clinical trial. *Circulation* **2002**, *105*, 788–793. [CrossRef]
27. Ruel, M.; Beanlands, R.S.; Lortie, M.; Chan, V.; Camack, N.; deKemp, R.A.; Suuronen, E.J.; Rubens, F.D.; DaSilva, J.N.; Sellke, F.W.; et al. Concomitant treatment with oral L-arginine improves the efficacy of surgical angiogenesis in patients with severe diffuse coronary artery disease: The Endothelial Modulation in Angiogenic Therapy randomized controlled trial. *J. Thorac. Cardiovasc. Surg.* **2008**, *135*, 762–770.e1. [CrossRef]
28. Lathi, K.G.; Cespedes, R.M.; Losordo, D.W.; Vale, P.R.; Symes, J.F.; Isner, J.M. Direct intramyocardial gene therapy with vegf for inoperable coronary artery disease: Preliminary clinical results. *Anesth. Analg.* **1999**, *88*, 73SCA. [CrossRef]
29. Hartikainen, J.; Hassinen, I.; Hedman, A.; Kivelä, A.; Saraste, A.; Knuuti, J.; Husso, M.; Mussalo, H.; Hedman, M.; Rissanen, T.T.; et al. Adenoviral intramyocardial VEGF-DΔNΔC gene transfer increases myocardial perfusion reserve in refractory angina patients: A phase I/IIa study with 1-year follow-up. *Eur. Heart J.* **2017**, *38*, 2547–2555. [CrossRef]
30. Stewart, D.J.; Hilton, J.D.; Arnold, J.M.O.; Gregoire, J.; Rivard, A.; Archer, S.L.; Charbonneau, F.; Cohen, E.; Curtis, M.; Buller, C.E.; et al. Angiogenic gene therapy in patients with nonrevascularizable ischemic heart disease: A phase 2 randomized, controlled trial of AdVEGF121 (AdVEGF121) versus maximum medical treatment. *Gene Ther.* **2006**, *13*, 1503–1511. [CrossRef] [PubMed]
31. Hedman, M.; Hartikainen, J.; Syvänne, M.; Stjernvall, J.; Hedman, A.; Kivelä, A.; Vanninen, E.; Mussalo, H.; Kauppila, E.; Simula, S.; et al. Safety and feasibility of catheter-based local intracoronary vascular endothelial growth factor gene transfer in the prevention of postangioplasty and in-stent restenosis and in the treatment of chronic myocardial ischemia: Phase II results of the Kuopio. *Circulation* **2003**, *107*, 2677–2683. [CrossRef]
32. Grines, C.L.; Watkins, M.W.; Helmer, G.; Penny, W.; Brinker, J.; Marmur, J.D.; West, A.; Rade, J.J.; Marrott, P.; Hammond, H.K.; et al. Angiogenic Gene Therapy (AGENT) trial in patients with stable angina pectoris. *Circulation* **2002**, *105*, 1291–1297. [CrossRef] [PubMed]

33. Nikol, S.; Baumgartner, I.; Van Belle, E.; Diehm, C.; Visoná, A.; Capogrossi, M.C.; Ferreira-Maldent, N.; Gallino, A.; Graham Wyatt, M.; Dinesh Wijesinghe, L.; et al. Therapeutic Angiogenesis With Intramuscular NV1FGF Improves Amputation-free Survival in Patients With Critical Limb Ischemia. *Mol. Ther.* **2008**, *16*, 972–978. [CrossRef]
34. Lunde, K.; Solheim, S.; Aakhus, S.; Arnesen, H.; Abdelnoor, M.; Egeland, T.; Endresen, K.; Ilebekk, A.; Mangschau, A.; Fjeld, J.G.; et al. Intracoronary injection of mononuclear bone marrow cells in acute myocardial infarction. *N. Engl. J. Med.* **2006**, *355*, 1199–1209. [CrossRef]
35. Perin, E.C.; Willerson, J.T.; Pepine, C.J.; Henry, T.D.; Ellis, S.G.; Zhao, D.X.M.; Silva, G.V.; Lai, D.; Thomas, J.D.; Kronenberg, M.W.; et al. Effect of Transendocardial Delivery of Autologous Bone Marrow Mononuclear Cells on Functional Capacity, Left Ventricular Function, and Perfusion in Chronic Heart Failure: The FOCUS-CCTRN Trial. *JAMA* **2012**, *307*, 1717–1726. [CrossRef] [PubMed]
36. Meyer, G.P.; Wollert, K.C.; Lotz, J.; Steffens, J.; Lippolt, P.; Fichtner, S.; Hecker, H.; Schaefer, A.; Arseniev, L.; Hertenstein, B.; et al. Intracoronary bone marrow cell transfer after myocardial infarction: Eighteen months' follow-up data from the randomized, controlled BOOST (BOne marrOw transfer to enhance ST-elevation infarct regeneration) trial. *Circulation* **2006**, *113*, 1287–1294. [CrossRef] [PubMed]
37. Bartunek, J.; Terzic, A.; Davison, B.A.; Filippatos, G.S.; Radovanovic, S.; Beleslin, B.; Merkely, B.; Musialek, P.; Wojakowski, W.; Andreka, P.; et al. Cardiopoietic cell therapy for advanced ischaemic heart failure: Results at 39 weeks of the prospective, randomized, double blind, sham-controlled CHART-1 clinical trial. *Eur. Heart J.* **2017**, *38*, 648–660. [CrossRef] [PubMed]
38. Bartunek, J.; Behfar, A.; Dolatabadi, D.; Vanderheyden, M.; Ostojic, M.; Dens, J.; El Nakadi, B.; Banovic, M.; Beleslin, B.; Vrolix, M.; et al. Cardiopoietic stem cell therapy in heart failure: The C-CURE (Cardiopoietic stem Cell therapy in heart failURE) multicenter randomized trial with lineage-specified biologics. *J. Am. Coll. Cardiol.* **2013**, *61*, 2329–2338. [CrossRef]
39. Assmus, B.; Honold, J.; Schächinger, V.; Britten, M.B.; Fischer-Rasokat, U.; Lehmann, R.; Teupe, C.; Pistorius, K.; Martin, H.; Abolmaali, N.D.; et al. Transcoronary transplantation of progenitor cells after myocardial infarction. *N. Engl. J. Med.* **2006**, *355*, 1222–1232. [CrossRef]
40. Henry, T.D.; Grines, C.L.; Watkins, M.W.; Dib, N.; Barbeau, G.; Moreadith, R.; Andrasfay, T.; Engler, R.L. Effects of Ad5FGF-4 in patients with angina: An analysis of pooled data from the AGENT-3 and AGENT-4 trials. *J. Am. Coll. Cardiol.* **2007**, *50*, 1038–1046. [CrossRef]
41. Huang, X.; Zhou, G.; Wu, W.; Duan, Y.; Ma, G.; Song, J.; Xiao, R.; Vandenberghe, L.; Zhang, F.; D'Amore, P.A.; et al. Genome editing abrogates angiogenesis in vivo. *Nat. Commun.* **2017**, *8*, 112. [CrossRef]
42. Suzuki, G.; Iyer, V.; Lee, T.C.; Canty, J.M., Jr. Autologous Mesenchymal Stem Cells Mobilize cKit+ and CD133+ Bone Marrow Progenitor Cells and Improve Regional Function in Hibernating Myocardium. *Circ. Res.* **2011**, *109*, 1044–1054. [CrossRef]
43. Weil, B.R.; Suzuki, G.; Leiker, M.M.; Fallavollita, J.A.; Canty, J.M., Jr. Comparative Efficacy of Intracoronary Allogeneic Mesenchymal Stem Cells and Cardiosphere-Derived Cells in Swine with Hibernating Myocardium. *Circ. Res.* **2015**, *117*, 634–644. [CrossRef] [PubMed]
44. Schaefer, A.; Zwadlo, C.; Fuchs, M.; Meyer, G.P.; Lippolt, P.; Wollert, K.C.; Drexler, H. Long-term effects of intracoronary bone marrow cell transfer on diastolic function in patients after acute myocardial infarction: 5-year results from the randomized-controlled BOOST trial–an echocardiographic study. *Eur. J. Echocardiogr.* **2010**, *11*, 165–171. [CrossRef] [PubMed]
45. De Noronha, N.C.; Mizukami, A.; Caliári-Oliveira, C.; Cominal, J.G.; Rocha, J.L.M.; Covas, D.T.; Swiech, K.; Malmegrim, K.C.R. Priming approaches to improve the efficacy of mesenchymal stromal cell-based therapies. *Stem Cell Res. Ther.* **2019**, *10*, 132. [CrossRef] [PubMed]
46. Chowdhury, S.M.; Abou-Elkacem, L.; Lee, T.; Dahl, J.; Lutz, A.M. Ultrasound and microbubble mediated therapeutic delivery: Underlying mechanisms and future outlook. *J. Control. Release* **2020**, *326*, 75–90. [CrossRef]
47. Gnecchi, M.; He, H.; Liang, O.D.; Melo, L.G.; Morello, F.; Mu, H.; Noiseux, N.; Zhang, L.; Pratt, R.E.; Ingwall, J.S.; et al. Paracrine action accounts for marked protection of ischemic heart by Akt-modified mesenchymal stem cells. *Nat. Med.* **2005**, *11*, 367–368. [CrossRef]
48. Gnecchi, M.; He, H.; Noiseux, N.; Liang, O.D.; Zhang, L.; Morello, F.; Mu, H.; Melo, L.G.; Pratt, R.E.; Ingwall, J.S.; et al. Evidence supporting paracrine hypothesis for Akt-modified mesenchymal stem cell-mediated cardiac protection and functional improvement. *FASEB J.* **2006**, *20*, 661–669. [CrossRef]
49. Alibhai, F.J.; Tobin, S.W.; Yeganeh, A.; Weisel, R.D.; Li, R.K. Emerging roles of extracellular vesicles in cardiac repair and rejuvenation. *Am. J. Physiol. Heart Circ. Physiol.* **2018**, *315*, H733–H744. [CrossRef]
50. Potz, B.A.; Scrimgeour, L.A.; Pavlov, V.I.; Sodha, N.R.; Abid, M.R.; Sellke, F.W. Extracellular Vesicle Injection Improves Myocardial Function and Increases Angiogenesis in a Swine Model of Chronic Ischemia. *J. Am. Heart Assoc.* **2018**, *7*, e008344. [CrossRef]
51. Anderson, J.D.; Johansson, H.J.; Graham, C.S.; Vesterlund, M.; Pham, M.T.; Bramlett, C.S.; Montgomery, E.N.; Mellema, M.S.; Bardini, R.L.; Contreras, Z.; et al. Comprehensive Proteomic Analysis of Mesenchymal Stem Cell Exosomes Reveals Modulation of Angiogenesis via Nuclear Factor-KappaB Signaling. *Stem Cells* **2016**, *34*, 601–613. [CrossRef]
52. Kim, H.-S.; Choi, D.-Y.; Yun, S.J.; Choi, S.-M.; Kang, J.W.; Jung, J.W.; Hwang, D.; Kim, K.P.; Kim, D.-W. Proteomic Analysis of Microvesicles Derived from Human Mesenchymal Stem Cells. *J. Proteome Res.* **2012**, *11*, 839–849. [CrossRef] [PubMed]
53. Ruel, M.; Wu, G.F.; Khan, T.A.; Voisine, P.; Bianchi, C.; Li, J.; Li, J.; Laham, R.J.; Sellke, F.W. Inhibition of the cardiac angiogenic response to surgical FGF-2 therapy in a Swine endothelial dysfunction model. *Circulation* **2003**, *108* (Suppl. 1), II335–II340. [CrossRef] [PubMed]

54. Voisine, P.; Bianchi, C.; Ruel, M.; Malik, T.; Rosinberg, A.; Feng, J.; Khan, T.A.; Xu, S.-H.; Sandmeyer, J.; Laham, R.J.; et al. Inhibition of the cardiac angiogenic response to exogenous vascular endothelial growth factor. *Surgery* **2004**, *136*, 407–415. [CrossRef] [PubMed]
55. Boodhwani, M.; Nakai, Y.; Voisine, P.; Feng, J.; Li, J.; Mieno, S.; Ramlawi, B.; Bianchi, C.; Laham, R.; Sellke, F.W. High-dose atorvastatin improves hypercholesterolemic coronary endothelial dysfunction without improving the angiogenic response. *Circulation* **2006**, *114*, I402–I408. [CrossRef] [PubMed]
56. Boodhwani, M.; Mieno, S.; Voisine, P.; Feng, J.; Sodha, N.; Li, J.; Sellke, F.W. High-dose atorvastatin is associated with impaired myocardial angiogenesis in response to vascular endothelial growth factor in hypercholesterolemic swine. *J. Thorac. Cardiovasc. Surg.* **2006**, *132*, 1299–1306. [CrossRef]
57. Klauber, N.; Browne, F.; Anand-Apte, B.; D'Amato, R.J. New Activity of Spironolactone. *Circulation* **1996**, *94*, 2566–2571. [CrossRef]
58. Volpert, O.V.; Ward, W.F.; Lingen, M.W.; Chesler, L.; Solt, D.B.; Johnson, M.D.; Molteni, A.; Polverini, P.J.; Bouck, N.P. Captopril inhibits angiogenesis and slows the growth of experimental tumors in rats. *J. Clin. Investig.* **1996**, *98*, 671–679. [CrossRef]
59. Dai, X.; Yan, J.; Fu, X.; Pan, Q.; Sun, D.; Xu, Y.; Wang, J.; Nie, L.; Tong, L.; Shen, A.; et al. Aspirin Inhibits Cancer Metastasis and Angiogenesis via Targeting Heparanase. *Clin. Cancer Res. Off. J. Am. Assoc. Cancer Res.* **2017**, *23*, 6267–6278. [CrossRef]
60. Hu, Y.; Lou, X.; Wang, R.; Sun, C.; Liu, X.; Liu, S.; Wang, Z.; Ni, C. Aspirin, a Potential GLUT1 Inhibitor in a Vascular Endothelial Cell Line. *Open Med.* **2019**, *14*, 552–560. [CrossRef]
61. Sun, H.; Davison, B.A.; Cotter, G.; Pencina, M.J.; Koch, G.G. Evaluating Treatment Efficacy by Multiple End Points in Phase II Acute Heart Failure Clinical Trials. *Circ. Heart Fail.* **2012**, *5*, 742–749. [CrossRef]
62. Centers for Disease Control and Prevention. *National Diabetes Statistics Report, 2020*; Centers for Disease Control and Prevention, US Department of Health and Human Services: Atlanta, GA, USA, 2020.
63. Hales, C.M.; Carroll, M.D.; Fryar, C.D.; Ogden, C.L. *Prevalence of obesity and severe obesity among adults: United States, 2017–2018*; Centers for Disease Control and Prevention: Atlanta, GA, USA, 2020; p. 360.
64. Sodha, N.R.; Boodhwani, M.; Clements, R.T.; Xu, S.-H.; Khabbaz, K.R.; Sellke, F.W. Increased antiangiogenic protein expression in the skeletal muscle of diabetic swine and patients. *Arch. Surg.* **2008**, *143*, 463–470. [CrossRef]
65. Boodhwani, M.; Nakai, Y.; Mieno, S.; Voisine, P.; Bianchi, C.; Araujo, E.G.; Feng, J.; Michael, K.; Li, J.; Sellke, F.W. Hypercholesterolemia impairs the myocardial angiogenic response in a swine model of chronic ischemia: Role of endostatin and oxidative stress. *Ann. Thorac. Surg.* **2006**, *81*, 634–641. [CrossRef] [PubMed]
66. Sodha, N.R.; Clements, R.T.; Boodhwani, M.; Xu, S.-H.; Laham, R.J.; Bianchi, C.; Sellke, F.W. Endostatin and angiostatin are increased in diabetic patients with coronary artery disease and associated with impaired coronary collateral formation. *Am. J. Physiol. Heart Circ. Physiol.* **2009**, *296*, H428–H434. [CrossRef]
67. Aboulgheit, A.; Potz, B.A.; Scrimgeour, L.A.; Karbasiafshar, C.; Shi, G.; Zhang, Z.; Machan, J.T.; Schorl, C.; Brodsky, A.S.; Braga, K.; et al. Effects of High Fat Versus Normal Diet on Extracellular Vesicle-Induced Angiogenesis in a Swine Model of Chronic Myocardial Ischemia. *J. Am. Heart Assoc.* **2021**, *10*, e017437. [CrossRef] [PubMed]
68. Boodhwani, M.; Sodha, N.R.; Mieno, S.; Xu, S.-H.; Feng, J.; Ramlawi, B.; Clements, R.T.; Sellke, F.W. Functional, cellular, and molecular characterization of the angiogenic response to chronic myocardial ischemia in diabetes. *Circulation* **2007**, *116*, 31–37. [CrossRef] [PubMed]
69. Boodhwani, M.; Sodha, N.R.; Mieno, S.; Ramlawi, B.; Xu, S.-H.; Feng, J.; Clements, R.T.; Ruel, M.; Sellke, F.W. Insulin treatment enhances the myocardial angiogenic response in diabetes. *J. Thorac. Cardiovasc. Surg.* **2007**, *134*, 1453–1460. [CrossRef] [PubMed]
70. Johnson, T.; Zhao, L.; Manuel, G.; Taylor, H.; Liu, D. Approaches to therapeutic angiogenesis for ischemic heart disease. *J. Mol. Med.* **2019**, *97*, 141–151. [CrossRef]
71. Bai, Y.; Leng, Y.; Yin, G.; Pu, X.; Huang, Z.; Liao, X.; Chen, X.; Yao, Y. Effects of combinations of BMP-2 with FGF-2 and/or VEGF on HUVECs angiogenesis in vitro and CAM angiogenesis in vivo. *Cell Tissue Res.* **2014**, *356*, 109–121. [CrossRef]
72. Park, B.-W.; Jung, S.-H.; Das, S.; Lee, S.M.; Park, J.-H.; Kim, H.; Hwang, J.-W.; Lee, S.; Kim, H.-J.; Kım, H.-Y.; et al. In vivo priming of human mesenchymal stem cells with hepatocyte growth factor–engineered mesenchymal stem cells promotes therapeutic potential for cardiac repair. *Sci. Adv.* **2020**, *6*, eaay6994. [CrossRef]
73. Bandara, N.; Gurusinghe, S.; Chen, H.; Chen, S.; Wang, L.; Lim, S.Y.; Strappe, P. Minicircle DNA-mediated endothelial nitric oxide synthase gene transfer enhances angiogenic responses of bone marrow-derived mesenchymal stem cells. *Stem Cell Res. Ther.* **2016**, *7*, 48. [CrossRef]
74. Sun, J.; Shen, H.; Shao, L.; Teng, X.; Chen, Y.; Liu, X.; Yang, Z.; Shen, Z. HIF-1α overexpression in mesenchymal stem cell-derived exosomes mediates cardioprotection in myocardial infarction by enhanced angiogenesis. *Stem Cell Res. Ther.* **2020**, *11*, 373. [CrossRef] [PubMed]
75. Vale, P.R.; Losordo, D.W.; Milliken, C.E.; McDonald, M.C.; Gravelin, L.M.; Curry, C.M.; Esakof, D.D.; Maysky, M.; Symes, J.F.; Isner, J.M. Randomized, single-blind, placebo-controlled pilot study of catheter-based myocardial gene transfer for therapeutic angiogenesis using left ventricular electromechanical mapping in patients with chronic myocardial ischemia. *Circulation* **2001**, *103*, 2138–2143. [CrossRef]
76. Chu, H.; Wang, Y. Therapeutic angiogenesis: Controlled delivery of angiogenic factors. *Ther. Deliv.* **2012**, *3*, 693–714. [CrossRef]
77. Silva, E.A.; Mooney, D.J. Spatiotemporal control of vascular endothelial growth factor delivery from injectable hydrogels enhances angiogenesis. *J. Thromb. Haemost.* **2007**, *5*, 590–598. [CrossRef]

78. Zahid, M.; Phillips, B.E.; Albers, S.M.; Giannoukakis, N.; Watkins, S.C.; Robbins, P.D. Identification of a cardiac specific protein transduction domain by in vivo biopanning using a M13 phage peptide display library in mice. *PLoS ONE* **2010**, *5*, e12252. [CrossRef] [PubMed]
79. Kanki, S.; Jaalouk, D.E.; Lee, S.; Yu, A.Y.C.; Gannon, J.; Lee, R.T. Identification of targeting peptides for ischemic myocardium by in vivo phage display. *J. Mol. Cell. Cardiol.* **2011**, *50*, 841–848. [CrossRef]
80. Vandergriff, A.; Huang, K.; Shen, D.; Hu, S.; Hensley, M.T.; Caranasos, T.G.; Qian, L.; Cheng, K. Targeting regenerative exosomes to myocardial infarction using cardiac homing peptide. *Theranostics* **2018**, *8*, 1869–1878. [CrossRef] [PubMed]
81. Wang, X.; Chen, Y.; Zhao, Z.; Meng, Q.; Yu, Y.; Sun, J.; Yang, Z.; Chen, Y.; Li, J.; Ma, T.; et al. Engineered Exosomes With Ischemic Myocardium-Targeting Peptide for Targeted Therapy in Myocardial Infarction. *J. Am. Heart Assoc.* **2018**, *7*, e008737. [CrossRef] [PubMed]
82. Chu, H.; Gao, J.; Chen, C.-W.; Huard, J.; Wang, Y. Injectable fibroblast growth factor-2 coacervate for persistent angiogenesis. *Proc. Natl. Acad. Sci. USA* **2011**, *108*, 13444–13449. [CrossRef]
83. Chu, H.; Johnson, N.R.; Mason, N.S.; Wang, Y. A [polycation:heparin] complex releases growth factors with enhanced bioactivity. *J. Control. Release* **2011**, *150*, 157–163. [CrossRef]
84. Wu, J.; Ye, J.; Zhu, J.; Xiao, Z.; He, C.; Shi, H.; Wang, Y.; Lin, C.; Zhang, H.; Zhao, Y.; et al. Heparin-Based Coacervate of FGF2 Improves Dermal Regeneration by Asserting a Synergistic Role with Cell Proliferation and Endogenous Facilitated VEGF for Cutaneous Wound Healing. *Biomacromolecules* **2016**, *17*, 2168–2177. [CrossRef] [PubMed]

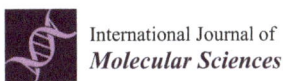

Review

Current Status of Angiogenic Cell Therapy and Related Strategies Applied in Critical Limb Ischemia

Lucía Beltrán-Camacho [1,2,†], Marta Rojas-Torres [1,2,†] and Mª Carmen Durán-Ruiz [1,2,*]

[1] Biomedicine, Biotechnology and Public Health Department, Cádiz University, 11519 Cadiz, Spain; lucia.beltrancamacho@alum.uca.es (L.B.-C.); marta.rojas@uca.es (M.R.-T.)
[2] Institute of Research and Innovation in Biomedical Sciences of Cadiz (INIBICA), 11009 Cádiz, Spain
* Correspondence: maricarmen.duran@gm.uca.es; Tel.: +34-956-012-727
† These authors contributed equally to this work.

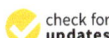

Citation: Beltrán-Camacho, L.; Rojas-Torres, M.; Durán-Ruiz, M.C. Current Status of Angiogenic Cell Therapy and Related Strategies Applied in Critical Limb Ischemia. *Int. J. Mol. Sci.* **2021**, *22*, 2335. https://doi.org/doi:10.3390/ijms22052335

Academic Editor: Paul Quax

Received: 7 January 2021
Accepted: 23 February 2021
Published: 26 February 2021

Publisher's Note: MDPI stays neutral with regard to jurisdictional claims in published maps and institutional affiliations.

Copyright: © 2021 by the authors. Licensee MDPI, Basel, Switzerland. This article is an open access article distributed under the terms and conditions of the Creative Commons Attribution (CC BY) license (https://creativecommons.org/licenses/by/4.0/).

Abstract: Critical limb ischemia (CLI) constitutes the most severe form of peripheral arterial disease (PAD), it is characterized by progressive blockade of arterial vessels, commonly correlated to atherosclerosis. Currently, revascularization strategies (bypass grafting, angioplasty) remain the first option for CLI patients, although less than 45% of them are eligible for surgical intervention mainly due to associated comorbidities. Moreover, patients usually require amputation in the short-term. Angiogenic cell therapy has arisen as a promising alternative for these "no-option" patients, with many studies demonstrating the potential of stem cells to enhance revascularization by promoting vessel formation and blood flow recovery in ischemic tissues. Herein, we provide an overview of studies focused on the use of angiogenic cell therapies in CLI in the last years, from approaches testing different cell types in animal/pre-clinical models of CLI, to the clinical trials currently under evaluation. Furthermore, recent alternatives related to stem cell therapies such as the use of secretomes, exosomes, or even microRNA, will be also described.

Keywords: critical limb ischemia; neovascularization; angiogenesis; arteriogenesis; cell therapy; secretomes

1. Critical Limb Ischemia

Critical Limb Ischemia (CLI) constitutes the most severe form of Peripheral Arterial Disease (PAD), a prevalent manifestation of atherosclerosis which involves the blockade of major systemic arteries other than those of the cerebral and coronary circulation [1], more common in legs than in arms [2]. PAD affects around 10–15% of adults, being an underestimated and underdiagnosed cardiovascular disease (CVD) due to its asymptomatic initial stages [3]. PAD is associated with risk factors such as older age, hypertension, dyslipidemia, or smoking [4], and it is more prevalent in diabetic people due to metabolic alterations such as angiogenesis impairment, inflammatory progression, or endothelial dysfunction [5–8]. CLI itself has an annual incidence of 0.35% and an average prevalence of 1.33%, affecting to 500–1000 people per 1 million population in Europe and the United States [9]. CLI patients are classified based on clinical criteria and hemodynamic parameters (i.e., pulse volume recordings, ankle and toe pressure values, rest pain, and tissue loss) [10–12] currently accepted in international consensus guidelines on PAD and CLI [12–16]. Overall, CLI patients suffer from chronic ischemic rest pain, ulcers, or gangrene, as well as an increased risk of cardiovascular events. CLI has a huge impact on the patients' quality of life, being associated with an increased risk of amputations (fingers, toes, or extremities) and, moreover, an increase in mortality rates [15,17–20]. This debilitating disease causes high dependency on caregivers, requiring permanent local wound treatment, and the chronic use of pain-relieving medications, considerably diminishing patient's quality of life [21].

Nowadays, the treatment of CLI remains highly variable and, in many situations, suboptimal [22]. Initial recommendations for CLI patients to prevent further cardiovascular events include smoking cessation, lipid lowering (statins mainly), antiplatelet therapies, or ACE inhibitors [16]. Alternatively, other medical strategies or pharmaceutical agents have been applied for the specific treatment of CLI patients (sympathectomy or spinal cord stimulation, iloprost) [23]. Unfortunately, these strategies do not seem to be totally effective in reducing limb-specific events [16], although larger studies/clinical trials are required in order to reach definitive conclusions.

The majority of CLI patients require revascularization interventions like bypass or angioplasty, having observed a significant improvement in the techniques and devices applied (cryoplasty, stent-grafts, drug-eluting balloons or stents, etc.) in the past decades. Nevertheless, the percentage of patients eligible for these strategies is not higher than 45% due to high comorbidity or surgical related issues such as difficult access due to narrow vessels, etc. Furthermore, patients that undergo surgery will usually require amputation at the short term [24]. Amputation rates are unacceptably high, typically exceeding 15–20% at 1 year and can vary by the presence of comorbid conditions [25] such as diabetes mellitus (DM), which elevates this rate up to 50% in CLI diabetic patients [26]. Diabetic patients have higher risk of suffering PAD/CLI and a negative outcome partly related to the abrogation of new vessel formation and remodeling of the pre-existing vasculature under hyperglycemic conditions [27]. Unfortunately, the increasing prevalence of PAD together with higher presence of other CLI risk factors (i.e., diabetes) and the rising number of people in advanced age provide little reason to believe that the number of patients suffering this disease will decrease in the near future [25]. The poor prognosis of CLI patients as well as their impaired quality of life makes compulsory to find effective and less invasive treatments. Moreover, the desirable treatment should be applicable to all CLI patients, because the actual percentage of ineligible patients is unacceptably high.

As an alternative to conventional treatments, therapeutic angiogenesis has arisen as a promising treatment for CLI patients, mainly those considered as "no-option", due to the potential of this strategy to promote revascularization of ischemic tissues [28–33]. To date, different approaches including angiogenic gene or cell-based therapies are currently under investigation.

In this review, we have mainly focused on the use of angiogenic cell therapy for CLI (Figure 1), from animal/pre-clinical models designed to study CLI and the tools applied to test for revascularization in response to cell therapy, to the angiogenic therapies currently under evaluation in clinical trials. Moreover, recent alternatives derived from stem cell therapies, such as the use of secretomes, exosomes, or even microRNAs, will be described.

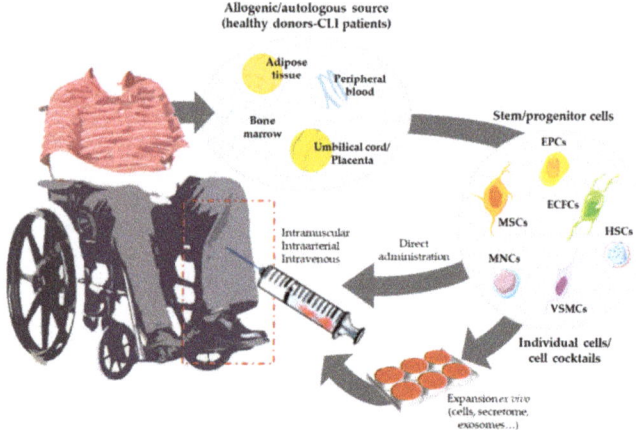

Figure 1. Overview of angiogenic cell therapy for Critical Limb Ischemia (CLI).

2. Animal Models of CLI

CLI animal models are not only used to study the disease itself [34,35], they also provide the appropriate scenario to evaluate strategies to induce neovascularization or to reduce inflammatory response. These models allow us to follow-up cell mobilization in response to ischemia [36–39]. Moreover, biodistribution assays are essential to determine the cell's fate [40,41] and more importantly, to evaluate the biosafety profile, being required by regulatory guidelines prior to initiating cell therapy into the clinic [42]. Furthermore, for treatments testing human components such as human cells, immunosuppressed animals (nude, athymic, etc.) are usually applied [43].

Thus, in order to pre-clinically evaluate the effect of cell therapy on revascularization, it becomes essential first to be able to achieve an optimal model of CLI capable to resemble as much as possible the characteristics found in humans. Until now, femoral artery ligation (FAL) remains the most common approach to induce CLI, which is usually performed in one limb, leaving the other as a non-ischemic control. Several studies performing single or double femoral ligation, or alternatively cutting the femoral artery in different sites or even excision of the artery (partly or in all branches) can be found, creating different grades of CLI [44,45] (Figure 2). Additionally, depending on the occlusion site, extent of the injury or the occlusion tools (suture knots, constrictors, electrocoagulation, etc.), it is possible to create different degrees of the disease, causing different ischemic stages and patterns of perfusion restoration [43,46].

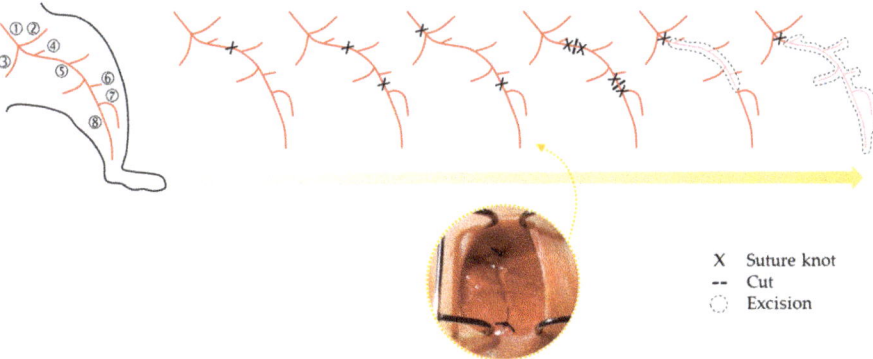

Figure 2. Schematic representation of femoral artery ligation (FAL) strategies usually applied to create PAD/CLI models, from the lowest (left) to the highest (right) severity models of the disease. A representative image of the FAL strategy followed in our research group is also shown [41,47]. Legend: ① Iliac artery, ② Iliacofemoral artery, ③ Internal iliac artery, ④ Pudendoepigastric trunk, ⑤ Femoral artery and its branches (lateral circumflex and proximal caudal), ⑥ Superficial caudal epigastric artery, ⑦ Popliteal artery, and ⑧ Saphenous artery. Arterial anatomy information was based on Kochi et al. [48].

The resulting CLI model not only depends on the methods described to promote ischemia, but also on the operator performing the interventions, the animals used (mouse, rat, rabbit, pig, etc.), or even the strain selected [49–51]. Moreover, it is difficult to reproduce an animal model that resembles 100% CLI in humans, as this disease courses with a very slow progression, without important or aggressive symptoms for years, until becomes chronic. In this regard, Lejay et al. proposed a sequential ligation process, ligating first the femoral artery and days after the iliac artery, in order to achieve a progressive model and with similar impaired functions than patients [52]. Krishna et al. performed a "two-stage model", with an initial arterial narrowing using ameroid constrictors over 14 days, prior to the induction of acute ischemia by FAL and excision [53]. Similarly, Han et al. created a model with local thrombosis in vessels by photochemical reaction triggered by the administration of erythrosine B, modifying endothelial function and occluding the vessels lumen by the blood clot, therefore getting closer to the human pathology than ligation [54].

On the other hand, the fact that most studies use healthy animals to generate CLI models constitutes an issue itself. CLI patients present, among other characteristics, endothelial dysfunction or reduced vascularity, which correlate with impaired vascular recovery. In FAL models, however, the vascular regeneration properties remain intact, which removes us from the reality of the patients' symptoms. Moreover, autologous cell therapy appears to be less effective than expected because cells show impaired functions under pathological conditions. For that reason, researchers have tried to combine FAL with additional strategies to replicate the pathophysiological characteristics found in CLI patients. Parikh et al. combined FAL with endothelial nitric oxide synthase (eNOS) inhibitor administration, increasing vasoconstriction and ischemia by blocking nitric oxide (NO) production [55]. Alternatively, animal models presenting risk factors associated with PAD, such as hyperlipidemia, hypercholesterolemia, or diabetes, have also been employed. Thus, CLI models generated in hyperlipidemic and diabetic mice generally coursed with reduced collateral formation and blood flow recovery, showing better correlation with human patients [56]. Apolipoprotein E (ApoE)-deficient mice, commonly accepted as a model of atherosclerosis [4], also show a decrease of muscle regeneration after FAL surgery [37].

Strategies Followed to Assess Neovascularization in CLI

The ultimate goal of any CLI treatment is to promote post-natal neovascularization, a repairing mechanism that takes place in response to ischemic events as an strategy to recover the damaged tissues and provide sufficient oxygen and nutrient supply to ensure tissue surveillance [57]. In adults, neovascularization comprises both angiogenesis and arteriogenesis, processes in which different types of vascular and immune cells participate [58]. Angiogenesis consists in the formation of new blood vessels from existing ones, while arteriogenesis involves collateral growth and remodeling of pre-existing arterioles to generate larger conductance vessels and to compensate for the loss of blood flow of occluded arteries (Figure 3a) [59]. Remarkably, FAL animal models and patients usually show similar neovascularization patterns, with enhanced arteriogenesis next to the occlusion site and increased angiogenesis in the distal ischemic tissue [49]. Thus, therapeutic strategies should seek the stimulation of both processes in order to promote neovascularization [58].

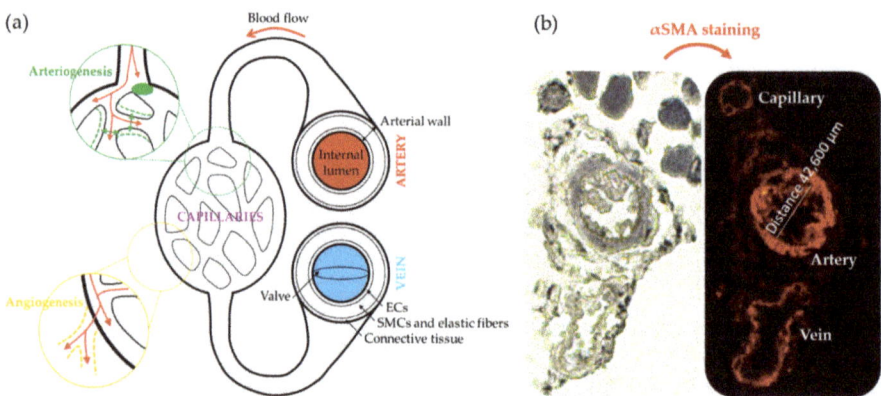

Figure 3. Mechanisms of neovascularization. (**a**) Schematic representation of the circulatory system in which angiogenesis and arteriogenesis processes are represented. (**b**) Representative immunohistochemistry image of blood vessels detected in the low back muscle of a CLI mouse [47], to evaluate vascular density and diameter size using anti-smooth muscle α-actin (α-SMA, red) antibody.

In studies involving CLI animal models (Table 1), different strategies are usually applied to analyze potential neovascularization. Blood flow recovery over time is often analyzed by Laser Doppler Perfusion (LDP). This technology is based on Doppler effect, consisting in the alteration of a wave's frequency as result of the movement between a laser light and circulating red blood cells. Alternatively, the LDP Imaging system creates images from blood perfusion values per pixel, getting a map of the blood flow in the region of interest [49]. In FAL-based studies, perfusion is measured before and after surgical intervention, and then registered during several days, usually 3–4 weeks. Perfusion data are normally shown as blood flow ratios (ischemic limb/healthy limb). Although there are other techniques to evaluate collateral formation and limb perfusion such as X-ray micro-angiography [49], LDP has been the most applied tool in recent publications due to the easy handling of the equipment and, moreover, because it constitutes a noninvasive method.

Histological analysis by immunohistochemistry (IHC) is also used to evaluate angiogenesis and arteriogenesis post-mortem. Most studies use anti-α smooth muscle actin antibodies to identify blood vessels in tissues (Figure 3b), together with antibodies against endothelial cells markers, such as CD31, von Willebrand factor, or lectins with specific affinity for endothelial cells, like *Ulex europaeus* agglutinin I in humans or *Griffonia simplicifolia* lectin I isolectin B4 in non-primates [47,49,60,61]. For angiogenesis, vascular density is calculated by counting the number of blood vessels, and capillary diameters are measured for arteriogenesis evaluation. The internal lumen's diameter is normally measured to evaluate arteriogenesis, although the arterial wall area is also interesting since arteriogenesis increases diameter and wall thickness [59,62]. Results are usually expressed as the number of blood vessels per mm^2 in angiogenesis and blood vessel diameter (μm) or area (μm^2) in arteriogenesis. Alternatively, another method to study angiogenesis is an in vivo matrigel plug assay, consisting in the injection of matrigel or similar hidrogels containing specific cell types into the subcutaneous space [63]. After several days of post-implantation, mice are sacrificed and the matrigel plugs are extracted and excised for further analysis. Sections can be then stained to identify capillary structures, and vasculature growth into matrigel provides information regarding angiogenesis [49].

3. Angiogenic Cell Therapy

Angiogenic therapy involves the use of angiogenic growth factors (VEGF, HIF-1a, FGF1, HGF, etc.) [33,64], gene transfer techniques using viral or non-viral vectors to transport a gene codifying for a therapeutic protein to the target tissues [65] or, alternatively, the use of angiogenic stem cells. All these strategies aim to improve revascularization by increasing the number/size of blood vessels, promoting blood flow recovery and therefore increasing tissue perfusion in the ischemic extremities [65]. Among them, cell-based therapies seem more efficient compared to protein- or gene-based approaches, not only because of their direct vasculogenic properties, but also due to their paracrine effect. Angiogenic cells can directly participate in the formation of new vessels, while in parallel they also provide endogenous growth factors, promoting vascular growth by paracrine fashion [66,67].

Thus, neovascularization can also be promoted by vasculogenesis, the novo formation of vessels mediated by circulating progenitors or stem cells [59]. Vasculogenesis was initially considered as an embryogenic process. However, post-natal vasculogenesis can also take place by incorporation of vascular stem or progenitor cells into vessel structures, allowing the formation of adult blood vessels [68]. To date, several strategies based on the use of stem and progenitor cells are being tested (Table 1), to promote vasculogenesis but also angiogenesis and arteriogenesis. The safety and efficacy of cell implantation therapies make of this less invasive treatment a feasible option for CLI patients.

Table 1. Classification of most important cell therapy pre-clinical studies. The table includes cell type used, first author and year of publication, reference number (ref), cell source, animal and strain, number of administered cells, route of administration, follow-up, and parameters checked to evaluate the therapy outcome. Abbreviations included (alphabetical order): a: autologous; AD: Arteriolar density; AI: Angiographic index; BFP: Blood flow perfusion; CBP: Calf Blood Pressure; CD: Capillary density; CVF: Collateral Vessel Formation; ESC-ECP: Stem cell-derived endothelial cell product; FS: Functional score; h: human; IA: Intraarterial; IC: Intracardiac; IM: Intramuscular; IV: Intravenous; MP: Matrigel plug; SC: Subcutaneous; TR: Tissue regeneration; VD: Vessel diameter; VIP: Vascular intersection percentage; VS: Visual Scale

Cell Type	Author (Year)	Ref.	Cell Source	Animal (Strain)	Administration (×10⁵ Cells)	Route of Administration	Follow-up (Weeks)	Outcome
aMSCs	Cunha (2013)	[69]	Bone marrow	Mice (Balb-C & C57/BL6)	5	IM	4	VS, CD, TR
hMSCs	García-Vázquez (2019)	[70]	Adipose tissue	Mice (Athymic nude)	6	IM	3	BFP, CD, VS
aMSCs	Nammian (2021)	[71]	Bone marrow & adipose tissue	Mice (C57/BL6)	5	IM	4	FS, CD
hMSCs + hECFCs	Rossi (2017)	[72]	Bone marrow & peripheral blood	Mice (Athymic nude)	N/A	IV	2	BFP, CD, VS
hCD34+	Lian (2018)	[73]	Peripheral blood	Mice (Balb-C Nude)	1	IM	3	FS, VS
hEPCs	Kalka (2000)	[74]	Peripheral blood	Mice (Athymic nude)	5	IC	4	BFP, CD, VS
hEPCs	Urbich (2003)	[75]	Peripheral blood	Mice (Athymic NMRI Nude)	5	IV	2	BFP, CD
hEPCs	Zhao (2016)	[76]	Fetal aorta	Rat (Goto-Kakizaki)	100	IM	8	BFP, CD, VS
hCACs	Beltrán-Camacho (2020)	[47]	Peripheral blood	Mice (Balb-C Nude)	5	IM	4 days	BFP, CD, FS, VD
hEPCs + hOECs	Yoon (2005)	[77]	Peripheral blood	Mice (Athymic nude)	2	IM	3	BFP, CD, VS, MP
hEPCs + hSMPCs	Foubert (2008)	[78]	Umbilical cord blood	Mice (Athymic nude)	5	IV	2	BFP, CD, AD
hESC-ECP	MacAskill (2018)	[40]	hESC line	Mice (CD1-STZ DM inductor)	10	IM	3	BFP, CD
aBM-MNCs	Shintani (2001)	[79]	Bone marrow	Rabbit (Male New Zealand White)	5	IM	4	BFP, CBP, CD, CVF
aBMCs	De Nigris (2007)	[80]	Bone marrow	Mice (ApoE−/−)	20	IV	2	BFP, CD, CVF
aBM-MNCs	Jeon (2007)	[81]	Bone marrow	Mice (C57/BL6)	20	IM	4	CD, CVF
aBM-MNCs	Gan (2009)	[82]	Bone marrow	Mice (C57/BL6)	30	IM	2	BFP, CD
hBM-NCs	Liu (2009)	[83]	Bone marrow	Mice (C57/BL6 ApoE−/−)	250	IA	4	BFP, CVF

Table 1. Cont.

Cell Type	Author (Year)	Ref.	Cell Source	Animal (Strain)	Administration (×10⁵ Cells)	Route of Administration	Follow-up (Weeks)	Outcome
aBM-MNCs	Brenes (2012)	[84]	Bone marrow	Mice (C57/BL6)	5, 10 & 20	IM	4	BFP, CD, FS
aBM-MNCs	Reis (2014)	[85]	Bone marrow	Mice (Balb-C)	5	IM	4	CD, TR, VS
hBM-MNCs	Rojas-Torres (2020)	[41]	Bone marrow	Mice (Balb-C Nude)	10	IM	3	BFP, CD, FS, VD
aBMC-derived macrophages	Kuwahara (2014)	[86]	Bone marrow	Mice (C57/BL6N)	1	IM	4	BFP, CD
hALDH high activity cells	Capoccia (2009)	[87]	Bone marrow	Mice (NOD/SCID b2M)	1–2	IM	3	BFP, CD
aMIAMI cells	Rahnemai-Azar (2011)	[88]	Bone marrow	Mice (Balb-C)	10	IM	4	BFP, CD, FS, VS
hPB-MNCs[1]	Li (2006)	[89]	Peripheral blood	Mice (Athymic nude)	10	IM	4	BFP, AI, CD, VS
aPB-MNCs + PRP	Padilla (2020)	[90]	Peripheral blood	Rat (Wistar)	15	IM	4	AI, VIP
aASCs	Liu (2020)	[91]	Adipose tissue	Mice (C57/BL6)	10	IM	3	BFP, CD, VS
aASCs + macrophages	Rybalko (2017)	[92]	Adipose tissue	Mice (C57/BL6)	2	IM	3	BFP, CD
hSVF	Jin (2017)	[93]	Adipose tissue	Mice (Nude)	10	IM	2	BFP, VS, CD, MP
PDX-PAD (adherent stromal cells)	Prather (2009)	[94]	Placenta	Mice (Balb-C)	10	IM	3	BFP, CD, FS
PLX-PAD (MSC like stromal cells)	Zahavi-Goldstein (2017)	[95]	Placenta	Mice (C57/BL6)	0.02–10	IM & SC	3	BFP, VS

[1] Cells mobilized with G-CSF.

3.1. Cell Therapies Based on Single or Combined Isolated Cells

Mesenchymal stem cells (MSCs) are the most used cells in advanced therapies for CVDs [96]. MSCs can be isolated from bone marrow, peripheral blood, or adipose tissues, and from them we can obtain osteoblasts, chondrocytes, adipocytes, neurons, endothelial cells (ECs), skeletal muscle cells, and vascular smooth muscle cells (VSMCs) [97]. MSCs are reported to promote angiogenesis because of their capacity to induce ECs proliferation, migration, and tube formation, while decreasing apoptosis and fibrosis [96,98,99]. Furthermore, MSCs support neoangiogenesis, releasing soluble factors that contribute to stimulate angiogenesis [100]. These cells are thought to improve hind limb ischemia by secreting cytokines that regulate macrophage differentiation to M2, an anti-inflammatory phenotype [101]. Likewise, apart from MSCs, endothelial progenitor cells (EPCs) also represent an important group of cells used in vascular regeneration. In 1997, Asahara et al. demonstrated that CD34+ cells can be isolated from peripheral blood mononuclear cells (PB-MNCs) and differentiated in vitro into ECs, showing the potential use for collateral vessel growth augmentation in ischemic tissues [102]. Although CD34 is not a specific marker of a single cell type, it is mostly associated to EPCs. Many researchers have explored the potential of using EPCs in tissue engineering as an angiogenic source for vascular repairing [103,104]. In the past years, several isolation and culturing techniques for EPCs have been described. Besides, the controversy regarding the definition of EPC phenotypes remains, with different studies still presenting a variety of results in terms of surface-based EPC markers [47,103,105,106]. At least, two different sub-populations have been accepted and clearly defined, based on their differentiation status and the capability to form colonies: early EPCs (eEPCs) also named circulating angiogenic cells (CACs) or myeloid angiogenic cells (MACs), with hematopoietic phenotype, and late EPCs or endothelial colony forming cells (ECFCs), with endothelial phenotype [106]. EPCs have been thought to derive from hematopoietic stem cells (HSCs), some EPCs could be derived from a niche close to the vasa vasorum in the macro-vascular wall [107]. Despite the controversy regarding the nature of these cells, no one denies the potential of EPCs to promote therapeutic angiogenesis and neovascularization of ischemic tissues [73,74,107]. Overall, in response to injury, cytokines and growth factors mobilize EPCs from the bone marrow into the peripheral blood, which will then participate in neovascularization [73]. Very recently, we have shown how, first days after administration of CACs to ischemic CLI mice, these cells migrate into the ischemic tissues, modulating immune cells recruitment and promoting an increase of angiogenesis and arteriogenesis [47]. However, the administered cells do not remain in the ischemic tissues over time suggesting that they may promote vasculogenesis in a paracrine form [47,108]. Moreover, early EPCs do not seem to differentiate to ECs, with this role being assigned to ECFCs [106,109]. Indeed, different studies support that the regenerative properties of eEPCs are mainly due to paracrine effects, while ECFCs present vessel-forming activity in vivo [47,109]. Thus, a cell therapy mediated by both cell types, early, and late EPCs, could be a good strategy for CVDs. Yoon et al. evaluated this combined cell therapy, demonstrating a synergistic neovascularization involving several cytokines and matrix metalloproteinases (MMPs) [77]. Very recently, our group has also corroborated the potential of CACs to promote angiogenesis of ECFCs in vitro, and such effect was impaired under an atherosclerotic environment [110]. In the same way, different cell combinations have been tested. Rossi et al. demonstrated that co-injection of MSCs with ECFCs in a murine model of CLI increased vessel density and foot perfusion in greater ratio than cells individually administered; corroborating the theory that MSCs support ECFC-mediated angiogenic processes [72]. Furthermore, their results indicated that MSCs accelerated muscle recovery via endoglin dependent mechanism. Similarly, the combination of EPCs and smooth muscle progenitor cells (SMPCs) has also been evaluated to treat CLI. This cell mixture improved vascular network formation, with both ECs and smooth muscle cells (SMCs) participating in vessel maturation and stability. Likewise, Foubert et al. demonstrated that co-administration of EPCs and SMPCs activates neovascularization resulting in a more effective therapy than these cells administered separately [78]. Some studies suggest that SMCs may also originate from bone marrow-derived cells as SMPCs have been identified in peripheral blood [111].

3.2. Cell Therapies Based on Cellular Cocktails

As an alternative to the injection of a single cell type or the combination of two previously isolated cells, the administration of cellular cocktails derived from different niches, such as bone marrow, peripheral blood, or adipose tissue, is also a frequent approach to treat CLI. Indeed, the regenerative properties of mononuclear cells (MNCs) derived from either bone marrow or peripheral blood have been largely studied in the last years. Therapies employing bone marrow mononuclear cells (BM-MNCs) constitute a promising alternative for CLI patients to avoid or delay the onset of amputation [112]. BM-MNCs consist of a heterogeneous mix of multipotent stem cells working cooperatively as MSCs, HSCs, EPCs, monocytes, lymphocytes, and pluripotent stem cells [41,113]. We and other researchers have reported the beneficial effects of different combinations of BM-MNCs, representing an effective approach in promoting new vessel formation, perfusion recovery, and CLI reversal [41,100,114–122]. In the ischemic tissue, BM-MNCs produce and secrete different cytokines and growth factors [123] and increase neovascularization and collateral vessel formation in limb ischemia [79]. Moreover, Kikuchi-Taura et al. have recently described that transplantation of BM-MNCs into a murine stroke model promoted ECs angiogenesis by gap junction mediated cell–cell interactions, elucidating a new theory of how cell-based therapies work, and suggesting that stem cells supply energy to injured cells [124]. This study suggested that, under hypoxic conditions, transplanted BM-MNCs are capable to transfer small molecules to ECs via gap junction interactions, leading to HIF-1α activation, which induced upregulation of VEGF uptake into ECs and ECs autophagy suppression [124].

Alternatively to BM-MNCs, PB-MNCs are formed by circulating cells with angiogenic potential, thereby several studies involving the administration of these cells to treat CLI have also shown promising results [125,126]. Li et al. made a comparison between CD34+ and CD34- cells in PB-MNCs, concluding that both induce neovascularization, but only CD34+ incorporate into new capillaries [89]. PB-MNCs promote revascularization in ischemic limbs, even more when they are combined with platelet-rich plasma (PRP) [90]. PRP, a source of platelets, cytokines, and growth factors, participates in ECs proliferation and differentiation, interacting with important cell receptors related with angiogenesis [90]. Furthermore, in order to achieve high stem cell concentrations, hematopoietic growth factors are frequently used to induce cell mobilization. For example, prior PB-MNCs harvesting, progenitor cells are usually mobilized injecting granulocyte colony-stimulating factor (G-CSF) [125–128]. BM-MNCs and PB-MNCs treatments have been compared, and no significant differences have been observed between them [129,130]. Remarkably, without previous mobilization, PB-MNCs show higher concentration of mature cells as red blood cells, platelets, lymphocytes, and monocytes, while BM-MNCs show higher levels of EPCs [131].

The use of adipose tissue-derived stem cells (ASCs) has increased in the last years, due to the easier accessibility, abundance, and less painful collection compared to other sources such as bone marrow [132]. The stromal vascular fraction (SVF) derived from adipose tissue contains heterogeneous cell populations such as mesenchymal progenitor/stem cells, pre-adipocytes, endothelial cells, pericytes, T cells, and M2 macrophages. SVF-derived mesenchymal progenitor/stem cells, usually referred as ASCs themselves, can be easily expanded in vitro and have the potential to differentiate into multiple lineages, including myogenic, osteogenic, neurogenic, and hematopoietic pathways [133–137]. The angiogenic properties of these cells have been correlated with a strong paracrine activity, secreting an important number of angiogenesis-related cytokines [136]. Moreover, the administration of ASCs to CLI mice promotes a significant recovery of blood flow in ASCs treated mice compared to ischemic, non-treated ones [133]. Very recently, Liu J et al. have shown that the regenerative properties of transplanted ASCs might correlate with an immunomodulatory effect promoted by these cells. In presence of ASCs, a higher number of macrophages can be found in the muscle, with increased presence of M2 macrophages [91], and its administration in a murine model of CLI induces an angiogenic process in the ischemic tissue [133]. The clear advantages of using these cells are easy access and isolation. ASCs are highly abundant in adipose tissue, making almost unnecessary culture expansion of these cells. Moreover, adipose tissue harvesting requires a minimally invasive intervention [138]. A pilot study using adipose-derived regenerative cells (ADRCs) in CLI patients has been recently published [139].

Finally, other cells with multi-differentiation potential such as amniotic fluid derived stem cells (AFSCs) or umbilical cord blood and placenta tissue derived stem/progenitor cells have also been considered. Placenta-derived MSCs stromal-like cells (PLX-PAD) in CLI mice are currently being tested in a Phase III trial (PACE Trial) with atherosclerotic CLI patients (NCT03006770) after promising results in animal assays [95]. Unfortunately, the low availability of these cells together with ethics concerns related to their use, has limited their translation as cell therapies.

4. Clinical Trials

The exciting results derived from pre-clinical studies fomented the initiation of numerous clinical trials: to date, over 50 studies have investigated a variety of cell therapies, usually employing BM- or PB-derived MNCs, showing modest but significant improvements of ischemic symptoms [140,141]. Patients enrolling these trials normally suffered from severe stages of PAD (Fontaine III-IV) with pain at rest due to atherosclerosis obliterans (ASO) rather than thrombo-angiitis obliterans (TAO) or Buerger's Disease. The first clinical trial that reported the efficacy of autologous BM-MNCs administration as cell therapy for CLI was published in 2002 [142]. The Therapeutic Angiogenesis using Cell Transplantation (TACT) trial conducted a pilot study first with 25 patients, followed by a randomized controlled trial in which 22 patients with bilateral leg ischemia were injected with BM-MNCs in one leg and PB-MNCs in the other as controls. Their findings indicated a significant improvement in ankle-brachial index (ABI), transcutaneous oxygen pressure (TcPO$_2$), and pain-free walking time sustained at 24 weeks, with a limb status improved in 39 out of 45 patients [142]. Table 2 includes a list, far from complete, of clinical studies already completed and with results published in the past decades, involving the use of different cell types, cell doses, and administration routes, with a minimum of 10 patients enrolled. Due to the huge interest in the field, the number of ongoing clinical trials using cell therapy in CLI is constantly growing, including examples such as the Phase III PACE trial (PLX-PAD cells, NCT03006770) [143], or the Phase III trial testing Rexmyelocel-T (REX-001), a solution enriched with human BM-derived MNCs (NCT03174522 and NCT03111238) in CLI Rutherford V and DM patients. Some of these studies are active and recruiting, therefore, their results are not yet available. Additional information regarding such trials can be found at www.clinicaltrials.gov (accessed on 14 December 2020).

Table 2. Classification of most important cell therapy clinical trials. The table shows first author and year of publication, reference number (ref), type of cell therapy, type of study, associated cause of PAD/CLI, disease stage, number of patients (T=Treated/C=Controls), control used, number of administered cells, route of administration, follow-up, and parameters checked to evaluate the cell therapy outcome. Parameters registering general improvement vs. baselines/controls are highlighted (**bold**). Abbreviations included (alphabetical order): ABI: Ankle-brachial index; AFS: Amputation-free survival; AR: Amputation rate; ASO: Arteriosclerosis obliterans; DR: Death rate; ECEPCs: enriched circulating endothelial progenitor cells; HD: High dose; LD: Low dose; MD: Medium dose; NC: Non-controlled; NR: Non-randomized; PFWD: Pain-free walking distance; RCT: Randomized controlled trial; RPS: Rest pain score; TAO: thromboangiitis obliterans; TcPO2: Transcutaneous oxygen pressure; UH: Ulcer healing.

Author (year)	Ref.	Type of Cell Therapy	Type of Study	Cause of PAD/CLI	Disease Stage	Nº Patients (T/C)	Control	Administration (x10^6 cells)	Route of Administration	Follow-up (Months)	Outcome
Huang (2005)	[125]	PB-MNCs[1]	RCT	ASO	Fontaine III-IV	28 (14/14)	Blank	3000	IM	3	**ABI, AR, DR, PFWD, RPS,** UH
Ozturk (2012)	[128]	PB-MNCs[1]	RCT	N/A	Fontaine III-IV	40 (20/20)	Blank	24.8/mL (CD34+)	IM	3	**ABI, AR, PFWD, RPS,** TcPO$_2$, UH
Mohammadzadeh (2013)	[127]	PB-MNCs[1]	RCT	N/A	Fontaine III-IV	21 (7/14)	Blank	900–1200	IM	3	**ABI, AR, UH, PFWD**
De Angelis (2015)	[144]	PB-MNCs	NR	ASO	Fontaine IV	86 (43/43)	Blank[5]	125.65	IM	4.5	AFS, **AR, DR, PFWD, RPS,** UH
Tateishi-Yuyama (2002) TACT	[142]	BM-MNCs / BM-MNCs	NR / R	ASO	Fontaine III-IV / Fontaine III-IV	25[2] / 22[3]	Blank / Placebo	700–2700 / 889–2800	IM / IM	6 / 6	**ABI, TcPO$_2$, RPS**
Arai (2006)	[145]	BM-MNCs	RCT	N/A	Fontaine III-IV	26 (13/13)	Blank	1000–3000	IM	1	**ABI, TcPO$_2$, RPS**
Dubsky (2013)	[129]	PB-MNCs / BM-MNCs	NR	N/A	Rutherford 4–6	33 (11/22)[4] / 39 (17/22)[4]	Blank	10400 / 1800	IM	6	**AR, TcPO$_2$, UH**
Huang (2007)	[146]	PB-MNCs / BM-MNCs	NC	ASO	N/A	76 / 74	N/A	7200 / 580	IM	3	**ABI, AR, PFWD, RPS,** TcPO2, UH
Matoba (2008)	[30]	BM-MNCs	NC	ASO & TAO	Fontaine III-IV	115	N/A	N/A	IM	25.3	ABI, AFS, **DR, PFWD, RPS,** TcPO2, UH
Ruiz-Salmeron (2011)	[120]	BM-MNCs	NC	ASO & others	Rutherford 4–6	20	N/A	100–400	IA	12	**ABI, AR, DR,** TcPO$_2$

Table 2. Cont.

Author (year)	Ref.	Type of Cell Therapy	Type of Study	Cause of PAD/CLI	Disease Stage	N° Patients (T/C)	Control	Administration (x10^6 cells)	Route of Administration	Follow-up (Months)	Outcome
Amann (2009) BONMONT-1	[114]	BM-MNCs / BM-TNCs	NC	N/A	Rutherford 4–6	12 / 39	N/A	1100 / 3000	IM	13.5	**ABI**, AFS, **PFWD**, TcPO$_2$
Walter (2011) PROVASA	[20]	BM-MNCs	RCT	ASO & TAO	Fontaine III–IV	40 (19/21)	Placebo	153	IA	3	ABI, AR, DR, **RPS**, TcPO$_2$, UH
Li (2013)	[147]	BM-MNCs	RCT	ASO	Fontaine III–IV	58 (29/29)	Placebo	10/mL	IM	6	**ABI**, AFS, AR, DR, RPS, UH
Teraa (2015) JUVENTAS	[148]	BM-MNCs	RCT	ASO	Fontaine IIB–IV	160 (81/79)	Placebo	500	IA	6	ABI, AR, DR, TcPO2, UH
Pignon (2017) BALI	[149]	BM-MNCs	RCT	ASO	Rutherford 4–5	36 (17/19)	Placebo	1300	IM	12	ABI, AR, RPS, TcPO2, UH
Guo (2018)	[116]	BM-MNCs	NR	TAO	N/A	59 (40/19)	Blank	3500	IM	129.5	**ABI**, AFS, AR, RPS, TcPO$_2$, UH
Lu (2011)	[150]	BM-MNCs / BM-MSCs	RCT	ASO	Fontaine IV	21^2 / 20^2	Blank	930 / 960	IM	6	**ABI**, AR, PFWT, RPS, TcPO$_2$, UH
Dash (2009)	[151]	BM-MSCs	RCT	ASO / Buerger	N/A	6 (3/3) / 18 (9/9)	Blank	N/A	IM	3	PFWD, UH
Gupta (2013)	[152]	BM-MSCs (allogenic)	RCT	ASO & TAO	Rutherford 4–6	20 (10/10)	Placebo	200	IM	6	ABI, AR, RPS, UH
Szabò (2013)	[153]	Ves-Cell	RCT / NC	N/A	Fontaine III–IV	20 (10/10)	Blank	66.4	IM	3 / 22.6	ABI, AR, DR, PFWD, RPS, TcPO$_2$, UH / **ABI**, AFS, **AR**, **DR**, PFWD, **RPS**, TcPO$_2$, UH
Raval (2014) SCRIPT-CLI	[154]	CD133+^{1}	RCT	ASO	N/A	10 (3/7)	Placebo	50–400	IM	12	AFS, AR, DR
Lara-Hernandez (2010)	[155]	EPCs^1	NC	ASO & TAO	Fontaine III–IV	28	N/A	N/A	IM	14.7	**ABI**, RPS, UH

Table 2. Cont.

Author (year)	Ref	Type of Cell Therapy	Type of Study	Cause of PAD/CLI	Disease Stage	N° Patients (T/C)	Control	Administration (x10^6 cells)	Route of Administration	Follow-up (Months)	Outcome
Kinoshita (2012)	[156]	CD34+[1]	NC	ASO & Buerger	Rutherford 4-5	17	N/A	0.1/kg (LD) 0.5/kg (MD) 1/kg (HD)	IM	12	**AR, DR, PFWD, RPS, TcPO$_2$, UH**
Dong (2013)	[157]	CD34+[1]	NC	ASO, TAO & others	Rutherford 4-5	25	N/A	0.1/kg (LD) 0.5/kg (MD) 1/kg (HD)	IM	6	**ABI, AR, DR, PFWT, RPS, TcPO$_2$, UH**
Fujita (2014)	[158]	CD34+[1]	NC	ASO & Buerger	Rutherford 4-5	11	N/A	1/kg	IM	12	**AR, PFWD, RPS, TcPO$_2$**
Powell (2012) RESTORE-CLI	[159]	Ixmyelocel-T	RCT	N/A	N/A	72 (48/24)	Placebo	35-295	IM	12	AFS, AR, DR
Losordo (2015)	[160]	CD34+[1]	RCT	N/A	Rutherford 4-5	28 (16/12)	Placebo	0.1/kg (LD) 1/kg (HD)	IM	12	ABI, AR, DR, PFWD, UH
Liotta (2018)	[161]	BM-MNCs ECEPCs	R	N/A	Rutherford 4-6	17 / 23	Blank[5]	50[6] / 250[6]	IM	12	**ABI, PFWD, RPS, TcPO2, UH**
Fang (2020)	[162]	PB-MNCs[1] CD34+[1]	RCT	TAO	Rutherford 4-5	78 / 82	PB-MNC	70, 37[7] / 31, 95[7]	IM	4,6	**ABI, AFS, PFWT, RPS, TcPO2**
Sharma (2021)	[163]	BM-MNCs	RCT	ASO & others	Fontaine IIC-IV	81 (41/40)	Placebo	71, 51	IA	6	**ABI, AR, PFWD, RPS, TcPO$_2$, UH**

[1] Cells mobilized with G-CSF; [2] The other limb was used as control, injected with saline serum; [3] Each limb was randomized for PB-MNCs/BM-MNCs; [4] Same control was used; [5] Retrospective; [6] Quantity referred to CD14+CD34^{low} cells; [7] Quantity referred to CD34+ cells.

One of the primary outcomes seen in clinical trials is hemodynamic improvement, represented as an absolute increase of ABI >10% [12,164]. Similarly, other researchers have reported an enhanced blood perfusion when administering either BM-MNCs, PB-MNCs, or MSCs [114,125,127,128,145,147,150,153]. Gupta et al. evaluated the effect of allogenic MSCs in patients (Rutherford grade 4–6) that suffered from CLI due to ASO and TAO. This study reported a significant increase of ABI ($p = 0.0018$) after 6 months of MSCs treatment (n:10) compared to patients transplanted with placebo (n:10), although no such significant changes could be observed in rest pain, ulcer healing, or amputation rates. Some authors debate about the selection of ABI as a primary endpoint, as this parameter is not considered a useful predictor for evaluating the long-term efficiency of the angiogenic therapy using bone marrow cells [20,142]. The PROVASA study, a randomized, double-blind, placebo-controlled intra-arterial progenitor cell transplantation of BM-MNCs for induction of neovascularization in patients with PAD, showed no significant differences in ABI primary outcome at 3 months. However, authors did observe significant improvements in other secondary endpoints, like ulcer healing and rest pain reduction in the BM-MSCs group [20].

Luckily, cell therapy has promoted an amelioration of the symptoms and therefore an improvement in the quality-of-life of these patients [158,160]. Thus, an improvement in rest pain is defined as a >50% decrease in pain scores, assessed with the visual analogue scale (VAS) at different time points [165]. In a non-randomized study, CLI-TAO patients (n:40) received autologous BM-MNCs, and after a mean follow-up of 129 months, a prominent improvement in VAS ($p = 0.0001$) was seen, also in their primary endpoint amputation-free survival and other secondary outcomes including ulcer status, ABI, toe-brachial index, and TcPO$_2$ [116]. This last hemodynamic measurement is employed in several clinical trials as secondary endpoint, and an augmentation in oxygen pressure has been observed in numerous studies using PB-MNCs, BM-MNCs, MSCs, as well as peripheral blood-derived angiogenic cell precursors (Ves-cells) [20,114,116,128,129,142,145,150,153].

Alternatively, CD34+ or CD133+ isolated cells have also been tested in CLI studies. In a randomized single-blinded non-inferiority trial, patients were divided 1:1 into those receiving either PB-MNCs or purified CD34+ cells. Although the number of patients included in this study was low, similar results were found in terms of limb salvage and quality of life improvements. No significant differences were found between both treatments in terms of amputation-free survival. On the other hand, the CD34+ group seemed to achieve faster rest-pain relief and overall earlier ischemia relief than the PB-MNCs group [166]. In the Stem Cell Revascularization for Patients with Critical Limb Ischemia (SCRIPT-CLI) trial, subjects with CLI due to ASO were divided in two groups in 2:1 proportion, receiving an active treatment with G-CSF for 5 days before leukapheresis and CD133+ injection in both legs, and a group receiving saline injections plus a sham leukapheresis and a placebo-buffered solution instead of cells. The safety of the procedure was proven 12 months after treatment, whereas a poor mobilization of CD133+ cells was found in several patients, together with higher rates of CD133+ senescent cells. These results reflected the need of studies with higher number of patients. Nevertheless, these authors suggested that this therapeutic approach might not be entirely successful with the patients selected [154]. Finally, other type of cells gaining popularity as a potential treatment for CLI patients are ASCs, SVF, or the very small embryonic-like stem cells (VSEL) [139,167,168].

Limitations in Cell-based Clinical Trials

Despite the promising results derived from the use of stem cells with CLI patients, the variability and heterogeneity found within the clinical trials is high. Remarkably, after 20 years of using stem cell therapy in CLI, it remains unclear which cell type or cell source triggers the highest benefits in terms of blood perfusion recovery or amelioration of ischemic symptoms. The first trials focused on using heterogeneous cell preparations from either bone marrow of peripheral blood. Such unpurified cell mixtures are often composed by a considerably low proportion of "active" cells, or cells with documented pro-angiogenic functions [109,125,142,169]. On the other hand, large amounts of cells are required during cell therapy, but proangiogenic progenitor cells are not present in high proportions in humans, being necessary to develop optimized and clinically applicable culture expansion methods for future perspectives. Cells could be efficiently selected by their expression of CD34, CD133, or also by their ALDH-activity, although this approach have detractors too, as extended culture is thought to negatively affect cell regenerative function [170,171]. However, the optimization of these cultures could solve the problematic associated with EPCs or MSCs dysfunctionality in CLI patients, as well as augmenting the angiogenic potency of cells through pre-stimulation prior transplantation [47,172]. In this sense, the next question relies in whether using an autologous or an allogenic strategy with these patients. Autologous administration avoids rejection-related issues, but also presents several disadvantages such as difficulties to recruit a significant number of cells from these donors, and moreover the already mentioned cellular dysfunction in response to atherosclerosis and/or related co-morbidities. The allogenic method complicates the therapy applicability by requiring HLA-matching [173–175].

Another matter of disparity is the cell dose to apply, depending on the cell type/source, as the number of MNCs and purified cells from MNCs always vary between patients and could be affected by the illness itself. Unfortunately, some studies did not even provide such information [30,170,174]. Similarly, the route of administration has not reached a consensus yet. The majority of trials have chosen an intramuscular cell delivery, considering this a more feasible and less invasive strategy [147,150]. Other authors postulate that an intra-arterial administration would better distribute the cells into areas with sufficient oxygen to prolong the pro-angiogenic function, trying to avoid the transient cell engraftment and integration after intramuscular injection [20,87,148]. In this regard, several studies have compared both intramuscular and intra-arterial strategies, showing similar results in terms of clinical outcome [176–178].

Overall, the comparison of the results derived from different trials comprises an arduous task in which meta-analysis are becoming increasingly useful to support evidence-based medicine, allowing to summarize the accumulated evidence and also to drive future research [179]. A meta-analysis performed by Rigato et al. includes robust statistical analysis of either randomized, controlled trials, and non-controlled studies. Their results showed that in patients not eligible for surgical revascularization, autologous cell therapy has the potential to reduce the risk of major amputation in 36%, improving also the probability of wound healing in 59%. Moreover, it appears to ameliorate several surrogate endpoints of limb perfusion, pain, and functional capacity [180]. Similarly, Gao et al. analyzed the results of over a thousand patients enrolling randomized controlled trials, indicating that cell implantation improved ulcer healing rate, ABI, $TcPO_2$, pain-free walking distance, and reduced amputation rate and rest pain score compared with standard care/conventional treatment [181]. Very recently, a review including 11 meta-analyses evaluated current evidence on cell-based therapy in PAD. Such study corroborates the effectiveness of using cell therapy with CLI patients, with a reduction in the number of major amputations and improved wound healing. Furthermore, for secondary outcomes such as ABI, $TcPO_2$, and RPS, a general improvement is seen [179]. Despite this, larger studies are required to increase statistical significance, together with the design of placebo-controlled studies, as clinical outcome differences are not clear when compared to the placebo effect [181,182].

The discrepancy found between the clinical trials reflects the fact that there is still a lot of work to do, as stated before, in order to reach a consensus regarding the optimal treatment. This, in turn, also requires of a better understanding of how cells work, in order to implement their use in clinical practice. Still, these studies share a common conclusion: the safety and feasibility of cell therapy in patients with no option of surgical revascularization, a population that represents half of the CLI patients diagnosed [120,144].

5. Strategies Derived from Cell Therapy

Due to increasing number of studies supporting that the regenerative power of stem cells is mainly due to their paracrine effect within the ischemic tissues, the use of the cells released factors (secretome) and, more recently, the so-called exosomes as an alternative to cell therapy, is currently being investigated. Secretomes are also named in different studies as conditioned medium (CM), referring to the factors released to the medium where cells have been cultured. The modulatory effect of these secretomes could depend on the presence of different growth factors, angiogenic factors, hormones, cytokines, extracellular matrix proteins and proteases, hormones, lipid mediators and genetic material secreted from stem or progenitor cells for cell communications, interfering in different biological functions such as growth, division, differentiation, apoptosis, and signaling [183,184]. The stem cell secretome has shown great potential and could mediate intracellular pathways in injured cells or activate adjacent tissues secretion [184].

Secretomes derived from different progenitor or stem cells are being studied, especially thanks to mass spectrometry approaches. In this way, Barberg et al. analyzed the MSCs secretome composition, identifying proteins related to cell growth, signal transduction and cell communication, as well as cytokines and growth factors involved in physiological regulation of hematopoiesis [185]. Likewise, Maffioli et al. described that, in a proinflammatory environment, MSCs increase the secretion of proteins related with immunomodulation and angiogenesis [186]. Although MSCs secretomes are the most studied ones, secretomes of other stem/progenitor cells are also showing promising results. Very recently, we analyzed by a proteomic approach the secretome of CACs, identifying a significant number of angiogenic factors, and moreover, we demonstrated that incubation ex vivo of ECFCs with this secretome enhances ECFCs angiogenesis, in agreement with previous studies [77,110]. Moreover, ASCs secretome contains multiple angiogenic factors, which appear to promote, among others, survival, proliferation, and migration of ECs, as well as vasculogenesis [187,188]. Indeed, ASCs conditioned medium has been shown to enhance proliferation and survival of endothelial cells in vitro [133]. Some of these secretomes have already been tested as therapy in vivo showing encouraging results, since they seem to be as effective as cell therapy [189–191]. The complete knowledge of the secretomes activity and their factors would allow us to reproduce them artificially by means of bioactive molecules to use in regenerative medicine. Finally, the administration of secretomes as an alternative approach to cell therapy eliminates disadvantages such as immune rejection or tumorigenicity [184]. Currently, novel strategies such as secretomes liberation approaches to enhance their angiogenic properties are being evaluated. For example, Felice et al. used nanoparticles to achieve a controlled EPCs secretome, demonstrating the potential of this system in FAL rat models [192]. Likewise, extracellular vesicles derived from stem or progenitor cells, also called "exosomes", seem to participate as well in the regenerative role of cellular secretomes. Exosomes derived from MSCs appear to promote bone regeneration and angiogenesis [193]. In the same way, exosomes derived from CD34+ cells have been shown to participate in angiogenesis and are essential for the repairing properties assigned to these cells [194].

Finally, microRNAs have recently arisen as a promising alternative therapy against ischemic diseases. MicroRNAs, short non-coding RNAs that inhibit translation of messenger RNAs, can regulate an entire network or pathway simultaneously, besides, in response to ischemia, they appear to be involved in the regulation of angiogenesis and arteriogenesis [58,195]. Different strategies against PAD are based on the modulation of factors related to the development of vasculature. However, modifications in a single factor do not seem to be sufficient for the treatment of this disease, and therefore the development of therapeutic strategies based on microRNAs are very promising, as this approach would allow to regulate several pathways at the same time. Some of the most studied microRNAs in CLI are miR-494, miR-487b, miR-329, and miR-495. Thus, the inhibition of some of these molecules, described as antiangiogenic microRNAs, seems to promote blood flow recovery in CLI mice [195,196]. Some studies suggest that microRNAs could be transferred by stem or progenitor cells through exosomes to ECs, promoting angiogenesis in these forms [197]. Although microRNAs are the best known and most studied RNA non-coding molecules for their therapeutic potential, there are other related types of RNA, such as circular or long noncoding RNAs, that also act in the regulation of gene expression and therefore should be also evaluated as therapeutic targets.

6. Conclusions

In the past decades, an enormous effort has been made to find appropriate strategies for the optimal treatment of CLI patients. Stem cell-based therapies have proven to be safe and efficient to achieve therapeutic angiogenesis and to promote blood flow recovery, representing an alternative for these patients. In this sense, the interest in the field is clear, and the number of clinical trials using cell therapy in CLI is constantly growing. Still, the variability seen between these trials is high, reflecting a lack of consensus regarding key factors such as cell doses, cell types or sources, administration routes, the parameters to define outcome efficacy, or the cohorts themselves. Moreover, further investigation is required in order to better understand how the cells, or the molecules/exosomes derived from them, exert such beneficial effects. Thus, a lot of work needs to be done before their translation into the clinical practice. Even so, the results are promising, and a therapy based on the administration of stem/progenitor cells and/or their derivatives could hopefully represent a good alternative for CLI patients, especially for those with no other options.

Author Contributions: Conceptualization: L.B.-C., M.R.-T., and M.C.D.-R.; data curation: L.B.-C., M.R.-T., and M.C.D.-R.; writing—original draft preparation: L.B.-C., M.R.-T., and M.C.D.-R.; writing—review and editing: L.B.-C., M.R.-T., and M.C.D.-R.; supervision, project administration, and funding acquisition: M.C.D.-R. All authors have read and agreed to the published version of the manuscript.

Funding: This work was supported by the Institute of Health Carlos III, ISCIII (PI16-00784, PI20-00716) and the Programa Operativo de Andalucia FEDER, Iniciativa Territorial Integrada ITI 2014-2020 Consejeria de Salud, Junta de Andalucia (PI0026-2017).

Institutional Review Board Statement: Not applicable.

Informed Consent Statement: Not applicable.

Data Availability Statement: Not applicable.

Conflicts of Interest: The authors declare no conflict of interest.

Abbreviations

a	Autologous
ABI	Ankle brachial index
aBMCs	Autologous bone marrow cell transplantation
AD	Arteriolar density
ADRCs	Adipose-derived regenerative cells
AFS	Amputation free survival
AFSCs	Amniotic fluid-derived stem cells
AI	Angiographic index
AR	Amputation rate
ASCs	Adipose tissue derived stem cells
ASO	Atherosclerosis obliterans
BM-MNCs	Bone marrow-derived mononuclear cells
BM-MSCs	Bone marrow mesenchymal stem cells
BM-TNCs	Bone marrow total nucleated cells
BFP	Blood flow perfusion
CACs	Circulating angiogenic cells
CBF	Calf blood pressure
CD	Capillary density

CM	Conditioned medium
CLI	Critical limb ischemia
CVDs	Cardiovascular diseases
CVF	Collateral vessel formation
DM	Diabetes mellitus
DR	Death rate
ECFCs	Endothelial colony forming cells
ECs	Endothelial cells
ECEPCs	Enriched circulating endothelial progenitor cells
EPCs	Endothelial progenitor cells
ESC-ECP	Stem cell-derived endothelial cell product
FAL	Femoral artery ligation
FGF1	Fibroblast growth factor 1
FS	Functional score
G-CSF	Granulocyte colony-stimulating factor
HD	High dose
HGF	Hepatocyte growth factor
HIF-1a	Hypoxia-inducible factor 1-alpha
HPCs	Hematopoietic progenitor cells
h	Human
IA	Intraarterial
IC	Intracardiac
IHC	Immunohistochemistry
IM	Intramuscular
IV	Intravenous
LD	Low dose
LDP	Laser Doppler Perfusion
MACs	Myeloid angioenic cells
MD	Medium dose
MMPs	Matrix metalloproteinases
MP	Matrigel plug
MSCs	Mesenchymal stem cells
NC	Non-controlled
NO	Nitric oxide
NR	Non-randomized
PAD	Peripheral arterial disease
PB-MNCs	Peripheral blood mononuclear cells
PFWD	Pain-free walking distance
PRP	Platelet-rich plasma
RCT	Randomized controlled trial
RPS	Rest pain score
SC	Subcutaneous
SMCs	Smooth muscle cells
SMPCs	Smooth muscle progenitor cells
SVF	Stromal vascular fraction
TAO	Thrombo-angiitis obliterans
$TcPO_2$	Transcutaneous oxygen pressure
TR	Tissue regeneration
UH	Ulcer healing
VAS	Visual analogue scale
VD	Vessel diameter
VEGF	Vascular endothelial growth factor
VIP	Vascular intersection percentage
VS	Visual Scale
VSEL	Very small embryonic-like stem cells

References

1. Conte, S.M.; Vale, P.R. Peripheral Arterial Disease. *Heart Lung Circ.* **2018**, *27*, 427–432. [CrossRef] [PubMed]
2. Balakumar, P.; Maung, U.K.; Jagadeesh, G. Prevalence and prevention of cardiovascular disease and diabetes mellitus. *Pharmacol. Res.* **2016**, *113 Pt A*, 600–609. [CrossRef] [PubMed]
3. van Weel, V.; van Tongeren, R.B.; van Hinsbergh, V.W.; van Bockel, J.H.; Quax, P.H. Vascular growth in ischemic limbs: A review of mechanisms and possible therapeutic stimulation. *Ann. Vasc. Surg.* **2008**, *22*, 582–597. [CrossRef]
4. Krishna, S.M.; Moxon, J.V.; Golledge, J. A review of the pathophysiology and potential biomarkers for peripheral artery disease. *Int. J. Mol. Sci.* **2015**, *16*, 11294–11322. [CrossRef]
5. Giacco, F.; Brownlee, M. Oxidative stress and diabetic complications. *Circ. Res.* **2010**, *107*, 1058–1070. [CrossRef]
6. Hao, C.; Shintani, S.; Shimizu, Y.; Kondo, K.; Ishii, M.; Wu, H.; Murohara, T. Therapeutic angiogenesis by autologous adipose-derived regenerative cells: Comparison with bone marrow mononuclear cells. *Am. J. Physiol. Heart Circ. Physiol.* **2014**, *307*, H869–H879. [CrossRef]
7. Jude, E.B.; Oyibo, S.O.; Chalmers, N.; Boulton, A.J. Peripheral arterial disease in diabetic and nondiabetic patients: A comparison of severity and outcome. *Diabetes Care* **2001**, *24*, 1433–1437. [CrossRef] [PubMed]
8. Pickup, J.C.; Chusney, G.D.; Thomas, S.M.; Burt, D. Plasma interleukin-6, tumour necrosis factor alpha and blood cytokine production in type 2 diabetes. *Life Sci.* **2000**, *67*, 291–300. [CrossRef]
9. Nehler, M.R.; Duval, S.; Diao, L.; Annex, B.H.; Hiatt, W.R.; Rogers, K.; Zakharyan, A.; Hirsch, A.T. Epidemiology of peripheral arterial disease and critical limb ischemia in an insured national population. *J. Vasc. Surg.* **2014**, *60*, 686–695 e2. [CrossRef]
10. Suggested standards for reports dealing with lower extremity ischemia. Prepared by the Ad Hoc Committee on Reporting Standards, Society for Vascular Surgery/North American Chapter, International Society for Cardiovascular Surgery. *J. Vasc. Surg.* **1986**, *4*, 80–94.
11. Fontaine, R.; Kim, M.; Kieny, R. [Surgical treatment of peripheral circulation disorders]. *Helv. Chir. Acta.* **1954**, *21*, 499–533.
12. Rutherford, R.B.; Baker, J.D.; Ernst, C.; Johnston, K.W.; Porter, J.M.; Ahn, S.; Jones, D.N. Recommended standards for reports dealing with lower extremity ischemia: Revised version. *J. Vasc. Surg.* **1997**, *26*, 517–538. [CrossRef]
13. Becker, F.; Robert-Ebadi, H.; Ricco, J.B.; Setacci, C.; Cao, P.; de Donato, G.; Eckstein, H.H.; De Rango, P.; Diehm, N.; Schmidli, J.; et al. Chapter I: Definitions, epidemiology, clinical presentation and prognosis. *Eur. J. Vasc. Endovasc. Surg.* **2011**, *42* (Suppl. 2), S4–S12. [CrossRef]
14. Dormandy, J.A.; Rutherford, R.B. Management of peripheral arterial disease (PAD). TASC Working Group. TransAtlantic Inter-Society Consensus (TASC). *J. Vasc. Surg.* **2000**, *31 Pt 2*, S1–S296. [PubMed]
15. Norgren, L.; Hiatt, W.R.; Dormandy, J.A.; Nehler, M.R.; Harris, K.A.; Fowkes, F.G.; Group, T.I.W. Inter-Society Consensus for the Management of Peripheral Arterial Disease (TASC II). *J. Vasc. Surg.* **2007**, *45* (Suppl. S), S5–S67. [CrossRef] [PubMed]
16. Teraa, M.; Conte, M.S.; Moll, F.L.; Verhaar, M.C. Critical Limb Ischemia: Current Trends and Future Directions. *J. Am. Heart Assoc.* **2016**, *5*, e002938. [CrossRef] [PubMed]
17. Conte, M.S.; Pomposelli, F.B. Society for Vascular Surgery Practice guidelines for atherosclerotic occlusive disease of the lower extremities management of asymptomatic disease and claudication. Introduction. *J. Vasc. Surg.* **2015**, *61* (Suppl. 3), 1S. [CrossRef]
18. Hirsch, A.T.; Haskal, Z.J.; Hertzer, N.R.; Bakal, C.W.; Creager, M.A.; Halperin, J.L.; Hiratzka, L.F.; Murphy, W.R.; Olin, J.W.; Puschett, J.B.; et al. ACC/AHA 2005 Practice Guidelines for the management of patients with peripheral arterial disease (lower extremity, renal, mesenteric, and abdominal aortic): A collaborative report from the American Association for Vascular Surgery/Society for Vascular Surgery, Society for Cardiovascular Angiography and Interventions, Society for Vascular Medicine and Biology, Society of Interventional Radiology, and the ACC/AHA Task Force on Practice Guidelines (Writing Committee to Develop Guidelines for the Management of Patients With Peripheral Arterial Disease): Endorsed by the American Association of Cardiovascular and Pulmonary Rehabilitation; National Heart, Lung, and Blood Institute; Society for Vascular Nursing; TransAtlantic Inter-Society Consensus; and Vascular Disease Foundation. *Circulation* **2006**, *113*, e463–e654.
19. Simpson, E.L.; Kearns, B.; Stevenson, M.D.; Cantrell, A.J.; Littlewood, C.; Michaels, J.A. Enhancements to angioplasty for peripheral arterial occlusive disease: Systematic review, cost-effectiveness assessment and expected value of information analysis. *Health Technol. Assess.* **2014**, *18*, 1–252. [CrossRef]
20. Walter, D.H.; Krankenberg, H.; Balzer, J.O.; Kalka, C.; Baumgartner, I.; Schluter, M.; Tonn, T.; Seeger, F.; Dimmeler, S.; Lindhoff-Last, E.; et al. Intraarterial administration of bone marrow mononuclear cells in patients with critical limb ischemia: A randomized-start, placebo-controlled pilot trial (PROVASA). *Circ. Cardiovasc. Interv.* **2011**, *4*, 26–37. [CrossRef]
21. Lawall, H.; Zemmrich, C.; Bramlage, P.; Amann, B. Health related quality of life in patients with critical limb ischemia. *Vasa* **2012**, *41*, 78–88. [CrossRef]
22. Patel, R.S. Team Approach to Critical Limb Ischemia Care and Research. *Tech. Vasc Interv. Radiol.* **2016**, *19*, 101–103. [CrossRef]
23. Setacci, C.; de Donato, G.; Teraa, M.; Moll, F.L.; Ricco, J.B.; Becker, F.; Robert-Ebadi, H.; Cao, P.; Eckstein, H.H.; De Rango, P.; et al. Chapter IV: Treatment of critical limb ischaemia. *Eur. J. Vasc. Endovasc. Surg.* **2011**, *42* (Suppl. 2), S43–S59. [CrossRef]
24. Lichtenberg, M.; Schreve, M.A.; Ferraresi, R.; van den Heuvel, D.A.F.; Unlu, C.; Cabane, V.; Kum, S. Surgical and endovascular venous arterialization for treatment of critical limb ischaemia. *Vasa* **2018**, *47*, 17–22. [CrossRef]
25. Duff, S.; Mafilios, M.S.; Bhounsule, P.; Hasegawa, J.T. The burden of critical limb ischemia: A review of recent literature. *Vasc Health Risk Manag.* **2019**, *15*, 187–208. [CrossRef] [PubMed]

26. Spreen, M.I.; Gremmels, H.; Teraa, M.; Sprengers, R.W.; Verhaar, M.C.; Statius van Eps, R.G.; de Vries, J.P.; Mali, W.P.; van Overhagen, H.; Padi; et al. Diabetes Is Associated with Decreased Limb Survival in Patients With Critical Limb Ischemia: Pooled Data From Two Randomized Controlled Trials. *Diabetes Care* **2016**, *39*, 2058–2064. [CrossRef]
27. Howangyin, K.Y.; Silvestre, J.S. Diabetes mellitus and ischemic diseases: Molecular mechanisms of vascular repair dysfunction. *Arterioscler. Thromb. Vasc. Biol.* **2014**, *34*, 1126–1135. [CrossRef] [PubMed]
28. Ouma, G.O.; Zafrir, B.; Mohler, E.R., 3rd; Flugelman, M.Y. Therapeutic angiogenesis in critical limb ischemia. *Angiology* **2013**, *64*, 466–480. [CrossRef] [PubMed]
29. Belch, J.; Hiatt, W.R.; Baumgartner, I.; Driver, I.V.; Nikol, S.; Norgren, L.; Van Belle, E.; TAMRIS Committees and Investigators. Effect of fibroblast growth factor NV1FGF on amputation and death: A randomised placebo-controlled trial of gene therapy in critical limb ischaemia. *Lancet* **2011**, *377*, 1929–1937. [CrossRef]
30. Matoba, S.; Tatsumi, T.; Murohara, T.; Imaizumi, T.; Katsuda, Y.; Ito, M.; Saito, Y.; Uemura, S.; Suzuki, H.; Fukumoto, S.; et al. Long-term clinical outcome after intramuscular implantation of bone marrow mononuclear cells (Therapeutic Angiogenesis by Cell Transplantation [TACT] trial) in patients with chronic limb ischemia. *Am. Heart J.* **2008**, *156*, 1010–1018. [CrossRef] [PubMed]
31. Powell, R.J.; Goodney, P.; Mendelsohn, F.O.; Moen, E.K.; Annex, B.H.; Investigators, H.G.F.T. Safety and efficacy of patient specific intramuscular injection of HGF plasmid gene therapy on limb perfusion and wound healing in patients with ischemic lower extremity ulceration: Results of the HGF-0205 trial. *J. Vasc. Surg.* **2010**, *52*, 1525–1530. [CrossRef]
32. van Royen, N.; Schirmer, S.H.; Atasever, B.; Behrens, C.Y.; Ubbink, D.; Buschmann, E.E.; Voskuil, M.; Bot, P.; Hoefer, I.; Schlingemann, R.O.; et al. START Trial: A pilot study on STimulation of ARTeriogenesis using subcutaneous application of granulocyte-macrophage colony-stimulating factor as a new treatment for peripheral vascular disease. *Circulation* **2005**, *112*, 1040–1046. [CrossRef] [PubMed]
33. Ko, S.H.; Bandyk, D.F. Therapeutic angiogenesis for critical limb ischemia. *Semin. Vasc. Surg.* **2014**, *27*, 23–31. [CrossRef]
34. Lee, C.W.; Stabile, E.; Kinnaird, T.; Shou, M.; Devaney, J.M.; Epstein, S.E.; Burnett, M.S. Temporal patterns of gene expression after acute hindlimb ischemia in mice: Insights into the genomic program for collateral vessel development. *J. Am. Coll. Cardiol.* **2004**, *43*, 474–482. [CrossRef]
35. Westvik, T.S.; Fitzgerald, T.N.; Muto, A.; Maloney, S.P.; Pimiento, J.M.; Fancher, T.T.; Magri, D.; Westvik, H.H.; Nishibe, T.; Velazquez, O.C.; et al. Limb ischemia after iliac ligation in aged mice stimulates angiogenesis without arteriogenesis. *J. Vasc. Surg.* **2009**, *49*, 464–473. [CrossRef] [PubMed]
36. Brechot, N.; Gomez, E.; Bignon, M.; Khallou-Laschet, J.; Dussiot, M.; Cazes, A.; Alanio-Brechot, C.; Durand, M.; Philippe, J.; Silvestre, J.S.; et al. Modulation of macrophage activation state protects tissue from necrosis during critical limb ischemia in thrombospondin-1-deficient mice. *PLoS ONE* **2008**, *3*, e3950. [CrossRef]
37. Crawford, R.S.; Albadawi, H.; Robaldo, A.; Peck, M.A.; Abularrage, C.J.; Yoo, H.J.; Lamuraglia, G.M.; Watkins, M.T. Divergent systemic and local inflammatory response to hind limb demand ischemia in wild-type and ApoE$^{-/-}$ mice. *J. Surg. Res.* **2013**, *183*, 952–962. [CrossRef]
38. Rishi, M.T.; Selvaraju, V.; Thirunavukkarasu, M.; Shaikh, I.A.; Takeda, K.; Fong, G.H.; Palesty, J.A.; Sanchez, J.A.; Maulik, N. Deletion of prolyl hydroxylase domain proteins (PHD1, PHD3) stabilizes hypoxia inducible factor-1 alpha, promotes neovascularization, and improves perfusion in a murine model of hind-limb ischemia. *Microvasc. Res.* **2015**, *97*, 181–188. [CrossRef] [PubMed]
39. Yan, J.; Tie, G.; Park, B.; Yan, Y.; Nowicki, P.T.; Messina, L.M. Recovery from hind limb ischemia is less effective in type 2 than in type 1 diabetic mice: Roles of endothelial nitric oxide synthase and endothelial progenitor cells. *J. Vasc. Surg.* **2009**, *50*, 1412–1422. [CrossRef] [PubMed]
40. MacAskill, M.G.; Saif, J.; Condie, A.; Jansen, M.A.; MacGillivray, T.J.; Tavares, A.A.S.; Fleisinger, L.; Spencer, H.L.; Besnier, M.; Martin, E.; et al. Robust Revascularization in Models of Limb Ischemia Using a Clinically Translatable Human Stem Cell-Derived Endothelial Cell Product. *Mol. Ther.* **2018**, *26*, 1669–1684. [CrossRef]
41. Rojas-Torres, M.; Jiménez-Palomares, M.; Martín-Ramírez, J.; Beltrán-Camacho, L.; Sánchez-Gomar, I.; Eslava-Alcon, S.; Rosal-Vela, A.; Gavaldá, S.; Durán-Ruiz, M.C. REX-001, a BM-MNC Enriched Solution, Induces Revascularization of Ischemic Tissues in a Murine Model of Chronic Limb-Threatening Ischemia. *Front. Cell Dev. Biol.* **2020**, *8*, 1546. [CrossRef]
42. Creane, M.; Howard, L.; O'Brien, T.; Coleman, C.M. Biodistribution and retention of locally administered human mesenchymal stromal cells: Quantitative polymerase chain reaction-based detection of human DNA in murine organs. *Cytotherapy* **2017**, *19*, 384–394. [CrossRef]
43. Thomas, D.; Thirumaran, A.; Mallard, B.; Chen, X.; Browne, S.; Wheatley, A.M.; O'Brien, T.; Pandit, A. Variability in Endogenous Perfusion Recovery of Immunocompromised Mouse Models of Limb Ischemia. *Tissue. Eng. Part C Methods* **2016**, *22*, 370–381. [CrossRef] [PubMed]
44. Goto, T.; Fukuyama, N.; Aki, A.; Kanabuchi, K.; Kimura, K.; Taira, H.; Tanaka, E.; Wakana, N.; Mori, H.; Inoue, H. Search for appropriate experimental methods to create stable hind-limb ischemia in mouse. *Tokai J. Exp. Clin. Med.* **2006**, *31*, 128–132.
45. Krishna, S.M.; Omer, S.M.; Golledge, J. Evaluation of the clinical relevance and limitations of current pre-clinical models of peripheral artery disease. *Clin. Sci.* **2016**, *130*, 127–150. [CrossRef] [PubMed]
46. Hellingman, A.A.; Bastiaansen, A.J.; de Vries, M.R.; Seghers, L.; Lijkwan, M.A.; Lowik, C.W.; Hamming, J.F.; Quax, P.H. Variations in surgical procedures for hind limb ischaemia mouse models result in differences in collateral formation. *Eur. J. Vasc. Endovasc. Surg.* **2010**, *40*, 796–803. [CrossRef] [PubMed]

47. Beltran-Camacho, L.; Jimenez-Palomares, M.; Rojas-Torres, M.; Sanchez-Gomar, I.; Rosal-Vela, A.; Eslava-Alcon, S.; Perez-Segura, M.C.; Serrano, A.; Antequera-Gonzalez, B.; Alonso-Pinero, J.A.; et al. Identification of the initial molecular changes in response to circulating angiogenic cells-mediated therapy in critical limb ischemia. *Stem. Cell. Res. Ther.* **2020**, *11*, 106. [CrossRef]
48. Kochi, T.; Imai, Y.; Takeda, A.; Watanabe, Y.; Mori, S.; Tachi, M.; Kodama, T. Characterization of the arterial anatomy of the murine hindlimb: Functional role in the design and understanding of ischemia models. *PLoS ONE* **2013**, *8*, e84047. [CrossRef]
49. Aref, Z.; de Vries, M.R.; Quax, P.H.A. Variations in Surgical Procedures for Inducing Hind Limb Ischemia in Mice and the Impact of These Variations on Neovascularization Assessment. *Int. J. Mol. Sci.* **2019**, *20*, 3704. [CrossRef]
50. Fukino, K.; Sata, M.; Seko, Y.; Hirata, Y.; Nagai, R. Genetic background influences therapeutic effectiveness of VEGF. *Biochem Biophys Res. Commun.* **2003**, *310*, 143–147. [CrossRef]
51. Nossent, A.Y.; Bastiaansen, A.J.; Peters, E.A.; de Vries, M.R.; Aref, Z.; Welten, S.M.; de Jager, S.C.; van der Pouw Kraan, T.C.; Quax, P.H. CCR7-CCL19/CCL21 Axis is Essential for Effective Arteriogenesis in a Murine Model of Hindlimb Ischemia. *J. Am. Heart Assoc.* **2017**, *6*, e005281. [CrossRef] [PubMed]
52. Lejay, A.; Choquet, P.; Thaveau, F.; Singh, F.; Schlagowski, A.; Charles, A.L.; Laverny, G.; Metzger, D.; Zoll, J.; Chakfe, N.; et al. A new murine model of sustainable and durable chronic critical limb ischemia fairly mimicking human pathology. *Eur. J. Vasc. Endovasc. Surg.* **2015**, *49*, 205–212. [CrossRef] [PubMed]
53. Krishna, S.M.; Omer, S.M.; Li, J.; Morton, S.K.; Jose, R.J.; Golledge, J. Development of a two-stage limb ischemia model to better simulate human peripheral artery disease. *Sci. Rep.* **2020**, *10*, 3449. [CrossRef]
54. Han, S.S.; Jin, Z.; Lee, B.S.; Han, J.S.; Choi, J.J.; Park, S.J.; Chung, H.M.; Mukhtar, A.S.; Moon, S.H.; Kang, S.W. Reproducible hindlimb ischemia model based on photochemically induced thrombosis to evaluate angiogenic effects. *Microvasc. Res.* **2019**, *126*, 103912. [CrossRef]
55. Parikh, P.P.; Castilla, D.; Lassance-Soares, R.M.; Shao, H.; Regueiro, M.; Li, Y.; Vazquez-Padron, R.; Webster, K.A.; Liu, Z.J.; Velazquez, O.C. A Reliable Mouse Model of Hind limb Gangrene. *Ann. Vasc. Surg.* **2018**, *48*, 222–232. [CrossRef]
56. Sligar, A.D.; Howe, G.; Goldman, J.; Felli, P.; Karanam, V.; Smalling, R.W.; Baker, A.B. Preclinical Model of Hind Limb Ischemia in Diabetic Rabbits. *J. Vis. Exp.* **2019**, *148*, e58964. [CrossRef] [PubMed]
57. Zampetaki, A.; Kirton, J.P.; Xu, Q. Vascular repair by endothelial progenitor cells. *Cardiovasc. Res.* **2008**, *78*, 413–421. [CrossRef]
58. van der Kwast, R.; Quax, P.H.A.; Nossent, A.Y. An Emerging Role for isomiRs and the microRNA Epitranscriptome in Neovascularization. *Cells.* **2019**, *9*, 61. [CrossRef]
59. Cooke, J.P.; Meng, S. Vascular Regeneration in Peripheral Artery Disease. *Arterioscler Thromb. Vasc. Biol.* **2020**, *40*, 1627–1634. [CrossRef]
60. Czapla, J.; Cichon, T.; Pilny, E.; Jarosz-Biej, M.; Matuszczak, S.; Drzyzga, A.; Krakowczyk, L.; Smolarczyk, R. Adipose tissue-derived stromal cells stimulated macrophages-endothelial cells interactions promote effective ischemic muscle neovascularization. *Eur. J. Pharmacol.* **2020**, *883*, 173354. [CrossRef]
61. Lin, R.Z.; Lee, C.N.; Moreno-Luna, R.; Neumeyer, J.; Piekarski, B.; Zhou, P.; Moses, M.A.; Sachdev, M.; Pu, W.T.; Emani, S.; et al. Host non-inflammatory neutrophils mediate the engraftment of bioengineered vascular networks. *Nat. Biomed. Eng.* **2017**, 1.
62. Limbourg, A.; von Felden, J.; Jagavelu, K.; Krishnasamy, K.; Napp, L.C.; Kapopara, P.R.; Gaestel, M.; Schieffer, B.; Bauersachs, J.; Limbourg, F.P.; et al. MAP-Kinase Activated Protein Kinase 2 Links Endothelial Activation and Monocyte/macrophage Recruitment in Arteriogenesis. *PLoS ONE* **2015**, *10*, e0138542. [CrossRef] [PubMed]
63. Lin, R.Z.; Chen, Y.C.; Moreno-Luna, R.; Khademhosseini, A.; Melero-Martin, J.M. Transdermal regulation of vascular network bioengineering using a photopolymerizable methacrylated gelatin hydrogel. *Biomaterials* **2013**, *34*, 6785–6796. [CrossRef]
64. Powell, R.J.; Simons, M.; Mendelsohn, F.O.; Daniel, G.; Henry, T.D.; Koga, M.; Morishita, R.; Annex, B.H. Results of a double-blind, placebo-controlled study to assess the safety of intramuscular injection of hepatocyte growth factor plasmid to improve limb perfusion in patients with critical limb ischemia. *Circulation* **2008**, *118*, 58–65. [CrossRef] [PubMed]
65. Yla-Herttuala, S.; Alitalo, K. Gene transfer as a tool to induce therapeutic vascular growth. *Nat. Med.* **2003**, *9*, 694–701. [CrossRef]
66. Menasche, P. Cell therapy for peripheral arterial disease. *Curr. Opin. Mol. Ther.* **2010**, *12*, 538–545. [PubMed]
67. Schmidt, C.A.; Amorese, A.J.; Ryan, T.E.; Goldberg, E.J.; Tarpey, M.D.; Green, T.D.; Karnekar, R.R.; Yamaguchi, D.J.; Spangenburg, E.E.; McClung, J.M. Strain-Dependent Variation in Acute Ischemic Muscle Injury. *Am. J. Pathol.* **2018**, *188*, 1246–1262. [CrossRef] [PubMed]
68. Asahara, T.; Kawamoto, A. Endothelial progenitor cells for postnatal vasculogenesis. *Am. J. Physiol. Cell Physiol.* **2004**, *287*, C572–C579. [CrossRef]
69. Cunha, F.F.; Martins, L.; Martin, P.K.; Stilhano, R.S.; Han, S.W. A comparison of the reparative and angiogenic properties of mesenchymal stem cells derived from the bone marrow of BALB/c and C57/BL6 mice in a model of limb ischemia. *Stem. Cell Res. Ther.* **2013**, *4*, 86. [CrossRef]
70. Garcia-Vazquez, M.D.; Herrero de la Parte, B.; Garcia-Alonso, I.; Morales, M.C. Analysis of Biological Properties of Human Adult Mesenchymal Stem Cells and Their Effect on Mouse Hind Limb Ischemia]. *J. Vasc. Res.* **2019**, *56*, 77–91. [CrossRef]
71. Nammian, P.; Asadi-Yousefabad, S.L.; Daneshi, S.; Sheikhha, M.H.; Tabei, S.M.B.; Razban, V. Comparative analysis of mouse bone marrow and adipose tissue mesenchymal stem cells for critical limb ischemia cell therapy. *Stem. Cell Res. Ther.* **2021**, *12*, 58. [CrossRef]

72. Rossi, E.; Smadja, D.; Goyard, C.; Cras, A.; Dizier, B.; Bacha, N.; Lokajczyk, A.; Guerin, C.L.; Gendron, N.; Planquette, B.; et al. Co-injection of mesenchymal stem cells with endothelial progenitor cells accelerates muscle recovery in hind limb ischemia through an endoglin-dependent mechanism. *Thromb. Haemost.* **2017**, *117*, 1908–1918. [CrossRef]
73. Lian, W.; Hu, X.; Pan, L.; Han, S.; Cao, C.; Jia, Z.; Li, M. Human primary CD34(+) cells transplantation for critical limb ischemia. *J. Clin. Lab. Anal.* **2018**, *32*, e22569. [CrossRef] [PubMed]
74. Kalka, C.; Masuda, H.; Takahashi, T.; Kalka-Moll, W.M.; Silver, M.; Kearney, M.; Li, T.; Isner, J.M.; Asahara, T. Transplantation of ex vivo expanded endothelial progenitor cells for therapeutic neovascularization. *Proc. Natl. Acad. Sci. USA* **2000**, *97*, 3422–3427. [CrossRef] [PubMed]
75. Urbich, C.; Heeschen, C.; Aicher, A.; Dernbach, E.; Zeiher, A.M.; Dimmeler, S. Relevance of monocytic features for neovascularization capacity of circulating endothelial progenitor cells. *Circulation* **2003**, *108*, 2511–2516. [CrossRef]
76. Zhao, W.N.; Xu, S.Q.; Liang, J.F.; Peng, L.; Liu, H.L.; Wang, Z.; Fang, Q.; Wang, M.; Yin, W.Q.; Zhang, W.J.; et al. Endothelial progenitor cells from human fetal aorta cure diabetic foot in a rat model. *Metabolism* **2016**, *65*, 1755–1767. [CrossRef] [PubMed]
77. Yoon, C.H.; Hur, J.; Park, K.W.; Kim, J.H.; Lee, C.S.; Oh, I.Y.; Kim, T.Y.; Cho, H.J.; Kang, H.J.; Chae, I.H.; et al. Synergistic neovascularization by mixed transplantation of early endothelial progenitor cells and late outgrowth endothelial cells: The role of angiogenic cytokines and matrix metalloproteinases. *Circulation* **2005**, *112*, 1618–1627. [CrossRef] [PubMed]
78. Foubert, P.; Matrone, G.; Souttou, B.; Lere-Dean, C.; Barateau, V.; Plouet, J.; Le Ricousse-Roussanne, S.; Levy, B.I.; Silvestre, J.S.; Tobelem, G. Coadministration of endothelial and smooth muscle progenitor cells enhances the efficiency of proangiogenic cell-based therapy. *Circ. Res.* **2008**, *103*, 751–760. [CrossRef]
79. Shintani, S.; Murohara, T.; Ikeda, H.; Ueno, T.; Sasaki, K.; Duan, J.; Imaizumi, T. Augmentation of postnatal neovascularization with autologous bone marrow transplantation. *Circulation* **2001**, *103*, 897–903. [CrossRef]
80. de Nigris, F.; Williams-Ignarro, S.; Sica, V.; D'Armiento, F.P.; Lerman, L.O.; Byrns, R.E.; Sica, G.; Fiorito, C.; Ignarro, L.J.; Napoli, C. Therapeutic effects of concurrent autologous bone marrow cell infusion and metabolic intervention in ischemia-induced angiogenesis in the hypercholesterolemic mouse hindlimb. *Int. J. Cardiol.* **2007**, *117*, 238–243. [CrossRef] [PubMed]
81. Jeon, O.; Song, S.J.; Bhang, S.H.; Choi, C.Y.; Kim, M.J.; Kim, B.S. Additive effect of endothelial progenitor cell mobilization and bone marrow mononuclear cell transplantation on angiogenesis in mouse ischemic limbs. *J. Biomed. Sci.* **2007**, *14*, 323–330. [CrossRef]
82. Gan, L.; Matsuura, H.; Ichiki, T.; Yin, X.; Miyazaki, R.; Hashimoto, T.; Cui, J.; Takeda, K.; Sunagawa, K. Improvement of neovascularization capacity of bone marrow mononuclear cells from diabetic mice by ex vivo pretreatment with resveratrol. *Hypertens. Res.* **2009**, *32*, 542–547. [CrossRef] [PubMed]
83. Liu, Q.; Chen, Z.; Terry, T.; McNatt, J.M.; Willerson, J.T.; Zoldhelyi, P. Intra-arterial transplantation of adult bone marrow cells restores blood flow and regenerates skeletal muscle in ischemic limbs. *Vasc. Endovascular. Surg.* **2009**, *43*, 433–443. [CrossRef]
84. Brenes, R.A.; Jadlowiec, C.C.; Bear, M.; Hashim, P.; Protack, C.D.; Li, X.; Lv, W.; Collins, M.J.; Dardik, A. Toward a mouse model of hind limb ischemia to test therapeutic angiogenesis. *J. Vasc. Surg.* **2012**, *56*, 1669–1679; discussion 1679. [CrossRef] [PubMed]
85. Reis, P.E.; de Carvalho, L.P.; Yasumura, Y.; da Silva, F.H.; Garcia, B.C.; Beutel, A.; Sacramento, C.B.; Baptista-Silva, J.C.; de Campos, R.R.; Takiya, C.M.; et al. Impact of angiogenic therapy in the treatment of critical lower limb ischemia in an animal model. *Vasc. Endovascular. Surg.* **2014**, *48*, 207–216. [CrossRef] [PubMed]
86. Kuwahara, G.; Nishinakamura, H.; Kojima, D.; Tashiro, T.; Kodama, S. GM-CSF treated F4/80+ BMCs improve murine hind limb ischemia similar to M-CSF differentiated macrophages. *PLoS ONE* **2014**, *9*, e106787. [CrossRef] [PubMed]
87. Capoccia, B.J.; Robson, D.L.; Levac, K.D.; Maxwell, D.J.; Hohm, S.A.; Neelamkavil, M.J.; Bell, G.I.; Xenocostas, A.; Link, D.C.; Piwnica-Worms, D.; et al. Revascularization of ischemic limbs after transplantation of human bone marrow cells with high aldehyde dehydrogenase activity. *Blood* **2009**, *113*, 5340–5351. [CrossRef]
88. Rahnemai-Azar, A.; D'Ippolito, G.; Gomez, L.A.; Reiner, T.; Vazquez-Padron, R.I.; Perez-Stable, C.; Roos, B.A.; Pham, S.M.; Schiller, P.C. Human marrow-isolated adult multilineage-inducible (MIAMI) cells protect against peripheral vascular ischemia in a mouse model. *Cytotherapy* **2011**, *13*, 179–192. [CrossRef]
89. Li, S.; Zhou, B.; Han, Z.C. Therapeutic neovascularization by transplantation of mobilized peripheral blood mononuclear cells for limb ischemia. A comparison between CD34+ and CD34- mononuclear cells. *Thromb. Haemost.* **2006**, *95*, 301–311. [PubMed]
90. Padilla, L.; Arguero-Sanchez, R.; Rodriguez-Trejo, J.M.; Carranza-Castro, P.H.; Suarez-Cuenca, J.A.; Polaco-Castillo, J.; DiSilvio-Lopez, M.; Lopez-Gutierrez, J.; Olguin-Juarez, H.; Hernandez-Patricio, A.; et al. Effect of autologous transplant of peripheral blood mononuclear cells in combination with proangiogenic factors during experimental revascularization of lower limb ischemia. *J. Tissue. Eng. Regen. Med.* **2020**, *14*, 600–608. [CrossRef]
91. Liu, J.; Qiu, P.; Qin, J.; Wu, X.; Wang, X.; Yang, X.; Li, B.; Zhang, W.; Ye, K.; Peng, Z.; et al. Allogeneic adipose-derived stem cells promote ischemic muscle repair by inducing M2 macrophage polarization via the HIF-1alpha/IL-10 pathway. *Stem. Cells* **2020**, *38*, 1307–1320. [PubMed]
92. Rybalko, V.; Hsieh, P.L.; Ricles, L.M.; Chung, E.; Farrar, R.P.; Suggs, L.J. Therapeutic potential of adipose-derived stem cells and macrophages for ischemic skeletal muscle repair. *Regen. Med.* **2017**, *12*, 153–167. [CrossRef] [PubMed]
93. Jin, E.; Chae, D.S.; Son, M.; Kim, S.W. Angiogenic characteristics of human stromal vascular fraction in ischemic hindlimb. *Int. J. Cardiol.* **2017**, *234*, 38–47. [CrossRef] [PubMed]
94. Prather, W.R.; Toren, A.; Meiron, M.; Ofir, R.; Tschope, C.; Horwitz, E.M. The role of placental-derived adherent stromal cell (PLX-PAD) in the treatment of critical limb ischemia. *Cytotherapy* **2009**, *11*, 427–434. [CrossRef] [PubMed]

95. Zahavi-Goldstein, E.; Blumenfeld, M.; Fuchs-Telem, D.; Pinzur, L.; Rubin, S.; Aberman, Z.; Sher, N.; Ofir, R. Placenta-derived PLX-PAD mesenchymal-like stromal cells are efficacious in rescuing blood flow in hind limb ischemia mouse model by a dose- and site-dependent mechanism of action. *Cytotherapy* **2017**, *19*, 1438–1446. [CrossRef] [PubMed]
96. Soria-Juan, B.; Escacena, N.; Capilla-Gonzalez, V.; Aguilera, Y.; Llanos, L.; Tejedo, J.R.; Bedoya, F.J.; Juan, V.; De la Cuesta, A.; Ruiz-Salmeron, R.; et al. Cost-Effective, Safe, and Personalized Cell Therapy for Critical Limb Ischemia in Type 2 Diabetes Mellitus. *Front Immunol.* **2019**, *10*, 1151. [CrossRef]
97. Kim, Y.; Kim, H.; Cho, H.; Bae, Y.; Suh, K.; Jung, J. Direct comparison of human mesenchymal stem cells derived from adipose tissues and bone marrow in mediating neovascularization in response to vascular ischemia. *Cell Physiol. Biochem.* **2007**, *20*, 867–876. [CrossRef]
98. Wang, Z.; Zheng, L.; Lian, C.; Qi, Y.; Li, W.; Wang, S. Human Umbilical Cord-Derived Mesenchymal Stem Cells Relieve Hind Limb Ischemia by Promoting Angiogenesis in Mice. *Stem. Cells Dev.* **2019**, *28*, 1384–1397. [CrossRef] [PubMed]
99. Mathew, S.A.; Naik, C.; Cahill, P.A.; Bhonde, R.R. Placental mesenchymal stromal cells as an alternative tool for therapeutic angiogenesis. *Cell Mol. Life Sci.* **2020**, *77*, 253–265. [CrossRef] [PubMed]
100. Cobellis, G.; Maione, C.; Botti, C.; Coppola, A.; Silvestroni, A.; Lillo, S.; Schiavone, V.; Molinari, A.M.; Sica, V. Beneficial effects of VEGF secreted from stromal cells in supporting endothelial cell functions: Therapeutic implications for critical limb ischemia. *Cell Transplant.* **2010**, *19*, 1425–1437. [CrossRef]
101. Song, Y.; Zhang, T.J.; Li, Y.; Gao, Y. Mesenchymal Stem Cells Decrease M1/M2 Ratio and Alleviate Inflammation to Improve Limb Ischemia in Mice. *Med. Sci. Monit.* **2020**, *26*, e923287. [CrossRef]
102. Asahara, T.; Murohara, T.; Sullivan, A.; Silver, M.; van der Zee, R.; Li, T.; Witzenbichler, B.; Schatteman, G.; Isner, J.M. Isolation of putative progenitor endothelial cells for angiogenesis. *Science* **1997**, *275*, 964–967. [CrossRef]
103. Patel, J.; Donovan, P.; Khosrotehrani, K. Concise Review: Functional Definition of Endothelial Progenitor Cells: A Molecular Perspective. *Stem Cells Transl. Med.* **2016**, *5*, 1302–1306. [CrossRef]
104. Edwards, N.; Langford-Smith, A.W.W.; Wilkinson, F.L.; Alexander, M.Y. Endothelial Progenitor Cells: New Targets for Therapeutics for Inflammatory Conditions with High Cardiovascular Risk. *Front. Med.* **2018**, *5*, 200. [CrossRef] [PubMed]
105. Chopra, H.H.M.K.; Kwong, D.L.; Zhang, C.F.; Pow, E.H.N. Insights into Endothelial Progenitor Cells: Origin, Classification, Potentials, and prospects. *Stem. Cell Int.* **2018**, *2018*, 24. [CrossRef]
106. Medina, R.J.; Barber, C.L.; Sabatier, F.; Dignat-George, F.; Melero-Martin, J.M.; Khosrotehrani, K.; Ohneda, O.; Randi, A.M.; Chan, J.K.Y.; Yamaguchi, T.; et al. Endothelial Progenitors: A Consensus Statement on Nomenclature. *Stem. Cells Transl. Med.* **2017**, *6*, 1316–1320. [CrossRef]
107. Stitt, A.W.; O'Neill, C.L.; O'Doherty, M.T.; Archer, D.B.; Gardiner, T.A.; Medina, R.J. Vascular stem cells and ischaemic retinopathies. *Prog. Retin. Eye. Res.* **2011**, *30*, 149–166. [CrossRef]
108. Ziegelhoeffer, T.; Fernandez, B.; Kostin, S.; Heil, M.; Voswinckel, R.; Helisch, A.; Schaper, W. Bone marrow-derived cells do not incorporate into the adult growing vasculature. *Circ. Res.* **2004**, *94*, 230–238. [CrossRef] [PubMed]
109. Yoder, M.C.; Mead, L.E.; Prater, D.; Krier, T.R.; Mroueh, K.N.; Li, F.; Krasich, R.; Temm, C.J.; Prchal, J.T.; Ingram, D.A. Redefining endothelial progenitor cells via clonal analysis and hematopoietic stem/progenitor cell principals. *Blood* **2007**, *109*, 1801–1809. [CrossRef] [PubMed]
110. Eslava-Alcon, S.; Extremera-Garcia, M.J.; Sanchez-Gomar, I.; Beltran-Camacho, L.; Rosal-Vela, A.; Munoz, J.; Ibarz, N.; Alonso-Pinero, J.A.; Rojas-Torres, M.; Jimenez-Palomares, M.; et al. Atherosclerotic Pre-Conditioning Affects the Paracrine Role of Circulating Angiogenic Cells Ex-Vivo. *Int. J. Mol. Sci.* **2020**, *21*, 5256. [CrossRef]
111. Le Ricousse-Roussanne, S.; Barateau, V.; Contreres, J.O.; Boval, B.; Kraus-Berthier, L.; Tobelem, G. Ex vivo differentiated endothelial and smooth muscle cells from human cord blood progenitors home to the angiogenic tumor vasculature. *Cardiovasc. Res.* **2004**, *62*, 176–184. [CrossRef]
112. Fowkes, F.G.; Aboyans, V.; Fowkes, F.J.; McDermott, M.M.; Sampson, U.K.; Criqui, M.H. Peripheral artery disease: Epidemiology and global perspectives. *Nat. Rev. Cardiol.* **2017**, *14*, 156–170. [CrossRef] [PubMed]
113. Ratajczak, M.Z.; Zuba-Surma, E.K.; Machalinski, B.; Ratajczak, J.; Kucia, M. Very small embryonic-like (VSEL) stem cells: Purification from adult organs, characterization, and biological significance. *Stem. Cell Rev.* **2008**, *4*, 89–99. [CrossRef] [PubMed]
114. Amann, B.; Luedemann, C.; Ratei, R.; Schmidt-Lucke, J.A. Autologous bone marrow cell transplantation increases leg perfusion and reduces amputations in patients with advanced critical limb ischemia due to peripheral artery disease. *Cell Transplant.* **2009**, *18*, 371–380. [CrossRef]
115. Fadini, G.P.; Agostini, C.; Avogaro, A. Autologous stem cell therapy for peripheral arterial disease meta-analysis and systematic review of the literature. *Atherosclerosis* **2010**, *209*, 10–17. [CrossRef]
116. Guo, J.; Guo, L.; Cui, S.; Tong, Z.; Dardik, A.; Gu, Y. Autologous bone marrow-derived mononuclear cell therapy in Chinese patients with critical limb ischemia due to thromboangiitis obliterans: 10-year results. *Stem. Cell Res. Ther.* **2018**, *9*, 43. [CrossRef]
117. Idei, N.; Soga, J.; Hata, T.; Fujii, Y.; Fujimura, N.; Mikami, S.; Maruhashi, T.; Nishioka, K.; Hidaka, T.; Kihara, Y.; et al. Limb ischemia: A comparison of atherosclerotic peripheral arterial disease and Buerger disease. *Circ. Cardiovasc. Interv.* **2011**, *4*, 15–25. [CrossRef]
118. Liang, T.W.; Jester, A.; Motaganahalli, R.L.; Wilson, M.G.; G'Sell, P.; Akingba, G.A.; Fajardo, A.; Murphy, M.P. Autologous bone marrow mononuclear cell therapy for critical limb ischemia is effective and durable. *J. Vasc. Surg.* **2016**, *63*, 1541–1545. [CrossRef]

119. Murphy, M.P.; Lawson, J.H.; Rapp, B.M.; Dalsing, M.C.; Klein, J.; Wilson, M.G.; Hutchins, G.D.; March, K.L. Autologous bone marrow mononuclear cell therapy is safe and promotes amputation-free survival in patients with critical limb ischemia. *J. Vasc. Surg.* **2011**, *53*, 1565–1574 e1. [CrossRef]
120. Ruiz-Salmeron, R.; de la Cuesta-Diaz, A.; Constantino-Bermejo, M.; Perez-Camacho, I.; Marcos-Sanchez, F.; Hmadcha, A.; Soria, B. Angiographic demonstration of neoangiogenesis after intra-arterial infusion of autologous bone marrow mononuclear cells in diabetic patients with critical limb ischemia. *Cell Transplant.* **2011**, *20*, 1629–1639. [CrossRef] [PubMed]
121. Wahid, F.S.A.; Ismail, N.A.; Wan Jamaludin, W.F.; Muhamad, N.A.; Mohamad Idris, M.A.; Lai, N.M. Efficacy and Safety of Autologous Cell-based Therapy in Patients with No-option Critical Limb Ischaemia: A Meta-Analysis. *Curr. Stem. Cell Res. Ther.* **2018**, *13*, 265–283. [CrossRef] [PubMed]
122. Yusoff, F.M.; Kajikawa, M.; Matsui, S.; Hashimoto, H.; Kishimoto, S.; Maruhashi, T.; Chowdhury, M.; Noma, K.; Nakashima, A.; Kihara, Y.; et al. Review of the Long-term Effects of Autologous Bone-Marrow Mononuclear Cell Implantation on Clinical Outcomes in Patients with Critical Limb Ischemia. *Sci. Rep.* **2019**, *9*, 7711. [CrossRef]
123. Kumar, A.; Prasad, M.; Jali, V.P.; Pandit, A.K.; Misra, A.; Kumar, P.; Chakravarty, K.; Kathuria, P.; Gulati, A. Bone marrow mononuclear cell therapy in ischaemic stroke: A systematic review. *Acta. Neurol. Scand.* **2017**, *135*, 496–506. [CrossRef]
124. Kikuchi-Taura, A.; Okinaka, Y.; Takeuchi, Y.; Ogawa, Y.; Maeda, M.; Kataoka, Y.; Yasui, T.; Kimura, T.; Gul, S.; Claussen, C.; et al. Bone Marrow Mononuclear Cells Activate Angiogenesis via Gap Junction-Mediated Cell-Cell Interaction. *Stroke* **2020**, *51*, 1279–1289. [CrossRef]
125. Huang, P.; Li, S.; Han, M.; Xiao, Z.; Yang, R.; Han, Z.C. Autologous transplantation of granulocyte colony-stimulating factor-mobilized peripheral blood mononuclear cells improves critical limb ischemia in diabetes. *Diabetes. Care* **2005**, *28*, 2155–2160. [CrossRef] [PubMed]
126. Kawamura, A.; Horie, T.; Tsuda, I.; Abe, Y.; Yamada, M.; Egawa, H.; Iida, J.; Sakata, K.; Onodera, K.; Tamaki, T.; et al. Clinical study of therapeutic angiogenesis by autologous peripheral blood stem cell (PBSC) transplantation in 92 patients with critically ischemic limbs. *J. Artif. Organs.* **2006**, *9*, 226–233. [CrossRef]
127. Mohammadzadeh, L.; Samedanifard, S.H.; Keshavarzi, A.; Alimoghaddam, K.; Larijani, B.; Ghavamzadeh, A.; Ahmadi, A.S.; Shojaeifard, A.; Ostadali, M.R.; Sharifi, A.M.; et al. Therapeutic outcomes of transplanting autologous granulocyte colony-stimulating factor-mobilised peripheral mononuclear cells in diabetic patients with critical limb ischaemia. *Exp. Clin. Endocrinol. Diabetes* **2013**, *121*, 48–53. [CrossRef] [PubMed]
128. Ozturk, A.; Kucukardali, Y.; Tangi, F.; Erikci, A.; Uzun, G.; Bashekim, C.; Sen, H.; Terekeci, H.; Narin, Y.; Ozyurt, M.; et al. Therapeutic potential of autologous peripheral blood mononuclear cell transplantation in patients with type 2 diabetic critical limb ischemia. *J. Diabetes Complicat.* **2012**, *26*, 29–33. [CrossRef] [PubMed]
129. Dubsky, M.; Jirkovska, A.; Bem, R.; Fejfarova, V.; Pagacova, L.; Sixta, B.; Varga, M.; Langkramer, S.; Sykova, E.; Jude, E.B. Both autologous bone marrow mononuclear cell and peripheral blood progenitor cell therapies similarly improve ischaemia in patients with diabetic foot in comparison with control treatment. *Diabetes Metab. Res. Rev.* **2013**, *29*, 369–376. [CrossRef] [PubMed]
130. Minamino, T.; Toko, H.; Tateno, K.; Nagai, T.; Komuro, I. Peripheral-blood or bone-marrow mononuclear cells for therapeutic angiogenesis? *Lancet* **2002**, *360*, 2083–2084; author reply 2084. [CrossRef]
131. Capiod, J.C.; Tournois, C.; Vitry, F.; Sevestre, M.A.; Daliphard, S.; Reix, T.; Nguyen, P.; Lefrere, J.J.; Pignon, B. Characterization and comparison of bone marrow and peripheral blood mononuclear cells used for cellular therapy in critical leg ischaemia: Towards a new cellular product. *Vox. Sang.* **2009**, *96*, 256–265. [CrossRef] [PubMed]
132. Mazini, L.; Rochette, L.; Amine, M.; Malka, G. Regenerative Capacity of Adipose Derived Stem Cells (ADSCs), Comparison with Mesenchymal Stem Cells (MSCs). *Int. J. Mol. Sci.* **2019**, *20*, 2523. [CrossRef]
133. Rehman, J.; Traktuev, D.; Li, J.; Merfeld-Clauss, S.; Temm-Grove, C.J.; Bovenkerk, J.E.; Pell, C.L.; Johnstone, B.H.; Considine, R.V.; March, K.L. Secretion of angiogenic and antiapoptotic factors by human adipose stromal cells. *Circulation* **2004**, *109*, 1292–1298. [CrossRef]
134. Safford, K.M.; Hicok, K.C.; Safford, S.D.; Halvorsen, Y.D.; Wilkison, W.O.; Gimble, J.M.; Rice, H.E. Neurogenic differentiation of murine and human adipose-derived stromal cells. *Biochem. Biophys. Res. Commun.* **2002**, *294*, 371–379. [CrossRef]
135. Dragoo, J.L.; Choi, J.Y.; Lieberman, J.R.; Huang, J.; Zuk, P.A.; Zhang, J.; Hedrick, M.H.; Benhaim, P. Bone induction by BMP-2 transduced stem cells derived from human fat. *J. Orthop. Res.* **2003**, *21*, 622–629. [CrossRef]
136. Zhi, K.; Gao, Z.; Bai, J.; Wu, Y.; Zhou, S.; Li, M.; Qu, L. Application of adipose-derived stem cells in critical limb ischemia. *Front Biosci.* **2014**, *19*, 768–776. [CrossRef] [PubMed]
137. Han, S.; Sun, H.M.; Hwang, K.C.; Kim, S.W. Adipose-Derived Stromal Vascular Fraction Cells: Update on Clinical Utility and Efficacy. *Crit. Rev. Eukaryot. Gene. Expr.* **2015**, *25*, 145–152. [CrossRef]
138. Hong, S.J.; Traktuev, D.O.; March, K.L. Therapeutic potential of adipose-derived stem cells in vascular growth and tissue repair. *Curr. Opin. Organ. Transplant.* **2010**, *15*, 86–91. [CrossRef] [PubMed]
139. Katagiri, T.; Kondo, K.; Shibata, R.; Hayashida, R.; Shintani, S.; Yamaguchi, S.; Shimizu, Y.; Unno, K.; Kikuchi, R.; Kodama, A.; et al. Therapeutic angiogenesis using autologous adipose-derived regenerative cells in patients with critical limb ischaemia in Japan: A clinical pilot study. *Sci. Rep.* **2020**, *10*, 16045. [CrossRef]
140. Qadura, M.; Terenzi, D.C.; Verma, S.; Al-Omran, M.; Hess, D.A. Concise Review: Cell Therapy for Critical Limb Ischemia: An Integrated Review of Preclinical and Clinical Studies. *Stem. Cells* **2018**, *36*, 161–171. [CrossRef] [PubMed]

141. Silvestre, J.S. Pro-angiogenic cell-based therapy for the treatment of ischemic cardiovascular diseases. *Thromb. Res.* **2012**, *130* (Suppl. 1), S90–S94. [CrossRef]
142. Tateishi-Yuyama, E.; Matsubara, H.; Murohara, T.; Ikeda, U.; Shintani, S.; Masaki, H.; Amano, K.; Kishimoto, Y.; Yoshimoto, K.; Akashi, H.; et al. Therapeutic angiogenesis for patients with limb ischaemia by autologous transplantation of bone-marrow cells: A pilot study and a randomised controlled trial. *Lancet* **2002**, *360*, 427–435. [CrossRef]
143. Norgren, L.; Weiss, N.; Nikol, S.; Hinchliffe, R.J.; Lantis, J.C.; Patel, M.R.; Reinecke, H.; Ofir, R.; Rosen, Y.; Peres, D.; et al. PLX-PAD Cell Treatment of Critical Limb Ischaemia: Rationale and Design of the PACE Trial. *Eur. J. Vasc. Endovasc. Surg.* **2019**, *57*, 538–545. [CrossRef]
144. De Angelis, B.; Gentile, P.; Orlandi, F.; Bocchini, I.; Di Pasquali, C.; Agovino, A.; Gizzi, C.; Patrizi, F.; Scioli, M.G.; Orlandi, A.; et al. Limb rescue: A new autologous-peripheral blood mononuclear cells technology in critical limb ischemia and chronic ulcers. *Tissue. Eng. Part C Methods* **2015**, *21*, 423–435. [CrossRef] [PubMed]
145. Arai, M.; Misao, Y.; Nagai, H.; Kawasaki, M.; Nagashima, K.; Suzuki, K.; Tsuchiya, K.; Otsuka, S.; Uno, Y.; Takemura, G.; et al. Granulocyte colony-stimulating factor: A noninvasive regeneration therapy for treating atherosclerotic peripheral artery disease. *Circ. J.* **2006**, *70*, 1093–1098. [CrossRef] [PubMed]
146. Huang, P.P.; Yang, X.F.; Li, S.Z.; Wen, J.C.; Zhang, Y.; Han, Z.C. Randomised comparison of G-CSF-mobilized peripheral blood mononuclear cells versus bone marrow-mononuclear cells for the treatment of patients with lower limb arteriosclerosis obliterans. *Thromb. Haemost.* **2007**, *98*, 1335–1342. [CrossRef] [PubMed]
147. Li, M.; Zhou, H.; Jin, X.; Wang, M.; Zhang, S.; Xu, L. Autologous bone marrow mononuclear cells transplant in patients with critical leg ischemia: Preliminary clinical results. *Exp. Clin. Transplant* **2013**, *11*, 435–439. [CrossRef]
148. Teraa, M.; Sprengers, R.W.; Schutgens, R.E.; Slaper-Cortenbach, I.C.; van der Graaf, Y.; Algra, A.; van der Tweel, I.; Doevendans, P.A.; Mali, W.P.; Moll, F.L.; et al. Effect of repetitive intra-arterial infusion of bone marrow mononuclear cells in patients with no-option limb ischemia: The randomized, double-blind, placebo-controlled Rejuvenating Endothelial Progenitor Cells via Transcutaneous Intra-arterial Supplementation (JUVENTAS) trial. *Circulation* **2015**, *131*, 851–860.
149. Pignon, B.; Sevestre, M.A.; Kanagaratnam, L.; Pernod, G.; Stephan, D.; Emmerich, J.; Clement, C.; Sarlon, G.; Boulon, C.; Tournois, C.; et al. Autologous Bone Marrow Mononuclear Cell Implantation and Its Impact on the Outcome of Patients With Critical Limb Ischemia- Results of a Randomized, Double-Blind, Placebo-Controlled Trial. *Circ. J.* **2017**, *81*, 1713–1720. [CrossRef] [PubMed]
150. Lu, D.; Chen, B.; Liang, Z.; Deng, W.; Jiang, Y.; Li, S.; Xu, J.; Wu, Q.; Zhang, Z.; Xie, B.; et al. Comparison of bone marrow mesenchymal stem cells with bone marrow-derived mononuclear cells for treatment of diabetic critical limb ischemia and foot ulcer: A double-blind, randomized, controlled trial. *Diabetes Res. Clin. Pract.* **2011**, *92*, 26–36. [CrossRef]
151. Dash, N.R.; Dash, S.N.; Routray, P.; Mohapatra, S.; Mohapatra, P.C. Targeting nonhealing ulcers of lower extremity in human through autologous bone marrow-derived mesenchymal stem cells. *Rejuvenation Res.* **2009**, *12*, 359–366. [CrossRef] [PubMed]
152. Gupta, P.K.; Chullikana, A.; Parakh, R.; Desai, S.; Das, A.; Gottipamula, S.; Krishnamurthy, S.; Anthony, N.; Pherwani, A.; Majumdar, A.S. A double blind randomized placebo controlled phase I/II study assessing the safety and efficacy of allogeneic bone marrow derived mesenchymal stem cell in critical limb ischemia. *J. Transl. Med.* **2013**, *11*, 143. [CrossRef]
153. Szabo, G.V.; Kovesd, Z.; Cserepes, J.; Daroczy, J.; Belkin, M.; Acsady, G. Peripheral blood-derived autologous stem cell therapy for the treatment of patients with late-stage peripheral artery disease-results of the short- and long-term follow-up. *Cytotherapy* **2013**, *15*, 1245–1252. [CrossRef]
154. Raval, A.N.; Schmuck, E.G.; Tefera, G.; Leitzke, C.; Ark, C.V.; Hei, D.; Centanni, J.M.; de Silva, R.; Koch, J.; Chappell, R.G.; et al. Bilateral administration of autologous CD133+ cells in ambulatory patients with refractory critical limb ischemia: Lessons learned from a pilot randomized, double-blind, placebo-controlled trial. *Cytotherapy* **2014**, *16*, 1720–1732. [CrossRef] [PubMed]
155. Lara-Hernandez, R.; Lozano-Vilardell, P.; Blanes, P.; Torreguitart-Mirada, N.; Galmes, A.; Besalduch, J. Safety and efficacy of therapeutic angiogenesis as a novel treatment in patients with critical limb ischemia. *Ann. Vasc. Surg.* **2010**, *24*, 287–294. [CrossRef] [PubMed]
156. Kinoshita, M.; Fujita, Y.; Katayama, M.; Baba, R.; Shibakawa, M.; Yoshikawa, K.; Katakami, N.; Furukawa, Y.; Tsukie, T.; Nagano, T.; et al. Long-term clinical outcome after intramuscular transplantation of granulocyte colony stimulating factor-mobilized CD34 positive cells in patients with critical limb ischemia. *Atherosclerosis* **2012**, *224*, 440–445. [CrossRef]
157. Dong, Z.; Chen, B.; Fu, W.; Wang, Y.; Guo, D.; Wei, Z.; Xu, X.; Mendelsohn, F.O. Transplantation of purified CD34+ cells in the treatment of critical limb ischemia. *J. Vasc. Surg.* **2013**, *58*, 404–411 e3. [CrossRef]
158. Fujita, Y.; Kinoshita, M.; Furukawa, Y.; Nagano, T.; Hashimoto, H.; Hirami, Y.; Kurimoto, Y.; Arakawa, K.; Yamazaki, K.; Okada, Y.; et al. Phase II clinical trial of CD34+ cell therapy to explore endpoint selection and timing in patients with critical limb ischemia. *Circ. J.* **2014**, *78*, 490–501. [CrossRef] [PubMed]
159. Powell, R.J.; Marston, W.A.; Berceli, S.A.; Guzman, R.; Henry, T.D.; Longcore, A.T.; Stern, T.P.; Watling, S.; Bartel, R.L. Cellular therapy with Ixmyelocel-T to treat critical limb ischemia: The randomized, double-blind, placebo-controlled RESTORE-CLI trial. *Mol. Ther.* **2012**, *20*, 1280–1286. [CrossRef]
160. Losordo, D.W.; Kibbe, M.R.; Mendelsohn, F.; Marston, W.; Driver, V.R.; Sharafuddin, M.; Teodorescu, V.; Wiechmann, B.N.; Thompson, C.; Kraiss, L.; et al. A randomized, controlled pilot study of autologous CD34+ cell therapy for critical limb ischemia. *Circ. Cardiovasc. Interv.* **2012**, *5*, 821–830. [CrossRef]

161. Liotta, F.; Annunziato, F.; Castellani, S.; Boddi, M.; Alterini, B.; Castellini, G.; Mazzanti, B.; Cosmi, L.; Acquafresca, M.; Bartalesi, F.; et al. Therapeutic Efficacy of Autologous Non-Mobilized Enriched Circulating Endothelial Progenitors in Patients With Critical Limb Ischemia- The SCELTA Trial. *Circ. J.* **2018**, *82*, 1688–1698. [CrossRef]
162. Fang, G.; Jiang, X.; Fang, Y.; Pan, T.; Liu, H.; Ren, B.; Wei, Z.; Gu, S.; Chen, B.; Jiang, J.; et al. Autologous peripheral blood-derived stem cells transplantation for treatment of no-option angiitis-induced critical limb ischemia: 10-year management experience. *Stem. Cell Res. Ther.* **2020**, *11*, 458. [CrossRef] [PubMed]
163. Sharma, S.; Pandey, N.N.; Sinha, M.; Kumar, S.; Jagia, P.; Gulati, G.S.; Gond, K.; Mohanty, S.; Bhargava, B. Randomized, Double-Blind, Placebo-Controlled Trial to Evaluate Safety and Therapeutic Efficacy of Angiogenesis Induced by Intraarterial Autologous Bone Marrow-Derived Stem Cells in Patients with Severe Peripheral Arterial Disease. *J. Vasc. Interv. Radiol.* **2021**, *32*, 157–163. [CrossRef] [PubMed]
164. Rutherford, R.B.; Becker, G.J. Standards for evaluating and reporting the results of surgical and percutaneous therapy for peripheral arterial disease. *Radiology* **1991**, *181*, 277–281. [CrossRef] [PubMed]
165. Kusumanto, Y.H.; van Weel, V.; Mulder, N.H.; Smit, A.J.; van den Dungen, J.J.; Hooymans, J.M.; Sluiter, W.J.; Tio, R.A.; Quax, P.H.; Gans, R.O.; et al. Treatment with intramuscular vascular endothelial growth factor gene compared with placebo for patients with diabetes mellitus and critical limb ischemia: A double-blind randomized trial. *Hum. Gene. Ther.* **2006**, *17*, 683–691. [CrossRef]
166. Dong, Z.; Pan, T.; Fang, Y.; Wei, Z.; Gu, S.; Fang, G.; Liu, Y.; Luo, Y.; Liu, H.; Zhang, T.; et al. Purified CD34(+) cells versus peripheral blood mononuclear cells in the treatment of angiitis-induced no-option critical limb ischaemia: 12-Month results of a prospective randomised single-blinded non-inferiority trial. *EBioMedicine* **2018**, *35*, 46–57. [CrossRef]
167. Carstens, M.H.; Zelaya, M.; Calero, D.; Rivera, C.; Correa, D. Adipose-derived stromal vascular fraction (SVF) cells for the treatment of non-reconstructable peripheral vascular disease in patients with critical limb ischemia: A 6-year follow-up showing durable effects. *Stem. Cell Res.* **2020**, *49*, 102071. [CrossRef] [PubMed]
168. Guerin, C.L.; Loyer, X.; Vilar, J.; Cras, A.; Mirault, T.; Gaussem, P.; Silvestre, J.S.; Smadja, D.M. Bone-marrow-derived very small embryonic-like stem cells in patients with critical leg ischaemia: Evidence of vasculogenic potential. *Thromb. Haemost.* **2015**, *113*, 1084–1094. [CrossRef] [PubMed]
169. Yoder, M.C.; Ingram, D.A. Endothelial progenitor cell: Ongoing controversy for defining these cells and their role in neoangiogenesis in the murine system. *Curr. Opin. Hematol.* **2009**, *16*, 269–273. [CrossRef]
170. Ohtake, T.; Mochida, Y.; Ishioka, K.; Oka, M.; Maesato, K.; Moriya, H.; Hidaka, S.; Higashide, S.; Ioji, T.; Fujita, Y.; et al. Autologous Granulocyte Colony-Stimulating Factor-Mobilized Peripheral Blood CD34 Positive Cell Transplantation for Hemodialysis Patients with Critical Limb Ischemia: A Prospective Phase II Clinical Trial. *Stem Cells Transl. Med.* **2018**, *7*, 774–782. [CrossRef] [PubMed]
171. Povsic, T.J.; Zavodni, K.L.; Kelly, F.L.; Zhu, S.; Goldschmidt-Clermont, P.J.; Dong, C.; Peterson, E.D. Circulating progenitor cells can be reliably identified on the basis of aldehyde dehydrogenase activity. *J. Am. Coll Cardiol.* **2007**, *50*, 2243–2248. [CrossRef]
172. Gremmels, H.; Teraa, M.; Quax, P.H.; den Ouden, K.; Fledderus, J.O.; Verhaar, M.C. Neovascularization capacity of mesenchymal stromal cells from critical limb ischemia patients is equivalent to healthy controls. *Mol. Ther.* **2014**, *22*, 1960–1970. [CrossRef]
173. Fadini, G.P.; Sartore, S.; Schiavon, M.; Albiero, M.; Baesso, I.; Cabrelle, A.; Agostini, C.; Avogaro, A. Diabetes impairs progenitor cell mobilisation after hindlimb ischaemia-reperfusion injury in rats. *Diabetologia* **2006**, *49*, 3075–3084. [CrossRef] [PubMed]
174. Jialal, I.; Devaraj, S.; Singh, U.; Huet, B.A. Decreased number and impaired functionality of endothelial progenitor cells in subjects with metabolic syndrome: Implications for increased cardiovascular risk. *Atherosclerosis* **2010**, *211*, 297–302. [CrossRef]
175. Sibal, L.; Aldibbiat, A.; Agarwal, S.C.; Mitchell, G.; Oates, C.; Razvi, S.; Weaver, J.U.; Shaw, J.A.; Home, P.D. Circulating endothelial progenitor cells, endothelial function, carotid intima-media thickness and circulating markers of endothelial dysfunction in people with type 1 diabetes without macrovascular disease or microalbuminuria. *Diabetologia* **2009**, *52*, 1464–1473. [CrossRef] [PubMed]
176. Gu, Y.Q.; Zhang, J.; Guo, L.R.; Qi, L.X.; Zhang, S.W.; Xu, J.; Li, J.X.; Luo, T.; Ji, B.X.; Li, X.F.; et al. Transplantation of autologous bone marrow mononuclear cells for patients with lower limb ischemia. *Chin. Med. J.* **2008**, *121*, 963–967. [CrossRef] [PubMed]
177. Van Tongeren, R.B.; Hamming, J.F.; Fibbe, W.E.; Van Weel, V.; Frerichs, S.J.; Stiggelbout, A.M.; Van Bockel, J.H.; Lindeman, J.H. Intramuscular or combined intramuscular/intra-arterial administration of bone marrow mononuclear cells: A clinical trial in patients with advanced limb ischemia. *J. Cardiovasc Surg.* **2008**, *49*, 51–58.
178. Madaric, J.; Klepanec, A.; Valachovicova, M.; Mistrik, M.; Bucova, M.; Olejarova, I.; Necpal, R.; Madaricova, T.; Paulis, L.; Vulev, I. Characteristics of responders to autologous bone marrow cell therapy for no-option critical limb ischemia. *Stem Cell Res. Ther.* **2016**, *7*, 116. [CrossRef]
179. Jaluvka, F.; Ihnat, P.; Madaric, J.; Vrtkova, A.; Janosek, J.; Prochazka, V. Current Status of Cell-Based Therapy in Patients with Critical Limb Ischemia. *Int. J. Mol. Sci.* **2020**, *21*, 8999. [CrossRef] [PubMed]
180. Rigato, M.; Monami, M.; Fadini, G.P. Autologous Cell Therapy for Peripheral Arterial Disease: Systematic Review and Meta-Analysis of Randomized, Nonrandomized, and Noncontrolled Studies. *Circ. Res.* **2017**, *120*, 1326–1340. [CrossRef]
181. Gao, W.; Chen, D.; Liu, G.; Ran, X. Autologous stem cell therapy for peripheral arterial disease: A systematic review and meta-analysis of randomized controlled trials. *Stem Cell Res. Ther.* **2019**, *10*, 140. [CrossRef] [PubMed]
182. Peeters Weem, S.M.; Teraa, M.; de Borst, G.J.; Verhaar, M.C.; Moll, F.L. Bone Marrow derived Cell Therapy in Critical Limb Ischemia: A Meta-analysis of Randomized Placebo Controlled Trials. *Eur. J. Vasc. Endovasc. Surg.* **2015**, *50*, 775–783. [CrossRef] [PubMed]

183. Makridakis, M.; Roubelakis, M.G.; Vlahou, A. Stem cells: Insights into the secretome. *Biochim. Biophys. Acta* **2013**, *1834*, 2380–2384. [CrossRef] [PubMed]
184. Xia, J.; Minamino, S.; Kuwabara, K.; Arai, S. Stem cell secretome as a new booster for regenerative medicine. *Biosci. Trends.* **2019**, *13*, 299–307. [CrossRef]
185. Baberg, F.; Geyh, S.; Waldera-Lupa, D.; Stefanski, A.; Zilkens, C.; Haas, R.; Schroeder, T.; Stuhler, K. Secretome analysis of human bone marrow derived mesenchymal stromal cells. *Biochim. Biophys. Acta Proteins. Proteom.* **2019**, *1867*, 434–441. [CrossRef] [PubMed]
186. Maffioli, E.; Nonnis, S.; Angioni, R.; Santagata, F.; Cali, B.; Zanotti, L.; Negri, A.; Viola, A.; Tedeschi, G. Proteomic analysis of the secretome of human bone marrow-derived mesenchymal stem cells primed by pro-inflammatory cytokines. *J. Proteomics.* **2017**, *166*, 115–126. [CrossRef] [PubMed]
187. Merfeld-Clauss, S.; Lupov, I.P.; Lu, H.; March, K.L.; Traktuev, D.O. Adipose Stromal Cell Contact with Endothelial Cells Results in Loss of Complementary Vasculogenic Activity Mediated by Induction of Activin A. *Stem Cells* **2015**, *33*, 3039–3051. [CrossRef]
188. Rubina, K.; Kalinina, N.; Efimenko, A.; Lopatina, T.; Melikhova, V.; Tsokolaeva, Z.; Sysoeva, V.; Tkachuk, V.; Parfyonova, Y. Adipose stromal cells stimulate angiogenesis via promoting progenitor cell differentiation, secretion of angiogenic factors, and enhancing vessel maturation. *Tissue. Eng. Part A* **2009**, *15*, 2039–2050. [CrossRef]
189. Bhang, S.H.; Lee, S.; Shin, J.Y.; Lee, T.J.; Jang, H.K.; Kim, B.S. Efficacious and clinically relevant conditioned medium of human adipose-derived stem cells for therapeutic angiogenesis. *Mol. Ther.* **2014**, *22*, 862–872. [CrossRef]
190. Di Santo, S.; Yang, Z.; Wyler von Ballmoos, M.; Voelzmann, J.; Diehm, N.; Baumgartner, I.; Kalka, C. Novel cell-free strategy for therapeutic angiogenesis: In vitro generated conditioned medium can replace progenitor cell transplantation. *PLoS ONE* **2009**, *4*, e5643. [CrossRef] [PubMed]
191. Shrestha, C.; Zhao, L.; Chen, K.; He, H.; Mo, Z. Enhanced healing of diabetic wounds by subcutaneous administration of human umbilical cord derived stem cells and their conditioned media. *Int. J. Endocrinol.* **2013**, *2013*, 592454. [CrossRef]
192. Felice, F.; Piras, A.M.; Rocchiccioli, S.; Barsotti, M.C.; Santoni, T.; Pucci, A.; Burchielli, S.; Chiellini, F.; Ucciferri, N.; Solaro, R.; et al. Endothelial progenitor cell secretome delivered by novel polymeric nanoparticles in ischemic hindlimb. *Int. J. Pharm.* **2018**, *542*, 82–89. [CrossRef]
193. Takeuchi, R.; Katagiri, W.; Endo, S.; Kobayashi, T. Exosomes from conditioned media of bone marrow-derived mesenchymal stem cells promote bone regeneration by enhancing angiogenesis. *PLoS ONE* **2019**, *14*, e0225472. [CrossRef]
194. Mathiyalagan, P.; Liang, Y.; Kim, D.; Misener, S.; Thorne, T.; Kamide, C.E.; Klyachko, E.; Losordo, D.W.; Hajjar, R.J.; Sahoo, S. Angiogenic Mechanisms of Human CD34(+) Stem Cell Exosomes in the Repair of Ischemic Hindlimb. *Circ. Res.* **2017**, *120*, 1466–1476. [CrossRef] [PubMed]
195. Kir, D.; Schnettler, E.; Modi, S.; Ramakrishnan, S. Regulation of angiogenesis by microRNAs in cardiovascular diseases. *Angiogenesis* **2018**, *21*, 699–710. [CrossRef]
196. Welten, S.M.; Bastiaansen, A.J.; de Jong, R.C.; de Vries, M.R.; Peters, E.A.; Boonstra, M.C.; Sheikh, S.P.; La Monica, N.; Kandimalla, E.R.; Quax, P.H.; et al. Inhibition of 14q32 MicroRNAs miR-329, miR-487b, miR-494, and miR-495 increases neovascularization and blood flow recovery after ischemia. *Circ Res.* **2014**, *115*, 696–708. [CrossRef] [PubMed]
197. Gong, M.; Yu, B.; Wang, J.; Wang, Y.; Liu, M.; Paul, C.; Millard, R.W.; Xiao, D.S.; Ashraf, M.; Xu, M. Mesenchymal stem cells release exosomes that transfer miRNAs to endothelial cells and promote angiogenesis. *Oncotarget* **2017**, *8*, 45200–45212. [CrossRef] [PubMed]

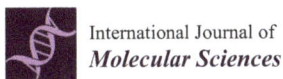

Review

Role of Vascular Smooth Muscle Cell Phenotype Switching in Arteriogenesis

Jasni Viralippurath Ashraf and Ayman Al Haj Zen *

College of Health & Life Sciences, Hamad Bin Khalifa University, Qatar Foundation, Doha 34110, Qatar; JAshraf@hbku.edu.qa
* Correspondence: aalhajzen@hbku.edu.qa; Tel.: +974-4454-6352

Abstract: Arteriogenesis is one of the primary physiological means by which the circulatory collateral system restores blood flow after significant arterial occlusion in peripheral arterial disease patients. Vascular smooth muscle cells (VSMCs) are the predominant cell type in collateral arteries and respond to altered blood flow and inflammatory conditions after an arterial occlusion by switching their phenotype between quiescent contractile and proliferative synthetic states. Maintaining the contractile state of VSMC is required for collateral vascular function to regulate blood vessel tone and blood flow during arteriogenesis, whereas synthetic SMCs are crucial in the growth and remodeling of the collateral media layer to establish more stable conduit arteries. Timely VSMC phenotype switching requires a set of coordinated actions of molecular and cellular mediators to result in an expansive remodeling of collaterals that restores the blood flow effectively into downstream ischemic tissues. This review overviews the role of VSMC phenotypic switching in the physiological arteriogenesis process and how the VSMC phenotype is affected by the primary triggers of arteriogenesis such as blood flow hemodynamic forces and inflammation. Better understanding the role of VSMC phenotype switching during arteriogenesis can identify novel therapeutic strategies to enhance revascularization in peripheral arterial disease.

Keywords: vascular smooth muscle cell; phenotypic switch; arteriogenesis; collateral arteries; peripheral arterial disease

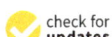

Citation: Ashraf, J.V.; Al Haj Zen, A. Role of Vascular Smooth Muscle Cell Phenotype Switching in Arteriogenesis. *Int. J. Mol. Sci.* **2021**, 22, 10585. https://doi.org/10.3390/ijms221910585

Academic Editor: Andrea Olschewski

Received: 29 August 2021
Accepted: 27 September 2021
Published: 30 September 2021

Publisher's Note: MDPI stays neutral with regard to jurisdictional claims in published maps and institutional affiliations.

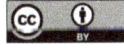

Copyright: © 2021 by the authors. Licensee MDPI, Basel, Switzerland. This article is an open access article distributed under the terms and conditions of the Creative Commons Attribution (CC BY) license (https://creativecommons.org/licenses/by/4.0/).

In peripheral arterial disease (PAD), atherosclerosis limits blood flow to the lower extremities and represents approximately 25% of the global burden of cardiovascular disease and 1.7% of the overall global burden of disease [1]. In people over 50 years of age, 40–50% will manifest atypical symptoms in lower extremities, 10–35% with classic intermittent claudication, and 1–2% with threatened limb amputation [2,3]. The current PAD prevalence figure is expected to increase with age. The current clinical guidelines suggest to manage PAD patients' control of cardiovascular risk factors through lifestyle modifications and vasodilators such as cilostazol to improve symptoms [4,5]. Patients who have symptoms not adequately controlled medically receive interventional endovascular treatment options or open surgery to revascularize and restore blood flow [6]. However, many patients are poor candidates for these interventions due to their comorbidities such as diabetes despite the availability of treatment options [7]. Moreover, 20% of treated patients develop recurrent symptoms that cannot further undergo vascular intervention [8,9]. Thus, the induction of endogenous revascularization has been attempted to establish an alternative strategy of revascularization that ensures efficient re-establishment of blood flow to ischemic tissues and improve PAD patients' clinical outcomes.

The endogenous revascularization after ischemic insult involves multiple biological processes including vasculogenesis, angiogenesis, and arteriogenesis. While vasculogenesis occurs mainly during embryonic life, experimental evidence has shown that vasculogenesis contributes to adult neovascularization at least to repair the damaged capillary networks. In vasculogenesis, blood vessels form de novo via the differentiation of progenitor vascular cells into discrete vascular cells such as endothelial cells [10,11], smooth muscle cells

(SMCs) [10], and pericytes [12]. Angiogenesis is a more effective blood vessel formation process in adults and is stimulated by the hypoxic inflammatory environment following arterial occlusion [13,14]. It involves sprouting new blood vessels from pre-existing capillaries to repair the vascular damage and restore tissue perfusion in distal ischemic tissues [15,16]. However, both vasculogenesis and angiogenesis are natural adaptive processes that do not bypass the blocked arteries instantly but require a long time to build a functional vascular network infiltrating ischemic tissues [17]. At the same time, innate collateral circulation mediates a quick adaptive response. Collaterals are the cross-connecting anastomoses between two feed arteries or crowns of adjacent arterial trees [18]. They are functionally and phenotypically different from arteries and veins as the blood flow along their length comes from opposite directions in the healthy tissue at baseline [19]. While significant variability exists between individuals and species in the extent of the pre-existing collateral trees [20–23], overwhelming findings demonstrate that these vascular tree arrangements can function as a natural bypass following significant arterial occlusions regardless of the extent of the pre-existing collaterals. That compensation is provided by dilating and enlarging these pre-existing vessels: this process is described as "arteriogenesis" [24,25]. Humans have progressive enlargement of pre-existing genicular arteries as collaterals from 2 to 8 weeks after femoral artery occlusion [26].

Nevertheless, most of our knowledge about the pathophysiology of arteriogenesis is based on experimental animal studies of arterial occlusion. The terms collateralization and arterialization are often confused with arteriogenesis and are poorly defined [19]. This review focuses on the arteriogenesis of collaterals as an arterial wall remodeling process where the pre-existing collaterals grow with an increase in diameter and wall thickness in response to an initial hemodynamic stimulus [27].

1. The Pathophysiology of Arteriogenesis after Ischemia

When a primary arterial trunk is occluded, it leads to a pressure drop downstream of the arterial network subsequently creating a pressure gradient across pre-existing collateral circulation and forcing the diversion of blood flow through the collaterals. The altered blood flow generates hemodynamic forces in collateral arterioles and arteries triggering two vascular responses: short-term vasodilation and long-term expansive vascular remodeling [28]. The short-term phase mediated by vasoactive molecules such as nitric oxide relax the smooth muscle cells leading to vasodilation [29]. The acute alteration of fluid shear stress induces the expression of chemokines and adhesion molecules by the endothelium [30]. Chemokines trigger the recruitment and attachment of circulating monocytes to activated endothelium that express adhesion molecules [31]. Monocytes transmigrate through the endothelium into the sub-intimal space where they transform into macrophages and produce inflammatory cytokines and growth factors such as transforming growth factor-β (TGFβ) [32], tumor necrosis factor-α (TNFα) [33], epidermal growth factor (EGF) [34], and fibroblast growth factor (FGF) [35]. The accumulation of macrophages has been reported in the perivascular area as well [36]. Eventually, these cytokines and growth factors diffuse into the medial layer of collaterals modulating the signaling pathways of SMC [37]. This results in SMC phenotypic switching that involves the SMC dedifferentiation from the quiescent contractile phenotype to a proliferative, migratory, and synthetic phenotype [38]. Growth factors and cytokines secreted from macrophages activate the proteolysis system for extracellular matrix (ECM) remodeling to further enhance SMC phenotypic switching [39].

Synthetic smooth muscle cells migrate from the media to the subendothelial space (intima) where they proliferate abundantly and produce ECM components including collagen, elastin, and proteoglycans to the subintimal space resulting in the formation of a new layer of SMC [38]. At this point, the collateral vessel has an approximately 25-fold larger diameter with a newly formed tunica intima, reconstituted tunica media, and thickened tunica adventitia that can restore blood flow up to 50% [40]. The increased vascular diameter is associated with the normalization of shear stress and mechanical strain on the vascular wall [41]. This reduced intravascular pressure in the collaterals impairs endothelial activation, attenuates inflammation, and causes synthetic SMCs to re-differentiate back into their contractile state, thus terminating the collateral growth process [42]. Concurrently, blood flow is reduced and gradually regresses in collaterals that fail to have mature arteriogenesis [43].

Upon successful arteriogenesis, the collaterals exhibit an extensive outward and hypertrophic remodeling, which is associated with the transformation of a small microvascular resistance vessel into a large conductance artery [44]. The smooth muscle cell is the primary cell type in this collateral remodeling [45] (Figure 1).

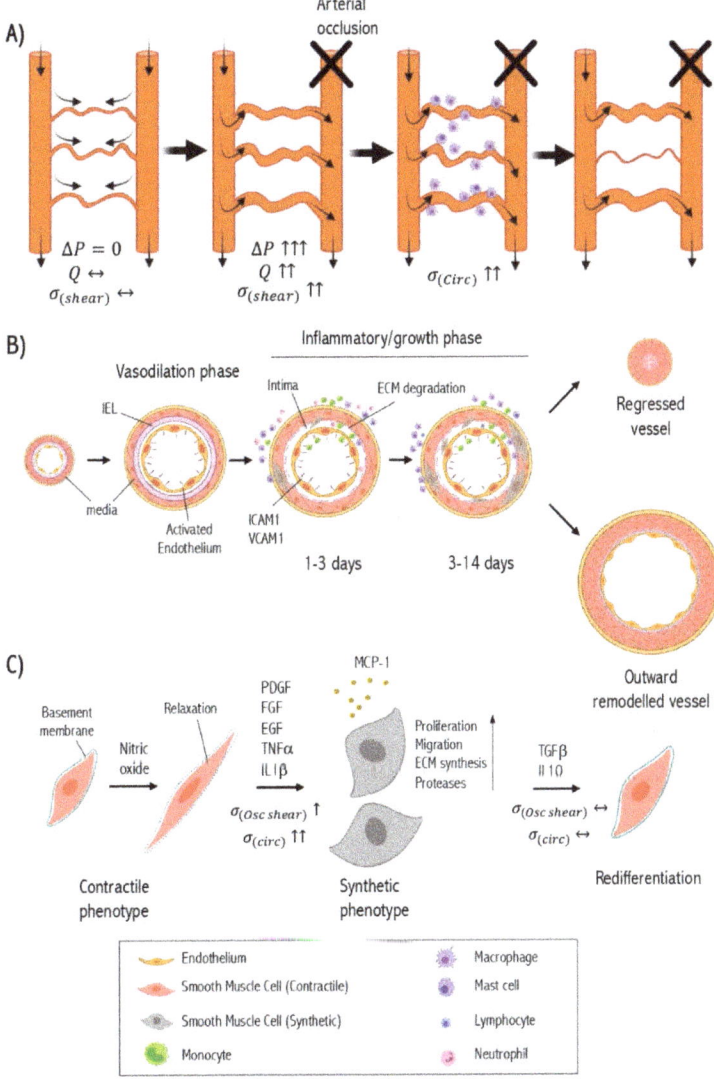

Figure 1. Pathophysiology of arteriogenesis. (**A**) Diagram illustrates the hemodynamic changes of collateral circulation after arterial occlusion. Pressure-gradient (ΔP); blood flow (Q); direction of blood flow (arrows); fluid shear stress ($\sigma_{(shear)}$); circumferential wall stress or tension ($\sigma_{(circ)}$).

(**B**) Cross-section of collateral arteries showing the different phases of the physiological arteriogenesis (IEL: internal elastic lamina). The presented time course of arteriogenesis phases is observed in the mouse model of limb ischemia. (**C**) The dynamics of the vascular smooth muscle cell (VSMC) phenotype switch during arteriogenesis. Oscillatory shear stress ($\sigma_{(shear)}$). The figure has been created with BioRender.com.

2. Molecular Regulation of SMC Phenotype Switching

Vascular smooth muscle cells in the adult vasculature are not terminally differentiated cells. They possess extensive plasticity such that it can be stimulated to undergo a structural and functional transition into proliferative/migratory/synthetic phenotype or undergo an extreme phenotypic change into osteochondrocyte-like cells [46], foam-like cells [47], and myofibroblasts [48] as detected in atherosclerotic lesions. Nevertheless, SMC plasticity enables de-differentiated SMCs to re-differentiate back to a quiescent and contractile state according to their microenvironment [49]. Many environmental factors of SMC phenotype are identified such as growth factors, cytokines, hormones, blood flow shear stress, cell-to-cell interactions, and cell-to-matrix interactions. SMCs phenotypic switching is a critical event in the pathogenesis of arterial wall diseases such as atherosclerosis [50], aneurysm [51], hypertension [52], and post-angioplasty restenosis [53].

The mature contractile phenotype of SMCs is morphologically characterized by low numbers of protein synthesis organelles, e.g., rough endoplasmic reticulum, Golgi apparatus, or free ribosomes [54]. They demonstrate high expression of proteins that are involved in muscle contraction and anchorage including α-smooth muscle actin (αSM actin) [55], smooth muscle-myosin heavy chain (SM-MHC) [56], h1-calponin [57], smooth muscle 22α (SM22α) [57], and smoothelin [58]. In contrast, synthetic SMCs have little or no contractile protein content and high active protein synthesis apparatus [59]. Synthetic SMCs produce pro-inflammatory factors such as TNF-α [60], C-C Motif Chemokine Ligand 2 (CCL2) or monocyte chemoattractant protein-1 (MCP-1) [61] and ECM remodeling proteins such as collagen I [62] and matrix-metalloproteinases [63]. Most of these proteins are involved in tissue repair and remodeling, which reflect the functional role of synthetic SMCs. Synthetic phenotypes are associated with abnormal mechanical forces.

The molecular basis of sustaining the SMC contractile state has been explained by maintaining CArG–SRF–Myocardin complex [64]. Any headway to disrupt this complex leads to down-regulation of genes encoding for contractile proteins, thus inducing a phenotypic switch to a synthetic pathways [65]. Indeed, the expression of the contractile genes is controlled by multiple CArG elements located within their promoter-enhancer regions [66]. The transcription factor serum response factor (SRF) binds to a general sequence motif in the CArG element (CC(A/T-rich)6GG) to regulate the expression of marker genes [67]. Myocardin (MYOCD) is a potent coactivator of SRF and acts as a mediator of environmental cues on the expression of SMC contractile genes [68]. Myocardin-related transcription factors (MRTFs) [69] and ternary complex factors (TCF) [70] have also been identified to be cofactors of SRF. Prior work has shown that MYOCD and MRTFs respond to pro-differentiation stimuli through Rho GTPases-actin signaling [71,72], whereas TCFs respond to dedifferentiation stimuli through mitogen-activated protein kinase (MAPK) signaling [73].

Several pathways transduce signals from cell surface receptors or integrins in response to the surrounding environmental factors to maintain the contractile phenotype. The RhoA/ROCK signaling triggers actin polymerization increases post-translational modification of MRTFs and releases it to the nucleus to induce contractile gene expression [69]. TGFβ enhances nuclear translocation of SMAD proteins. Interaction with SMAD-binding elements (SBEs) in turn upregulates the expression of differentiation marker genes [74]. Insulin growth factor (IGF) acts through PI3 K/AKT signaling which relieves FOXO4-repressive effect on the CArG–SRF–myocardin complex leading to stable expression of contractile genes [75,76].

The loss of the contractile phenotype occurs via growth factors such as Platelet-derived growth factor-BB (PDGF-BB), FGF, and EGF that activate MAPK cascade via the Ras/Raf/MEK/ERK pathway. The MAPK activation can phosphorylate and activate TCF proteins such as Elk-1 to displace MYOCD or induce SRF-dependent transcription of early response growth, dedifferentiation genes, and repression of smooth muscle contractile genes [77]. ERK can phosphorylate MRTFs in the cytoplasm and prevent nuclear translocation [78]. PDGF-BB induces Kruppel Like Factor 4 (KLF-4) by binding to G/C repressor elements or by competing with SRF for CArG elements to disrupt CArG–SRF–myocardin [79,80] (Figure 2). Epigenetic regulation has been reported to control SMC phenotype switching [81]. For instance, the overexpression of histone acetyltransferase (HAT) enhances TGF β1-regulated SMC marker gene expression and its inhibitors such as Twist1 and E1A. Histone deacetylase (HDAC) expression converses this effect of TGF β1 in SMC [82]. Decreased DNA methyltransferase activity and DNA hypomethylation was observed in the proliferating intimal SMC present in the atherosclerotic lesions both in vivo and in vitro [83,84]. Although some recent advancement sheds light on to the influence of environmental cues in modifying epigenome, deeper research involving genome-wide profiling with epigenetic markers are warranted to completely understand its role in SMC phenotype switching in arteriogenesis.

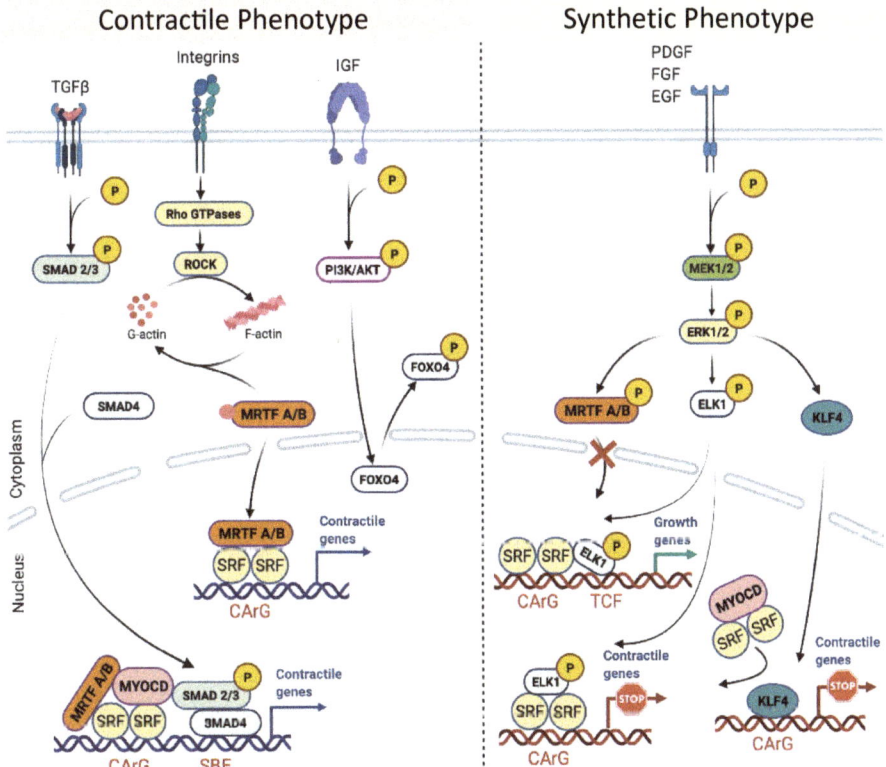

Figure 2. Molecular regulation of vascular smooth muscle phenotype. TGFβ induces the formation of pSMAD2/3-SMAD4 complex, which is translocated into the nucleus, where it binds to SMAD-binding elements (SBE), leading to the expression of early contractile SMC genes. The SMAD interaction with myocardin (MYOCD) or MRTFs enforces SMC differentiation and maturation. Rho/ROCK activates the actin polymerization, which release G-actin monomers from MRTFs, enabling MRTFs to translocate into the nucleus. There, they bind to the SRF/CArG, inducing the expression of SMC contractile genes. IGF activates the PI3 K/AKT signaling pathway that phosphorylates the nuclear FOXO4 facilitating the nuclear export

of FOXO4 to release the repression on the CArG/SRF/MYOCD complex. Growth factors (e.g., FGF, PDGF, EGF) through the MEK/ERK pathway represses SMC contractile genes by phosphorylation of the ternary complex factor (TCF) Elk-1 and MRTFs, and by increasing KLF4 level. Phospho-Elk-1 abolishes the SRF interaction with MYOCD or induces SRF-dependent transcription of early growth genes. The phosphorylation of MRTFs prevents their translocation into the nucleus. The figure has been created with BioRender.com.

3. The Effect of Hemodynamics on Smooth Muscle Cell Phenotype during Arteriogenesis

Upon arterial occlusion, the increase of blood flow and intravascular pressure in the bypass collaterals can generate two primary forces: fluid shear stress and circumferential wall tension [43]. The fluid shear stress force directly affects the endothelium [85]. Circumferential wall tension affects both endothelium and medial smooth muscle cells [86]. However, the fluid shear stress can indirectly affect the smooth muscle cells through diffusible vasoactive molecules secreted from activated endothelium, inflammation-induced shear stress factors, and shear stress generated by secondary interstitial flow [87]. Multiple in vitro studies have shown that both generated physical hemodynamic forces can influence the SMC phenotype [85]. Under physiological conditions, collaterals typically have little or no blood flow, and the fluid shear stress is minimal with little influence on the SMC phenotype [19]. Here, the phenotype of contractile SMCs in the collaterals is maintained mainly by the kinetic energy of flow, which is converted to potential energy that maintains the high circumferential wall stress of collaterals [88]. This also leads to an intense SMC investment of the collaterals unlike distal arterioles.

In contrast, after arterial occlusion, early vasodilation of collaterals leads to a rapid decrease in the intra-luminal pressure. Thus, according to Laplace's formula, we expect that the circumferential wall stress would not change significantly in the early stage. In addition, the diminished blood pressure in downstream vessels is much lower than the proximal arterial pressure; thus, this pressure is unlikely to cause a significant stretch force on medial SMC at this phase. Indeed, the SMC in small arteries and arterioles generally react to the acute rise of intraluminal pressure by contraction (myogenic response) to regulate the tissue blood flow [89,90]. However, the collaterals are dilated after the arterial occlusion indicating that shear-mediated responses predominate the intravascular pressure-mediated responses or this could be partially explained by the fact that collaterals lack myogenic responsiveness and have less SMC tone at baseline than the arteries/arterioles they interconnect [88]. Endothelial-smooth muscle cell co-culture studies have shown sustained exposure of endothelial cells to laminar shear stress inhibits SMC proliferation and induces a transition from a synthetic to a contractile phenotype [91]. These observations agree with in vivo animal studies showing an absence of SMC proliferation of the SMC phenotype switching at early stage (up to 48 hours after arterial occlusion) [92]. In summary, the increase in fluid shear stress is the dominant factor at the very beginnings where the SMCs are relaxed while maintaining their contractile phenotype.

The increase in fluid shear stress force is transmitted to the SMC by diffusible molecules such as nitric oxide (NO) [93]. NO is synthesized by endothelial nitric oxide synthase (eNOS) or inducible nitric oxide synthase (iNOS) [94]. NO can diffuse into the smooth muscle cells where it binds with soluble guanylate cyclase (cGC) to produce cyclic guanosine monophosphate (cGMP), which is a crucial factor to activate protein kinase G (PKG) that relaxes the smooth muscle cells leading to vasodilatation [95]. NO inhibits SMC proliferation through the extracellular signal-regulated kinase (ERK) pathway leading to increased protein levels of the cyclin-dependent kinase inhibitor p21 Waf1/Cip1 [96]. cGMP-dependent protein kinase (PKG) overexpression in synthetic SMC results in phenotypic switching of SMC to a contractile phenotype that expresses contractile markers [97] (SM-MHC, calponin, α-SM actin) with reduced expression of synthetic phenotype markers (osteopontin, thrombospondin) [98–101]. Despite the continuous production of NO through the process of arteriogenesis, the effect of NO on SMC phenotype is not predominant in the next stages of arteriogenesis and is overridden by other factors such as cytokines, growth factors, and the increase of circumferential wall tension. All these factors tend to induce the SMC synthetic phenotype. Mees et al. used the distal femoral artery ligation model that only causes marginal ischemia in the lower limb to specifically study arteriogenesis. Their findings demonstrate that tissue blood flow recovery was impaired in eNOS-knockout mice due to the inability to sufficiently vasodilate collaterals and not because of impaired arteriogenesis [102]. These findings were supported by several studies using mathematical modeling that showed that collateral vasodilation is a critical triggering factor for significant blood flow compensation to occur following arterial occlusion [103,104].

Most collaterals tend to be tortuous small arteries [105]. The steady low shear stress is transformed rapidly to turbulent shear stress when blood flow increases after proximal arterial occlusion. The sudden changes in fluid shear stress naturally promote acute activation of endothelial cells and inflammatory pathways [106]. Endothelial cells sense the change of fluid shear stress via mechanosensors and covert this into paracrine chemical signals that influence the medial SMC [107]. The mechanosensation process involves multiple endothelial cell components. For instance, the activation of volume-regulated endothelial chloride channels is one of the earliest responses to endothelial cell swelling resulting from an acute increase in fluid shear stress [108]. Other early responses led to mechanically gated channels such as transient receptor potential cation channel V4 (TRPV4) and Piezo1. These are sensitive to changes in the endothelial cell membrane's tension resulting from fluid shear stress [109].

Endothelial surface glycocalyx and its components can act as a mechanoreceptor and can transmit mechanical stimuli to the cytoskeleton, which can then activate downstream signaling pathways such as PI3K/AKT/eNOS and NFκB [110]. The platelet endothelial cell adhesion molecule-1 (PECAM-1), vascular endothelial-cadherin (VE-cadherin), and vascular endothelial growth factor receptor 2 (VEGFR2) can collectively act as mechanosensory complex in response to the fluid shear stress [111]. In vivo, the genetic deletion of the PECAM-1 component attenuates the NF-kB activation and downstream inflammatory response in collateral arteries following limb ischemia [112]. This was associated with partial recovery of blood flow and reduced collateral remodeling.

In contrast, the alterations in the intraluminal pressure in the later stages of arteriogenesis can be extended to exert a mechanical force on the cellular components of VSMCs, which act as a mechanosensor to initiate subsequent signal transduction events [43]. Medial SMC can also be indirectly exposed to the fluid shear stress and blood flow pressure through the (transmural) interstitial flow. This flow shear stress is driven by the transmural pressure differential between the intra-arterial and tissue pressure [113] and can exhibit a direct shear stress force on SMCs that their mechanosensors can sense. Many mechanosensors were identified on VSMCs to sense the surrounding mechanical stimuli such as membrane-like receptors, ion channels and pumps, glycocalyx, primary cilium, and integrins [114,115]. These mechanosensors could transmit signals from the surroundings to affect the SMC phenotype as an adaptive response [116]. Hu et al. demonstrated that the adaptor molecules of membrane mechanosensors are inactive in the quiescent SMC. The altered mechanical stress initially induces a conformational change in the plasma membrane leading to autophosphorylation of PDGFα receptors and sequential activation of MAPK cascades [117].

Additionally, activation of integrin receptors, stretch activated cation channels, and G proteins are also observed in SMC membranes of collateral vessels in response to stretch forces [118]. These forces play a pivotal role in SMC proliferation and differentiation [117]. SMCs are aligned circumferentially in the media layer. SMCs stretch along their central axis when the collaterals vasodilate due to the hemodynamic changes. The vasodilation might elevate circumferential wall stress via thinning of the pressure-bearing vessel wall leading to increased SMC wall mass as negative feedback of circumferential wall stress regulation [119]. This process requires VSMC proliferation, matrix degradation, and migration, which drives the ability to sense and adapt to mechanical stresses. In vitro studies have demonstrated that cyclic stretching activates ERK1/2 signaling bringing down the expression of SM-MHC, smoothelin, and calponin in VSMCs [120]. Downregulation of SMC marker genes mediates phenotypic modulation and sustained phosphorylation of ERK1/2 and contributes to the SMC medial layer's growth during arteriogenesis [121].

Cyclic stretching is a critical inducer of MCP-1 expression in SMC of remodeling collaterals [122]. It governs the recruitment of circulating monocytes and stimulates SMC's proliferation and inflammatory state through differential activation of the transcription factors NF-kB and AP-1 [123]. Ephrin B2 is another well-known inducer of arteriogenesis and is controlled by cyclic stretch. Ephrin B2 is an arterial marker that is upregulated in endothelial cells during collateral remodeling and plays a vital role in arteriogenesis by limiting SMC migration within defined borders and controlling monocyte extravasation [124]. Exposure of SMCs to cyclic stretch also increases collagen and fibronectin production, metalloproteinase activity, and TGFβ expression, thus modulating the arterial remodeling outcome [125].

The arterial wall strain is chronically elevated in systemic hypertension conditions. The small arteries and arterioles remodel inwardly through a eutrophic process of rearrangement of the same SMC around a smaller lumen [126]. Conversely, collateral arteries undergo robust anatomic outward remodeling [127]. The inflammatory profile plays a pivotal shift in the remodeling outcome towards expansive remodeling in response to the initial shear stress changes after arterial occlusion. There is a tight association between fluid shear stress and wall stretch dynamics according to a theoretical model simulating hemodynamic alterations-stimulated vascular remodeling responses [128]. Maintaining the relationship between the two forces is regarded a design principle for adequate collateral circulation [41].

4. The Role of Inflammation in SMC Phenotypic Change

The initial phase of collateral vasodilation is driven by fluid shear stress and occurs within the early stage of post-occlusion. However, this vessel enlargement accounts for a small proportion of final vessel expansion, and it slows following shear stress normalization [85]. The appearance of synthetic SMCs or a reduction in contractile SMCs occurs after the vasodilation phase in coincidence with increased inflammatory intensity. The inflammatory process is triggered by shear stress alterations and is an amplifying factor that drives the vessel expansion beyond this point to influence SMC phenotype [129]. Similar to the formation of atherosclerotic plaque in which inflammation sought to play an important role in SMC phenotypic modulation [130], a complex inflammation process leads to cell-to-cell crosstalk between VSMCs, endothelial cells, and immune cells for their phenotypic transition in the context of collateral remodeling [131]. The shear stress-induced inflammation offers a beneficial effect on arteriogenesis only if it remains transient. Indeed, that prolonged inflammation leads to ineffective arteriogenesis [132]. Hence, the factors affecting the time required to trigger inflammation must be well evaluated because the variability in individuals accounts for the variation in the extent of arteriogenesis between individuals and species.

Endothelial cells in pre-existing collaterals are the first effectors to initialize an inflammatory process following arterial occlusion [133]. In response to fluid shear stress alterations, endothelial cells express cell adhesion molecules, chemokines, and cytokines. Chemokines are vital mediators that recruit circulating monocytes into the subendothelial space of collaterals [134]. Additionally, significant accumulation of monocytes/macrophages in the perivascular area peaked within the first three days of arterial occlusion [31]. SMCs express many chemokine receptors on their surface, and they are responsive to accumulated chemokines in the collaterals. Therefore, chemokines can directly contribute to the modulation of SMC phenotypes during arteriogenesis. Exogenous MCP-1 is a potent chemokine in enhancing arteriogenesis and stimulates SMC proliferation [135]. In vitro forced expression of MCP-1 in SMCs leads to dedifferentiation [136]. The role of other chemokines involved in arteriogenesis and SMC phenotype changes remains unclear.

Medial SMCs also contributes to initiating or amplifying stretch-induced inflammation in collateral remodeling [137]. They produce multiple cytokines and chemokines, e.g., interleukin IL-1, IL-6, CCL2, and C-X-C Motif Chemokine Ligand 10 (CXCL10) in response to changes in intravascular pressure [138]. However, the collateral media often remains spared from immune cell infiltration. Monocytes/macrophages can mainly regulate the SMC phenotype through paracrine effects during arteriogenesis [139]. Monocytes are divided into a subset of populations based on the expression levels of cell surface markers and chemokine receptors: pro-inflammatory (Ly6 $C^{high}CCR2^{high}CX3\,CR1^{low}$) and tissue repair (Ly6 $C^{low}CCR2^{low}CX3\,CR1^{high}$) in *mouse* [140]. The infiltrated pro-inflammatory monocytes (Ly6C^{high}) are detected mainly in the collaterals during the early phase of arteriogenesis whereas the anti-inflammatory monocytes (Ly6 C^{low}) predominate the collaterals during the growth and expansion phase of arteriogenesis [141]. Ly6 C^{high} monocytes are more likely to differentiate into M1 macrophages, which secrete various pro-inflammatory cytokines such as interleukin (IL)-1, IL-6, IL-12, and TNFα. They exhibit high proteolytic activity [142]. In contrast, Ly6 C^{low} monocytes may differentiate into M2 macrophages, which secrete anti-inflammatory cytokines such as IL-10 and TGFβ1 and express growth factors such as vascular endothelial growth factor (VEGF) and basic fibroblast growth factor (bFGF), thus promoting collateral remodeling and expansion [143]. Many of the factors produced by macrophages have been linked with SMC growth and loss of contractile phenotype [144–146]. In vitro co-culture studies have shown that macrophage-derived PDGF enhances SMC proliferation and suppresses the expression of SMC contractile markers: SM α-actin and SM-MHC. IL-6 released by macrophages promotes Matrix metalloproteinase-1 (MMP-1) production by SMC [147]. Other factors such as TGF-β1 that is secreted by the M2 macrophage induces a contractile SMC phenotype [148,149].

Monocytes and macrophages are an important source of metalloproteinases and other proteases such as cathepsins during vascular repair process [150]. During arteriogenesis, metalloproteinases contribute actively to extracellular matrix breakdown to facilitate SMC migration and rearrangement. MMP-2 and MMP-9 stimulates the interaction of VSMCs with newly formed ECM to trigger intracellular signaling via integrins to induce a phenotypic switch and persistent migration [151]. SMCs develop an intercellular signaling system de novo: connexin-37 is a highly specific marker for developing collateral vessels [152]. All of these changes contribute to the release of constraints imposed by the structural scaffold of extracellular matrix. In turn, this directs collateral remodeling towards an outward remodeling. Metalloproteinases can increase the bioavailability of growth factors and cytokines by processing the bound species into an extracellular matrix, thus enhancing their capacity to regulate SMC phenotype in a spatial and temporal manner during the different phases of arteriogenesis [153].

Other inflammatory cell populations have been reported to infiltrate the collateral sites during arteriogenesis, e.g., neutrophils [154], mast cells [155], and lymphocytes [156]. Mast cells residing in the perivascular tissues of arteries are activated during arteriogenesis. Chillo et al. demonstrated that shear stress-induced mast cell activation is mediated by activated neutrophil and platelet-derived effectors such as reactive oxidative stress [157]. Degranulation occurs when mast cells are activated, and thus the bioactive granule content is released to the extracellular space leading to a powerful inflammatory reaction. Mast cell granules contain many bioactive constituents including vasoactive molecules, amines, cytokines, proteases, and proteoglycans that can diffuse into the media and influence the SMC function and phenotype [157]. T lymphocytes contribute to the inflammation process during arteriogenesis. Specifically, T cells positively regulate arteriogenesis as demonstrated by the impaired arteriogenesis observed in CD4+ knockout mice model for acute hindlimb ischemia [158]. Upregulation of CCR-7 and its ligands CCL19 and CCL21 were observed within 22 hours post-ischemia leading to a transient retention of CD4+ T lymphocytes in the tissue to mediate a positive role in the initial phase of arteriogenesis [132]. Additionally, the depletion of natural killer (NK) cells severely impairs arteriogenesis in C57BL/6 NK-cell-deficient transgenic mice [159]. Nevertheless, the significance of mast cells or lymphocyte role in SMC phenotype switching remains undefined in vascular pathologies including ischemia-induced arteriogenesis.

5. Conclusions Remarks on Targeting SMC Phenotype Switching as Therapeutic Arteriogenesis

Arteriogenesis is a physiological remodeling response of the collateral arteries in the occlusive arterial diseases. Despite the dramatic outward remodeling of collaterals, blood flow is restored only up to 40–50% of the unblocked artery without intervention. One reason for the limited restoration of blood flow is the premature normalization of fluid shear stress (primary trigger of arteriogenesis). This natural compensatory capacity is diminished even further in subjects with co-morbid diseases such as diabetes [160]. Using an experimental shunting procedure, the induction of high continuous fluid shear stress in collateral circulation led to an increase in the maximal collateral conductance up to 80% of the maximal blood flow of the arterial tree before occlusion [161]. Indeed, this experiment is a clear proof-of-concept that a therapeutic intervention is feasible to enhance the natural arteriogenesis and overcome the anatomical and physiological limits of blood flow recovery after acute ischemia.

Vascular smooth muscle cells play a central role during arteriogenesis due to their plasticity. Phenotypic switching of the contractile VSMC to a synthetic state is a critical cellular event that sustains the growth and outward remodeling of collaterals. In contrast, VSMC re-differentiation back to their contractile state is important to regain vascular functions and prevent inappropriate hypertrophic remodeling of collaterals that could perturb the blood flow for distal ischemic tissues. The physiological normalization of fluid shear can lead to a premature switch of synthetic VSMC to a contractile quiescent phenotype; this switch eventually attenuates the collateral wall growth and remodeling. It has been shown that growth factor therapy can stimulate angiogenesis and also is able to stimulate arteriogenesis [162,163]. Many of the used growth factors such as FGF2 and PDGF are involved in the induction of SMC phenotype switching into synthetic phenotype. However, the single growth factor therapy was never able to completely restore the conductance capacity of a larger artery [164]. Thus, administration of vasodilators combined with agents inducing synthetic SMC as therapeutic strategy could increase the maximal collateral conductance in occlusive artery disease.

Targeting vascular smooth muscle cell phenotype switching has been suggested to be a therapeutic approach for tackling other vascular diseases such as atherosclerosis and hypertension. However, since the dynamics of VSMC phenotype switching are different in arteriogenesis, the timing of intervention would be challenging to achieve effective therapy. Another challenge of targeting VSMC in arteriogenesis is that several cellular events of atherosclerotic plaque development are also involved in arteriogenesis. For instance, extracellular matrix degradation, VSMC migration, and proliferation are activated in both arteriogenesis and atherogenesis. The stimulation of arteriogenesis through agents that promote VSMC proliferation or positive arterial remodeling could have side effects on the aggravation of atherosclerotic plaques in PAD patients who typically suffer from atherosclerosis. While many experimental studies have been conducted to investigate the molecular mechanisms of VSMC phenotype regulation in the context of atherosclerosis, the molecular mechanisms of VSMC phenotype switching that specifically control arteriogenesis in ischemic vascular disease remain largely unknown. Previous studies have been carried out to trace the VSMC phenotype dynamics in vascular repair and atherosclerosis models. Further studies are required for VSMC lineage tracing studies during arteriogenesis. These can help to identify novel specific molecular targets for therapeutic arteriogenesis of peripheral arterial disease patients.

Author Contributions: Conceptualization, J.V.A. and A.A.H.Z.; Writing—original draft preparation, J.V.A.; writing—review and editing, A.A.H.Z.; supervision, A.A.H.Z. Both authors have read and agreed to the published version of the manuscript.

Funding: This research received no external funding.

Data Availability Statement: Not applicable.

Acknowledgments: J.V.A. is supported by a graduate scholarship from the College of Health and Life Sciences at Hamad Bin Khalifa University.

Conflicts of Interest: The authors declare that they have no conflict of interest.

References

1. Bauersachs, R.; Zeymer, U.; Briere, J.-B.; Marre, C.; Bowrin, K.; Huelsebeck, M. Burden of Coronary Artery Disease and Peripheral Artery Disease: A Literature Review. *Cardiovasc. Ther.* **2019**, *2019*, 8295054. [CrossRef] [PubMed]
2. Hirsch, A.T.; Haskal, Z.J.; Hertzer, N.R.; Bakal, C.W.; Creager, M.A.; Halperin, J.L.; Hiratzka, L.F.; Murphy, W.R.; Olin, J.W.; Puschett, J.B.; et al. ACC/AHA 2005 practice guidelines for the management of patients with peripheral arterial disease (lower extremity, renal, mesenteric, and abdominal aortic): A collaborative report from the American Association for Vascular Surgery/Society for Vascular Surgery, Society for Cardiovascular Angiography and Interventions, Society for Vascular Medicine and Biology, Society of Interventional Radiology, and the ACC/AHA task force on practice guidelines (writing committee to develop guidelines for the management of patients with peripheral arterial disease): Endorsed by the American Association of Cardiovascular and Pulmonary Rehabilitation; National Heart, Lung, and Blood Institute; Society for Vascular Nursing; TransAtlantic Inter-Society Consensus; and Vascular Disease Foundation. *Circulation* **2006**, *113*, e463–e654. [PubMed]
3. Johannesson, A.; Larsson, G.-U.; Ramstrand, N.; Turkiewicz, A.; Wiréhn, A.-B.; Atroshi, I. Incidence of Lower-Limb Amputation in the Diabetic and Nondiabetic General Population: A 10-year population-based cohort study of initial unilateral and contralateral amputations and reamputations. *Diabetes Care* **2009**, *32*, 275–280. [CrossRef] [PubMed]
4. Gerhard-Herman, M.D.; Gornik, H.L.; Barrett, C.; Barshes, N.R.; Corriere, M.A.; Drachman, D.E.; Fleisher, L.A.; Fowkes, F.G.; Hamburg, N.M.; Kinlay, S.; et al. 2016 AHA/ACC guideline on the management of patients with lower extremity peripheral artery disease: A report of the american college of cardiology/american heart association task force on clinical practice guidelines. *Circulation* **2017**, *135*, e726–e779. [PubMed]
5. Mohammed, M.; Gosch, K.; Safley, D.; Jelani, Q.-U.-A.; Aronow, H.D.; Mena, C.; Shishehbor, M.H.; Spertus, J.A.; Abbott, J.D.; Smolderen, K.G. Cilostazol and peripheral artery disease-specific health status in ambulatory patients with symptomatic PAD. *Int. J. Cardiol.* **2020**, *316*, 222–228. [CrossRef] [PubMed]
6. Lichtenberg, M. Peripheral artery disease: Endovascular therapy. *Med. Mon. Pharm.* **2017**, *40*, 102–106.
7. Yao, H.Q.; Wang, F.J.; Kang, Z. Effects of endovascular interventions on vWF and Fb levels in type 2 diabetic patients with peripheral artery disease. *Ann. Vasc. Surg.* **2016**, *33*, 159–166. [CrossRef] [PubMed]
8. Bae, M.J.; Lee, J.G.; Chung, S.W.; Lee, C.W.; Kim, C.W. The factors affecting recurrence of symptoms after infrainguinal arterial endovascular angioplasty. *Korean J. Thorac. Cardiovasc. Surg.* **2014**, *47*, 517–522. [CrossRef]
9. Meloni, M.; Izzo, V.; Giurato, L.; Del Giudice, C.; Da Ros, V.; Cervelli, V.; Gandini, R.; Uccioli, L. Recurrence of critical limb ischemia after endovascular intervention in patients with diabetic foot ulcers. *Adv. Wound Care* **2018**, *7*, 171–176. [CrossRef]
10. Ingram, D.A.; Mead, L.E.; Moore, D.B.; Woodard, W.; Fenoglio, A.; Yoder, M.C. Vessel wall–derived endothelial cells rapidly proliferate because they contain a complete hierarchy of endothelial progenitor cells. *Blood* **2005**, *105*, 2783–2786. [CrossRef]
11. Zengin, E.; Chalajour, F.; Gehling, U.M.; Ito, W.D.; Treede, H.; Lauke, H.; Weil, J.; Reichenspurner, H.; Kilic, N.; Ergün, S. Vascular wall resident progenitor cells: A source for postnatal vasculogenesis. *Development* **2006**, *133*, 1543–1551. [CrossRef]
12. Higuchi, M.; Kato, T.; Yoshida, S.; Ueharu, H.; Nishimura, N.; Kato, Y. PRRX1- and PRRX2-positive mesenchymal stem/progenitor cells are involved in vasculogenesis during rat embryonic pituitary development. *Cell Tissue Res.* **2015**, *361*, 557–565. [CrossRef] [PubMed]
13. Carmeliet, P. Angiogenesis in health and disease. *Nat. Med.* **2003**, *9*, 653–660. [CrossRef] [PubMed]
14. Pugh, C.W.; Ratcliffe, P.J. Regulation of angiogenesis by hypoxia: Role of the HIF system. *Nat. Med.* **2003**, *9*, 677–684. [CrossRef] [PubMed]
15. Ribatti, D.; Crivellato, E. "Sprouting angiogenesis", a reappraisal. *Dev. Biol.* **2012**, *372*, 157–165. [CrossRef]
16. Emanueli, C.; Madeddu, P. Angiogenesis gene therapy to rescue ischaemic tissues: Achievements and future directions. *Br. J. Pharmacol.* **2001**, *133*, 951–958. [CrossRef]
17. Simons, M. Angiogenesis: Where do we stand now? *Circulation* **2005**, *111*, 1556–1566. [CrossRef]
18. Buschmann, I.; Schaper, W. The pathophysiology of the collateral circulation (arteriogenesis). *J. Pathol.* **2000**, *190*, 338–342. [CrossRef]
19. Faber, J.E.; Chilian, W.M.; Deindl, E.; van Royen, N.; Simons, M. A Brief Etymology of the Collateral Circulation. *Arter. Thromb. Vasc. Biol.* **2014**, *34*, 1854–1859. [CrossRef] [PubMed]
20. Schaper, W. Collateral circulation: Past and present. *Basic Res. Cardiol.* **2009**, *104*, 5–21. [CrossRef] [PubMed]
21. Sherman, J.A.; Hall, A.; Malenka, D.J.; De Muinck, E.D.; Simons, M. Humoral and cellular factors responsible for coronary collateral formation. *Am. J. Cardiol.* **2006**, *98*, 1194–1197. [CrossRef]
22. Clayton, J.A.; Chalothorn, D.; Faber, J.E. Vascular endothelial growth factor-a specifies formation of native collaterals and regulates collateral growth in Ischemia. *Circ. Res.* **2008**, *103*, 1027–1036. [CrossRef] [PubMed]

23. Zhang, H.; Prabhakar, P.; Sealock, R.; E Faber, J. Wide genetic variation in the native pial collateral circulation is a major determinant of variation in severity of stroke. *J. Cereb. Blood Flow Metab.* **2010**, *30*, 923–934. [CrossRef] [PubMed]
24. Helisch, A.; Schaper, W. Arteriogenesis: The development and growth of collateral arteries. *Microcirculation* **2003**, *10*, 83–97. [CrossRef] [PubMed]
25. Scholz, D.; Ziegelhoeffer, T.; Helisch, A.; Wagner, S.; Friedrich, C.; Podzuweit, T.; Schaper, W. Contribution of arteriogenesis and angiogenesis to postocclusive hindlimb perfusion in mice. *J. Mol. Cell. Cardiol.* **2002**, *34*, 775–787. [CrossRef] [PubMed]
26. Ziegler, M.A.; DiStasi, M.R.; Bills, R.G.; Miller, S.J.; Alloosh, M.; Murphy, M.P.; Akingba, A.G.; Sturek, M.; Dalsing, M.C.; Unthank, J.L. Marvels, mysteries, and misconceptions of vascular compensation to peripheral artery occlusion. *Microcirculation* **2010**, *17*, 3–20. [CrossRef] [PubMed]
27. Herzog, S.; Sager, H.; Khmelevski, E.; Deylig, A.; Ito, W.D. Collateral arteries grow from preexisting anastomoses in the rat hindlimb. *Am. J. Physiol. Heart Circ. Physiol.* **2002**, *283*, H2012–H2020. [CrossRef]
28. Resnick, N.; Einav, S.; Chen-Konak, L.; Zilberman, M.; Yahav, H.; Shay-Salit, A. Hemodynamic forces as a stimulus for arteriogenesis. *Endothelium* **2003**, *10*, 197–206. [CrossRef]
29. Park, B.; Hoffman, A.; Yang, Y.; Yan, J.; Tie, G.; Bagshahi, H.; Nowicki, P.T.; Messina, L.M. Endothelial nitric oxide synthase affects both early and late collateral arterial adaptation and blood flow recovery after induction of hind limb ischemia in mice. *J. Vasc. Surg.* **2010**, *51*, 165–173. [CrossRef]
30. van Royen, N.; Piek, J.J.; Buschmann, I.; Hoefer, I.; Voskuil, M.; Schaper, W. Stimulation of arteriogenesis; a new concept for the treatment of arterial occlusive disease. *Cardiovasc. Res.* **2001**, *49*, 543–553. [CrossRef]
31. Bruce, A.C.; Kelly-Goss, M.R.; Heuslein, J.L.; Meisner, J.K.; Price, R.J.; Peirce, S.M. Monocytes are recruited from venules during arteriogenesis in the murine spinotrapezius ligation model. *Arter. Thromb. Vasc. Biol.* **2014**, *34*, 2012–2022. [CrossRef]
32. van Royen, N.; Hoefer, I.; Buschmann, I.; Heil, M.; Kostin, S.; Deindl, E.; Vogel, S.; Korff, T.; Augustin, H.; Bode, C.; et al. Exogenous application of transforming growth factor beta 1 stimulates arteriogenesis in the peripheral circulation. *FASEB J.* **2002**, *16*, 432–434. [CrossRef]
33. Hoefer, I.E.; Van Royen, N.; Rectenwald, J.E.; Bray, E.J.; Abouhamze, Z.; Moldawer, L.L.; Voskuil, M.; Piek, J.J.; Buschmann, I.R.; Ozaki, C.K. Direct evidence for tumor necrosis factor-α signaling in arteriogenesis. *Circulation* **2002**, *105*, 1639–1641. [CrossRef]
34. Belmadani, S.; Matrougui, K.; Kolz, C.; Pung, Y.F.; Palen, D.; Prockop, D.J.; Chilian, W.M. Amplification of coronary arteriogenic capacity of multipotent stromal cells by epidermal growth factor. *Arter. Thromb. Vasc. Biol.* **2009**, *29*, 802–808. [CrossRef] [PubMed]
35. Deindl, E.; Hoefer, I.E.; Fernandez, B.; Barancik, M.; Heil, M.; Strniskova, M.; Schaper, W. Involvement of the fibroblast growth factor system in adaptive and chemokine-induced arteriogenesis. *Circ. Res.* **2003**, *92*, 561–568. [CrossRef]
36. Vågesjö, E.; Parv, K.; Ahl, D.; Seignez, C.; Hidalgo, C.H.; Giraud, A.; Amoêdo-Leite, C.; Korsgren, O.; Wallén, H.; Juusola, G.; et al. Perivascular macrophages regulate blood flow following tissue damage. *Circ. Res.* **2021**, *128*, 1694–1707. [CrossRef] [PubMed]
37. Buschmann, I.; Heil, M.; Jost, M.; Schaper, W. Influence of inflammatory cytokines on arteriogenesis. *Microcirculation* **2003**, *10*, 371–379. [CrossRef] [PubMed]
38. Scholz, D.; Ito, W.; Fleming, I.; Deindl, E.; Sauer, A.; Wiesnet, M.; Busse, R.; Schaper, J. Ultrastructure and molecular histology of rabbit hind-limb collateral artery growth (arteriogenesis). *Virchows Archiv.* **2000**, *436*, 257–270. [CrossRef]
39. Ungerleider, J.L.; Johnson, T.D.; Hernandez, M.J.; Elhag, D.I.; Braden, R.L.; Dzieciatkowska, M.; Osborn, K.G.; Hansen, K.C.; Mahmud, E.; Christman, K.L. Extracellular matrix hydrogel promotes tissue remodeling, arteriogenesis, and perfusion in a rat hindlimb ischemia model. *JACC Basic Transl. Sci.* **2016**, *1*, 32–44. [CrossRef]
40. Scholz, D.; Cai, W.; Schaper, W. Arteriogenesis, a new concept of vascular adaptation in occlusive disease. *Angiogenesis* **2001**, *4*, 247–257. [CrossRef]
41. Ma, T.; Bai, Y.P. The hydromechanics in arteriogenesis. *Aging Med.* **2020**, *3*, 169–177. [CrossRef]
42. Rzucidlo, E.M.; Martin, K.A.; Powell, R.J. Regulation of vascular smooth muscle cell differentiation. *J. Vasc. Surg.* **2007**, *45*, A25–A32. [CrossRef]
43. Heil, M.; Schaper, W. Influence of mechanical, cellular, and molecular factors on collateral artery growth (arteriogenesis). *Circ. Res.* **2004**, *95*, 449–458. [CrossRef]
44. Hoefer, I.E.; Van Royen, N.; Buschmann, I.R.; Piek, J.J.; Schaper, W. Time course of arteriogenesis following femoral artery occlusion in the rabbit. *Cardiovasc. Res.* **2001**, *49*, 609–617. [CrossRef]
45. Shi, N.; Mei, X.; Chen, S.Y. Smooth muscle cells in vascular remodeling. *Arterioscler. Thromb. Vasc. Biol.* **2019**, *39*, e247–e252. [CrossRef] [PubMed]
46. Leopold, J.A. Vascular calcification: Mechanisms of vascular smooth muscle cell calcification. *Trends Cardiovasc. Med.* **2015**, *25*, 267–274. [CrossRef] [PubMed]
47. Yan, P.; Xia, C.; Duan, C.; Li, S.; Mei, Z. Biological characteristics of foam cell formation in smooth muscle cells derived from bone marrow stem cells. *Int. J. Biol. Sci.* **2011**, *7*, 937–946. [CrossRef]
48. Hegner, B.; Schaub, T.; Catar, R.; Kusch, A.; Wagner, P.; Essin, K.; Lange, C.; Riemekasten, G.; Dragun, D. Intrinsic deregulation of vascular smooth muscle and myofibroblast differentiation in mesenchymal stromal cells from patients with systemic sclerosis. *PLoS ONE* **2016**, *11*, e0153101. [CrossRef]
49. Owens, G.K.; Kumar, M.S.; Wamhoff, B.R. Molecular regulation of vascular smooth muscle cell differentiation in development and disease. *Physiol. Rev.* **2004**, *84*, 767–801. [CrossRef]

50. Bennett, M.R.; Sinha, S.; Owens, G.K. Vascular smooth muscle cells in atherosclerosis. *Circ. Res.* **2016**, *118*, 692–702. [CrossRef]
51. Chen, P.Y.; Qin, L.; Li, G.; Malagon-Lopez, J.; Wang, Z.; Bergaya, S.; Gujja, S.; Caulk, A.W.; Murtada, S.-I.; Zhang, X.; et al. Smooth muscle cell reprogramming in aortic aneurysms. *Cell Stem Cell* **2020**, *26*, 542–557. [CrossRef]
52. Régent, A.; Ly, K.H.; Lofek, S.; Clary, G.; Tamby, M.; Tamas, N.; Federici, C.; Broussard, C.; Chafey, P.; Liaudet-Coopman, E.; et al. Proteomic analysis of vascular smooth muscle cells in physiological condition and in pulmonary arterial hypertension: Toward contractile versus synthetic phenotypes. *Proteomics* **2016**, *16*, 2637–2649. [CrossRef]
53. Acampora, K.B.; Nagatomi, J.; Langan E.M., III; LaBerge, M. Increased synthetic phenotype behavior of smooth muscle cells in response to in vitro balloon angioplasty injury model. *Ann. Vasc. Surg.* **2010**, *24*, 116–126. [CrossRef]
54. Wang, G.; Jacquet, L.; Karamariti, E.; Xu, Q. Origin and differentiation of vascular smooth muscle cells. *J. Physiol.* **2015**, *593*, 3013–3030. [CrossRef] [PubMed]
55. Gabbiani, G.; Schmid, E.; Winter, S.; Chaponnier, C.; de Ckhastonay, C.; Vandekerckhove, J.; Weber, K.; Franke, W.W. Vascular smooth muscle cells differ from other smooth muscle cells: Predominance of vimentin filaments and a specific alpha-type actin. *Proc. Natl. Acad. Sci. USA* **1981**, *78*, 298–302. [CrossRef] [PubMed]
56. Miano, J.; Cserjesi, P.; Ligon, K.L.; Periasamy, M.; Olson, E.N. Smooth muscle myosin heavy chain exclusively marks the smooth muscle lineage during mouse embryogenesis. *Circ. Res.* **1994**, *75*, 803–812. [CrossRef] [PubMed]
57. Duband, J.-L.; Gimona, M.; Scatena, M.; Sartore, S.; Small, J.V. Calponin and SM22 as differentiation markers of smooth muscle: Spatiotemporal distribution during avian embryonic development. *Differentiation* **1993**, *55*, 1–11. [CrossRef]
58. van der Loop, F.T.; Schaart, G.; Timmer, E.D.; Ramaekers, F.C.; van Eys, G.J. Smoothelin, a novel cytoskeletal protein specific for smooth muscle cells. *J. Cell Biol.* **1996**, *134*, 401–411. [CrossRef]
59. Chamley-Campbell, J.; Campbell, G.R.; Ross, R. The smooth muscle cell in culture. *Physiol. Rev.* **1979**, *59*, 1–61. [CrossRef]
60. García-Miguel, M.; Riquelme, J.A.; Norambuena-Soto, I.; Morales, P.E.; Sanhueza-Olivares, F.; Núñez-Soto, C.; Mondaca-Ruff, D.; Cancino-Arenas, N.; Martín, A.S.; Chiong, M. Autophagy mediates tumor necrosis factor-α-induced phenotype switching in vascular smooth muscle A7r5 cell line. *PLoS ONE* **2018**, *13*, e0197210. [CrossRef]
61. Yu, B.; Wong, M.M.; Potter, C.M.F.; Simpson, R.M.L.; Karamariti, E.; Zhang, Z.; Zeng, L.; Warren, D.; Hu, Y.; Wang, W.; et al. Vascular stem/progenitor cell migration induced by smooth muscle cell-derived chemokine (C-C Motif) ligand 2 and chemokine (C-X-C motif) ligand 1 contributes to neointima formation. *Stem Cells* **2016**, *34*, 2368–2380. [CrossRef]
62. Okada, Y.; Katsuda, S.; Matsui, Y.; Watanabe, H.; Nakanishi, I. Collagen Synthesis by Cultured Arterial Smooth Muscle Cells during Spontaneous Phenotypic Modulation. *Pathol. Int.* **1990**, *40*, 157–164. [CrossRef] [PubMed]
63. Weinreb, R.N.; Kashiwagi, K.; Kashiwagi, F.; Tsukahara, S.; Lindsey, J.D. Prostaglandins increase matrix metalloproteinase release from human ciliary smooth muscle cells. *Investig. Ophthalmol. Vis. Sci.* **1997**, *38*, 2772–2780.
64. Yoshida, T.; Sinha, S.; Dandre, F.; Wamhoff, B.R.; Hoofnagle, M.H.; Kremer, B.E.; Wang, D.Z.; Olson, E.N.; Owens, G.K. Myocardin is a key regulator of CArG-dependent transcription of multiple smooth muscle marker genes. *Circ. Res.* **2003**, *92*, 856–864. [CrossRef] [PubMed]
65. Mack, C.P.; Hinson, J.S. Regulation of smooth muscle differentiation by the myocardin family of serum response factor co-factors. *J. Thromb. Haemost.* **2005**, *3*, 1976–1984. [CrossRef]
66. Mack, C.P.; Owens, G.K. Regulation of smooth muscle alpha-actin expression in vivo is dependent on CArG elements within the 5′ and first intron promoter regions. *Circ. Res.* **1999**, *84*, 852–861. [CrossRef] [PubMed]
67. Miano, J.M. Serum response factor: Toggling between disparate programs of gene expression. *J. Mol. Cell. Cardiol.* **2003**, *35*, 577–593. [CrossRef]
68. Wang, D.Z.; Chang, P.S.; Wang, Z.; Sutherland, L.; Richardson, J.A.; Small, E.; Krieg, P.A.; Olson, E.N. Activation of cardiac gene expression by myocardin, a transcriptional cofactor for serum response factor. *Cell* **2001**, *105*, 851–862. [CrossRef]
69. Cenik, B.K.; Liu, N.; Chen, B.; Bezprozvannaya, S.; Olson, E.N.; Bassel-Duby, R. Myocardin-related transcription factors are required for skeletal muscle development. *Development* **2016**, *143*, 2853–2861. [CrossRef]
70. Esnault, C.; Gualdrini, F.; Horswell, S.; Kelly, G.; Stewart, A.; East, P.; Matthews, N.; Treisman, R. ERK-induced activation of TCF family of SRF cofactors initiates a chromatin modification cascade associated with transcription. *Mol. Cell* **2017**, *65*, 1081–1095. [CrossRef]
71. Yang, Q.; Shi, W. Rho/ROCK-MYOCD in regulating airway smooth muscle growth and remodeling. *Am. J. Physiol. Lung Cell Mol. Physiol.* **2021**, *321*, L1–L5. [CrossRef]
72. Esnault, C.; Stewart, A.; Gualdrini, F.; East, P.; Horswell, S.; Matthews, N.; Treisman, R. Rho-actin signaling to the MRTF coactivators dominates the immediate transcriptional response to serum in fibroblasts. *Genes Dev.* **2014**, *28*, 943–958. [CrossRef]
73. A Hipskind, R.; Buscher, D.; Nordheim, A.; Baccarini, M. Ras/MAP kinase-dependent and -independent signaling pathways target distinct ternary complex factors. *Genes Dev.* **1994**, *8*, 1803–1816. [CrossRef]
74. Dennler, S.; Itoh, S.; Vivien, D.; ten Dijke, P.; Huet, S.; Gauthier, J.M. Direct binding of Smad3 and Smad4 to critical TGF beta-inducible elements in the promoter of human plasminogen activator inhibitor-type 1 gene. *EMBO J.* **1998**, *17*, 3091–3100. [CrossRef]
75. Jia, G.; Mitra, A.K.; Gangahar, D.M.; Agrawal, D.K. Insulin-like growth factor-1 induces phosphorylation of PI3K-Akt/PKB to potentiate proliferation of smooth muscle cells in human saphenous vein. *Exp. Mol. Pathol.* **2010**, *89*, 20–26. [CrossRef] [PubMed]
76. Liu, Z.-P.; Wang, Z.; Yanagisawa, H.; Olson, E.N. Phenotypic modulation of smooth muscle cells through interaction of Foxo4 and myocardin. *Dev. Cell* **2005**, *9*, 261–270. [CrossRef] [PubMed]

77. Dandre, F.; Owens, G.K. Platelet-derived growth factor-BB and Ets-1 transcription factor negatively regulate transcription of multiple smooth muscle cell differentiation marker genes. *Am. J. Physiol. Heart Circ. Physiol.* **2004**, *286*, H2042–H2051. [CrossRef] [PubMed]
78. Wang, Z.; Wang, D.-Z.; Hockemeyer, D.; McAnally, J.; Nordheim, A.; Olson, E.N. Myocardin and ternary complex factors compete for SRF to control smooth muscle gene expression. *Nat. Cell Biol.* **2004**, *428*, 185–189. [CrossRef] [PubMed]
79. Salmon, M.; Gomez, D.; Greene, E.; Shankman, L.; Owens, G.K. Cooperative binding of KLF4, pELK-1, and HDAC2 to a G/C repressor element in the SM22α promoter mediates transcriptional silencing during SMC phenotypic switching in vivo. *Circ. Res.* **2012**, *111*, 685–696. [CrossRef]
80. Kawai-Kowase, K.; Owens, G.K. Multiple repressor pathways contribute to phenotypic switching of vascular smooth muscle cells. *Am. J. Physiol. Cell Physiol.* **2007**, *292*, C59–C69. [CrossRef]
81. Alexander, M.R.; Owens, G.K. Epigenetic control of smooth muscle cell differentiation and phenotypic switching in vascular development and disease. *Annu. Rev. Physiol.* **2012**, *74*, 13–40. [CrossRef]
82. Qiu, P.; Ritchie, R.P.; Gong, X.Q.; Hamamori, Y.; Li, L. Dynamic changes in chromatin acetylation and the expression of histone acetyltransferases and histone deacetylases regulate the SM22alpha transcription in response to Smad3-mediated TGFbeta1 signaling. *Biochem. Biophys. Res. Commun.* **2006**, *348*, 351–358. [CrossRef]
83. Hiltunen, M.O.; Turunen, M.P.; Häkkinen, T.P.; Rutanen, J.; Hedman, M.; Mäkinen, K.; Turunen, A.M.; Aalto-Setalä, K.; Ylä-Herttuala, S. DNA hypomethylation and methyltransferase expression in atherosclerotic lesions. *Vasc. Med.* **2002**, *7*, 5–11. [CrossRef]
84. Connelly, J.J.; Cherepanova, O.A.; Doss, J.F.; Karaoli, T.; Lillard, T.S.; Markunas, C.; Nelson, S.; Wang, T.; Ellis, P.D.; Langford, C.F.; et al. Epigenetic regulation of COL15A1 in smooth muscle cell replicative aging and atherosclerosis. *Hum. Mol. Genet.* **2013**, *22*, 5107–5120. [CrossRef]
85. Pipp, F.; Boehm, S.; Cai, W.-J.; Adili, F.; Ziegler, B.; Karanovic, G.; Ritter, R.; Balzer, J.; Scheler, C.; Schaper, W.; et al. Elevated fluid shear stress enhances postocclusive collateral artery growth and gene expression in the pig hind limb. *Arter. Thromb. Vasc. Biol.* **2004**, *24*, 1664–1668. [CrossRef]
86. Gruionu, G.; Hoying, J.B.; Pries, A.R.; Secomb, T. Structural remodeling of the mouse gracilis artery: Coordinated changes in diameter and medial area maintain circumferential stress. *Microcirculation* **2012**, *19*, 610–618. [CrossRef]
87. Sakamoto, N.; Ohashi, T.; Sato, M. Effect of fluid shear stress on migration of vascular smooth muscle cells in cocultured model. *Ann. Biomed. Eng.* **2006**, *34*, 408–415. [CrossRef]
88. Zhang, H.; Chalothorn, D.; Faber, J.E. Collateral vessels have unique endothelial and smooth muscle cell phenotypes. *Int. J. Mol. Sci.* **2019**, *20*, 3608. [CrossRef] [PubMed]
89. Bagher, P.; Beleznai, T.; Kansui, Y.; Mitchell, R.; Garland, C.J.; Dora, K.A. Low intravascular pressure activates endothelial cell TRPV4 channels, local Ca2+ events, and IKCa channels, reducing arteriolar tone. *Proc. Natl. Acad. Sci. USA* **2012**, *109*, 18174–18179. [CrossRef] [PubMed]
90. Chen, Y.; Rivers, R.J. Measurement of membrane potential and intracellular Ca(2+) of arteriolar endothelium and smooth muscle in vivo. *Microvasc. Res.* **2001**, *62*, 55–62. [CrossRef] [PubMed]
91. Kim, S.A.; Sung, J.Y.; Woo, C.-H.; Choi, H.C. Laminar shear stress suppresses vascular smooth muscle cell proliferation through nitric oxide-AMPK pathway. *Biochem. Biophys. Res. Commun.* **2017**, *490*, 1369–1374. [CrossRef] [PubMed]
92. Tsai, M.-C.; Chen, L.; Zhou, J.; Tang, Z.; Hsu, T.-F.; Wang, Y.; Shih, Y.-T.; Peng, H.-H.; Wang, N.; Guan, Y.; et al. Shear stress induces synthetic-to-contractile phenotypic modulation in smooth muscle cells via peroxisome proliferator-activated receptor alpha/delta activations by prostacyclin released by sheared endothelial cells. *Circ. Res.* **2009**, *105*, 471–480. [CrossRef] [PubMed]
93. Li, Y.; Talotta-Altenburg, L.M.; Silimperi, K.A.; Ciabattoni, G.O.; Lowe-Krentz, L.J. Endothelial nitric oxide synthase activation is required for heparin receptor effects on vascular smooth muscle cells. *Am. J. Physiol. Physiol.* **2020**, *318*, C463–C475. [CrossRef] [PubMed]
94. Lowry, J.L.; Brovkovych, V.; Zhang, Y.; Skidgel, R.A. Endothelial nitric-oxide synthase activation generates an inducible nitric-oxide synthase-like output of nitric oxide in inflamed endothelium. *J. Biol. Chem.* **2013**, *288*, 4174–4193. [CrossRef]
95. Tabatabaei, S.N.; Girouard, H. Nitric oxide and cerebrovascular regulation. *Vitam. Horm.* **2014**, *96*, 347–385. [PubMed]
96. Zuckerbraun, B.S.; Stoyanovsky, D.A.; Sengupta, R.; Shapiro, R.A.; Ozanich, B.A.; Rao, J.; Barbato, J.E.; Tzeng, E. Nitric oxide-induced inhibition of smooth muscle cell proliferation involves S-nitrosation and inactivation of RhoA. *Am. J. Physiol. Physiol.* **2007**, *292*, C824–C831. [CrossRef] [PubMed]
97. Itoh, S.; Katoh, Y.; Konishi, H.; Takaya, N.; Kimura, T.; Periasamy, M.; Yamaguchi, H. Nitric oxide regulates smooth-muscle-specific myosin heavy chain gene expression at the transcriptional level—Possible role of SRF and YY1 through CArG element. *J. Mol. Cell. Cardiol.* **2001**, *33*, 95–107. [CrossRef] [PubMed]
98. Boerth, N.J.; Dey, N.B.; Cornwell, T.L.; Lincoln, T.M. Cyclic GMP-dependent protein kinase regulates vascular smooth muscle cell phenotype. *J. Vasc. Res.* **1997**, *34*, 245–259. [CrossRef]
99. Lincoln, T.M.; Sellak, H.; Dey, N.; Browner, N.; Choi, C.S.; Dostmann, W.W. Regulation of vascular smooth muscle cell gene expression and phenotype by cyclic GMP and cyclic GMP-dependent protein kinase. *BMC News Views* **2003**, *3*, 356–367. [CrossRef]
100. Dey, N.B.; Foley, K.F.; Lincoln, T.M.; Dostmann, W.R. Inhibition of cGMP-dependent protein kinase reverses phenotypic modulation of vascular smooth muscle cells. *J. Cardiovasc. Pharmacol.* **2005**, *45*, 404–413. [CrossRef]

101. Zhou, W.; Dasgupta, C.; Negash, S.; Raj, J.U. Modulation of pulmonary vascular smooth muscle cell phenotype in hypoxia: Role of cGMP-dependent protein kinase. *Am. J. Physiol. Lung Cell Mol. Physiol.* **2007**, *292*, L1459–L1466. [CrossRef] [PubMed]
102. Mees, B.; Wagner, S.; Ninci, E.; Tribulova, S.; Martin, S.; Van Haperen, R.; Kostin, S.; Heil, M.; De Crom, R.; Schaper, W. Endothelial nitric oxide synthase activity is essential for vasodilation during blood flow recovery but not for arteriogenesis. *Arter. Thromb. Vasc. Biol.* **2007**, *27*, 1926–1933. [CrossRef]
103. Wilstein, Z.; Alligood, D.M.; McLure, V.L.; Miller, A.C. Mathematical model of hypertension-induced arterial remodeling: A chemo-mechanical approach. *Math. Biosci.* **2018**, *303*, 10–25. [CrossRef] [PubMed]
104. Yang, J.; Clark, J.W.; Bryan, R.M.; Robertson, C.S. Mathematical modeling of the nitric oxide/cGMP pathway in the vascular smooth muscle cell. *Am. J. Physiol. Circ. Physiol.* **2005**, *289*, H886–H897. [CrossRef] [PubMed]
105. Kaufman, S.L.; Kan, J.S.; Mitchell, S.E.; Flaherty, J.T.; White, R.I. Embolization of systemic to pulmonary artery collaterals in the management of hemoptysis in pulmonary atresia. *Am. J. Cardiol.* **1986**, *58*, 1130–1132. [CrossRef]
106. Davies, P.F. Hemodynamic shear stress and the endothelium in cardiovascular pathophysiology. *Nat. Clin. Pr. Neurol.* **2008**, *6*, 16–26. [CrossRef]
107. Shi, Z.D.; Tarbell, J.M. Fluid flow mechanotransduction in vascular smooth muscle cells and fibroblasts. *Ann. Biomed. Eng.* **2011**, *39*, 1608–1619. [CrossRef]
108. Ziegelhoeffer, T.; Scholz, D.; Friedrich, C.; Helisch, A.; Wagner, S.; Fernandez, B.; Schaper, W. Inhibition of collateral artery growth by mibefradil: Possible role of volume-regulated chloride channels. *Endothelium* **2003**, *10*, 237–246. [CrossRef]
109. Swain, S.M.; Liddle, R.A. Piezo1 acts upstream of TRPV4 to induce pathological changes in endothelial cells due to shear stress. *J. Biol. Chem.* **2021**, *296*, 100171. [CrossRef]
110. Sieve, I.; Münster-Kühnel, A.K.; Hilfiker-Kleiner, D. Regulation and function of endothelial glycocalyx layer in vascular diseases. *Vasc. Pharmacol.* **2018**, *100*, 26–33. [CrossRef]
111. Pahakis, M.Y.; Kosky, J.R.; Dull, R.; Tarbell, J.M. The role of endothelial glycocalyx components in mechanotransduction of fluid shear stress. *Biochem. Biophys. Res. Commun.* **2007**, *355*, 228–233. [CrossRef]
112. Chen, Z.; Rubin, J.; Tzima, E. Role of PECAM-1 in arteriogenesis and specification of preexisting collaterals. *Circ. Res.* **2010**, *107*, 1355–1363. [CrossRef] [PubMed]
113. Shi, Z.D.; Ji, X.Y.; Berardi, D.E.; Qazi, H.; Tarbell, J.M. Interstitial flow induces MMP-1 expression and vascular SMC migration in collagen I gels via an ERK1/2-dependent and c-Jun-mediated mechanism. *Am. J. Physiol. Heart Circ. Physiol.* **2010**, *298*, H127–H135. [CrossRef] [PubMed]
114. Kang, H.; Liu, J.; Sun, A.; Liu, X.; Fan, Y.; Deng, X. Vascular smooth muscle cell glycocalyx mediates shear stress-induced contractile responses via a Rho kinase (ROCK)-myosin light chain phosphatase (MLCP) pathway. *Sci. Rep.* **2017**, *7*, 42092. [CrossRef] [PubMed]
115. Schwartz, M.A.; Schaller, M.D.; Ginsberg, M.H. Integrins: Emerging paradigms of signal transduction. *Annu Rev. Cell Dev. Biol.* **1995**, *11*, 549–599. [CrossRef] [PubMed]
116. Chen, J.; Zhou, Y.; Liu, S.; Li, C. Biomechanical signal communication in vascular smooth muscle cells. *J. Cell Commun. Signal.* **2020**, *14*, 357–376. [CrossRef] [PubMed]
117. Hu, Y.; Böck, G.; Wick, G.; Xu, Q. Activation of PDGF receptor α in vascular smooth muscle cells by mechanical stress. *FASEB J.* **1998**, *12*, 1135–1142. [CrossRef]
118. Li, C.; Xu, Q. Mechanical stress-initiated signal transductions in vascular smooth muscle cells. *Cell Signal.* **2000**, *12*, 435–445. [CrossRef]
119. Arnold, C.; Feldner, A.; Pfisterer, L.; Hödebeck, M.; Troidl, K.; Genové, G.; Wieland, T.; Hecker, M.; Korff, T. RGS 5 promotes arterial growth during arteriogenesis. *EMBO Mol. Med.* **2014**, *6*, 1075–1089. [CrossRef]
120. Shi, Z.D.; Abraham, G.; Tarbell, J.M. Shear stress modulation of smooth muscle cell marker genes in 2-D and 3-D depends on mechanotransduction by heparan sulfate proteoglycans and ERK1/2. *PLoS ONE* **2010**, *5*, e12196. [CrossRef]
121. Dardik, A.; Yamashita, A.; Aziz, F.; Asada, H.; Sumpio, B.E. Shear stress-stimulated endothelial cells induce smooth muscle cell chemotaxis via platelet-derived growth factor-BB and interleukin-1α. *J. Vasc. Surg.* **2005**, *41*, 321–331. [CrossRef] [PubMed]
122. Okada, M.; Matsumori, A.; Ono, K.; Furukawa, Y.; Shioi, T.; Iwasaki, A.; Matsushima, K.; Sasayama, S. Cyclic stretch upregulates production of interleukin-8 and monocyte chemotactic and activating factor/monocyte chemoattractant protein-1 in human endothelial cells. *Arter. Thromb. Vasc. Biol.* **1998**, *18*, 894–901. [CrossRef] [PubMed]
123. Demicheva, E.; Hecker, M.; Korff, T. Stretch-induced activation of the transcription factor activator protein-1 controls monocyte chemoattractant protein-1 expression during arteriogenesis. *Circ. Res.* **2008**, *103*, 477–484. [CrossRef] [PubMed]
124. Korff, T.; Braun, J.; Pfaff, D.; Augustin, H.G.; Hecker, M. Role of ephrinB2 expression in endothelial cells during arteriogenesis: Impact on smooth muscle cell migration and monocyte recruitment. *Blood* **2008**, *112*, 73–81. [CrossRef]
125. O'Callaghan, C.J.; Williams, B. Mechanical strain-induced extracellular matrix production by human vascular smooth muscle cells: Role of TGF-beta(1). *Hypertension* **2000**, *36*, 319–324. [CrossRef]
126. Parker, S.B.; Dobrian, A.D.; Wade, S.S.; Prewitt, R.L. AT1 receptor inhibition does not reduce arterial wall hypertrophy or PDGF-A expression in renal hypertension. *Am. J. Physiol. Circ. Physiol.* **2000**, *278*, H613–H622. [CrossRef]
127. Etz, C.D.; Kari, F.A.; Mueller, C.S.; Brenner, R.M.; Lin, H.-M.; Griepp, R.B. The collateral network concept: Remodeling of the arterial collateral network after experimental segmental artery sacrifice. *J. Thorac. Cardiovasc. Surg.* **2011**, *141*, 1029–1036. [CrossRef]

128. Amaya, R.; Pierides, A.; Tarbell, J.M. The interaction between fluid wall shear stress and solid circumferential strain affects endothelial gene expression. *PLoS ONE* **2015**, *10*, e0129952. [CrossRef]
129. Orr, A.; Hastings, N.E.; Blackman, B.R.; Wamhoff, B.R. Complex regulation and function of the inflammatory smooth muscle cell phenotype in atherosclerosis. *J. Vasc. Res.* **2010**, *47*, 168–180. [CrossRef]
130. Doran, A.C.; Meller, N.; McNamara, C.A. Role of smooth muscle cells in the initiation and early progression of atherosclerosis. *Arter. Thromb. Vasc. Biol.* **2008**, *28*, 812–819. [CrossRef]
131. Sorokin, V.; Vickneson, K.; Kofidis, T.; Woo, C.C.; Lin, X.Y.; Foo, R.; Shanahan, C.M. Role of vascular smooth muscle cell plasticity and interactions in vessel wall inflammation. *Front. Immunol.* **2020**, *11*, 3053. [CrossRef]
132. Nossent, A.Y.; Bastiaansen, A.J.N.M.; Peters, E.A.B.; de Vries, M.R.; Aref, Z.; Welten, S.M.J.; de Jager, S.C.A.; van der Pouw Kraan, T.C.T.M.; Quax, P.H.A. CCR7-CCL19/CCL21 axis is essential for effective arteriogenesis in a murine model of hindlimb ischemia. *J. Am. Heart Assoc.* **2017**, *6*, e005281. [CrossRef]
133. Kadl, A.; Leitinger, N. The role of endothelial cells in the resolution of acute inflammation. *Antioxid. Redox Signal.* **2005**, *7*, 1744–1754. [CrossRef]
134. Moraes, F.; Paye, J.; Mac Gabhann, F.; Zhuang, Z.W.; Zhang, J.; Lanahan, A.A.; Simons, M. Endothelial cell–dependent regulation of arteriogenesis. *Circ. Res.* **2013**, *113*, 1076–1086. [CrossRef]
135. Lin, X.C.; Pan, M.; Zhu, L.P.; Sun, Q.; Zhou, Z.S.; Li, C.C.; Zhang, G.G. NFAT5 promotes arteriogenesis via MCP-1-dependent monocyte recruitment. *J. Cell Mol. Med.* **2020**, *24*, 2052–2063. [CrossRef] [PubMed]
136. Denger, S.; Jahn, L.; Wende, P.; Watson, L.; Gerber, S.H.; Kübler, W.; Kreuzer, J. Expression of monocyte chemoattractant protein-1 cDNA in vascular smooth muscle cells: Induction of the synthetic phenotype: A possible clue to SMC differentiation in the process of atherogenesis. *Atherosclerosis* **1999**, *144*, 15–23. [CrossRef]
137. Li, C.; Xu, Q. Mechanical stress-initiated signal transduction in vascular smooth muscle cells in vitro and in vivo. *Cell Signal.* **2007**, *19*, 881–891. [CrossRef] [PubMed]
138. Heil, M.; Ziegelhoeffer, T.; Wagner, S.; Fernández, B.; Helisch, A.; Martin, S.; Tribulova, S.; Kuziel, W.A.; Bachmann, G.; Schaper, W. Collateral artery growth (arteriogenesis) after experimental arterial occlusion is impaired in mice lacking CC-chemokine receptor-2. *Circ. Res.* **2004**, *94*, 671–677. [CrossRef] [PubMed]
139. Fung, E.; Helisch, A. Macrophages in collateral arteriogenesis. *Front. Physiol.* **2012**, *3*, 353. [CrossRef] [PubMed]
140. Kratofil, R.M.; Kubes, P.; Deniset, J.F. Monocyte conversion during inflammation and injury. *Arter. Thromb. Vasc. Biol.* **2017**, *37*, 35–42. [CrossRef] [PubMed]
141. Cochain, C.; Rodero, M.; Vilar, J.; Recalde, A.; Richart, A.L.; Loinard, C.; Zouggari, Y.; Guérin, C.; Duriez, M.; Combadière, B.; et al. Regulation of monocyte subset systemic levels by distinct chemokine receptors controls post-ischaemic neovascularization. *Cardiovasc. Res.* **2010**, *88*, 186–195. [CrossRef] [PubMed]
142. O'Rourke, S.A.; Dunne, A.; Monaghan, M. The role of macrophages in the infarcted myocardium: Orchestrators of ECM remodeling. *Front. Cardiovasc. Med.* **2019**, *6*, 101. [CrossRef] [PubMed]
143. Nahrendorf, M.; Swirski, F.K.; Aikawa, E.; Stangenberg, L.; Wurdinger, T.; Figueiredo, J.-L.; Libby, P.; Weissleder, R.; Pittet, M.J. The healing myocardium sequentially mobilizes two monocyte subsets with divergent and complementary functions. *J. Exp. Med.* **2007**, *204*, 3037–3047. [CrossRef]
144. Rappolee, D.A.; Werb, Z. Macrophage-derived growth factors. *Curr. Top. Microbiol. Immunol.* **1992**, *181*, 87–140. [PubMed]
145. Macarie, R.D.; Vadana, M.; Ciortan, L.; Tucureanu, M.M.; Ciobanu, A.; Vinereanu, D.; Manduteanu, I.; Simionescu, M.; Butoi, E. The expression of MMP-1 and MMP-9 is up-regulated by smooth muscle cells after their cross-talk with macrophages in high glucose conditions. *J. Cell Mol. Med.* **2018**, *22*, 4366–4376. [CrossRef] [PubMed]
146. Butoi, E.; Gan, A.; Tucureanu, M.; Stan, D.; Macarie, R.; Constantinescu, C.; Calin, M.; Simionescu, M.; Manduteanu, I. Cross-talk between macrophages and smooth muscle cells impairs collagen and metalloprotease synthesis and promotes angiogenesis. *Biochim. Biophys. Acta (BBA) Bioenerg.* **2016**, *1863*, 1568–1578. [CrossRef]
147. Ntokou, A.; Dave, J.M.; Kauffman, A.C.; Sauler, M.; Ryu, C.; Hwa, J.; Herzog, E.L.; Singh, I.; Saltzman, W.M.; Greif, D.M. Macrophage-derived PDGF-B induces muscularization in murine and human pulmonary hypertension. *JCI Insight* **2021**, *6*, e139167. [CrossRef]
148. Xiong, W.; Frasch, S.C.; Thomas, S.M.; Bratton, D.L.; Henson, P.M. Induction of TGF-beta1 synthesis by macrophages in response to apoptotic cells requires activation of the scavenger receptor CD36. *PLoS ONE* **2013**, *8*, e72772. [CrossRef]
149. Ji, Y.; Lisabeth, E.M.; Neubig, R.R. Transforming growth factor beta1 increases expression of contractile genes in human pulmonary arterial smooth muscle cells by potentiating sphingosine-1-phosphate signaling. *Mol. Pharmacol.* **2021**, *100*, 53–60. [CrossRef]
150. Elkington, P.T.; Green, J.A.; Friedland, J.S. Analysis of Matrix Metalloproteinase Secretion by Macrophages. *Adv. Struct. Saf. Stud.* **2009**, *531*, 253–265.
151. Hobeika, M.J.; Edlin, R.S.; Muhs, B.E.; Sadek, M.; Gagne, P.J. Matrix metalloproteinases in critical limb ischemia. *J. Surg. Res.* **2008**, *149*, 148–154. [CrossRef] [PubMed]
152. Cai, W.-J.; Koltai, S.; Kocsis, E.; Scholz, D.; Schaper, W.; Schaper, J. Connexin37, not Cx40 and Cx43, is induced in vascular smooth muscle cells during coronary arteriogenesis. *J. Mol. Cell. Cardiol.* **2001**, *33*, 957–967. [CrossRef] [PubMed]
153. Johnson, J.L. Matrix metalloproteinases: Influence on smooth muscle cells and atherosclerotic plaque stability. *Expert Rev. Cardiovasc. Ther.* **2007**, *5*, 265–282. [CrossRef] [PubMed]

154. Bagi, Z. Impaired coronary collateral growth: miR-shaken neutrophils caught in the act. *Am. J. Physiol. Heart Circ. Physiol.* **2015**, *308*, H1321–H1322. [CrossRef]
155. Bot, I.; Velden, D.V.; Bouwman, M.; Kroner, M.J.; Kuiper, J.; Quax, P.H.A.; de Vries, M.R. Local mast cell activation promotes neovascularization. *Cells* **2020**, *9*, 701. [CrossRef]
156. Stabile, E.; Kinnaird, T.; la Sala, A.; Hanson, S.K.; Watkins, C.; Campia, U.; Shou, M.; Zbinden, S.; Fuchs, S.; Kornfeld, H.; et al. CD8 + T lymphocytes regulate the arteriogenic response to ischemia by infiltrating the site of collateral vessel development and recruiting CD4 + mononuclear cells through the expression of interleukin-16. *Circulation* **2006**, *113*, 118–124. [CrossRef]
157. Chillo, O.; Kleinert, E.C.; Lautz, T.; Lasch, M.; Pagel, J.-I.; Heun, Y.; Troidl, K.; Fischer, S.; Caballero-Martinez, A.; Mauer, A.; et al. Perivascular mast cells govern shear stress-induced arteriogenesis by orchestrating leukocyte function. *Cell Rep.* **2016**, *16*, 2197–2207. [CrossRef]
158. Stabile, E.; Burnett, M.S.; Watkins, C.; Kinnaird, T.; Bachis, A.; la Sala, A.; Miller, J.M.; Shou, M.; Epstein, S.E.; Fuchs, S. Impaired arteriogenic response to acute hindlimb ischemia in CD4-knockout mice. *Circulation* **2003**, *108*, 205–210. [CrossRef]
159. van Weel, V.; Toes, R.E.; Seghers, L.; Deckers, M.M.; de Vries, M.R.; Eilers, P.H.; Sipkens, J.; Schepers, A.; Eefting, D.; van Hinsbergh, V.W.; et al. Natural killer cells and CD4+ T-cells modulate collateral artery development. *Arterioscler Thromb. Vasc Biol.* **2007**, *27*, 2310–2318. [CrossRef] [PubMed]
160. Ruiter, M.S.; Van Golde, J.M.; Schaper, N.; Stehouwer, C.D.; Huijberts, M.S. Diabetes impairs arteriogenesis in the peripheral circulation: Review of molecular mechanisms. *Clin. Sci.* **2010**, *119*, 225–238. [CrossRef] [PubMed]
161. Eitenmüller, I.; Volger, O.; Kluge, A.; Troidl, K.; Barancik, M.; Cai, W.-J.; Heil, M.; Pipp, F.; Fischer, S.; Horrevoets, A.J.G.; et al. The range of adaptation by collateral vessels after femoral artery occlusion. *Circ. Res.* **2006**, *99*, 656–662. [CrossRef] [PubMed]
162. Unger, E.F.; Banai, S.; Shou, M.; Lazarous, D.F.; Jaklitsch, M.T.; Scheinowitz, M.; Correa, R.; Klingbeil, C.; Epstein, S.E. Basic fibroblast growth factor enhances myocardial collateral flow in a canine model. *Am. J. Physiol. Circ. Physiol.* **1994**, *266*, H1588–H1595. [CrossRef] [PubMed]
163. Yamada, N.; Li, W.; Ihaya, A.; Kimura, T.; Morioka, K.; Uesaka, T.; Takamori, A.; Handa, M.; Tanabe, S.; Tanaka, K. Platelet-derived endothelial cell growth factor gene therapy for limb ischemia. *J. Vasc. Surg.* **2006**, *44*, 1322–1328. [CrossRef] [PubMed]
164. Schierling, W.; Troidl, K.; Troidl, C.; Schmitz-Rixen, T.; Schaper, W.; Eitenmüller, I.K. The role of angiogenic growth factors in arteriogenesis. *J. Vasc. Res.* **2009**, *46*, 365–374. [CrossRef]

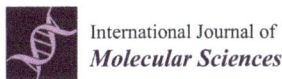

Article

In Vivo Matrigel Plug Assay as a Potent Method to Investigate Specific Individual Contribution of Angiogenesis to Blood Flow Recovery in Mice

Zeen Aref and Paul H. A. Quax *

Department of Surgery, Einthoven Laboratory for Experimental Vascular Medicine, Leiden University Medical Center, 2300 RC Leiden, The Netherlands; z.aref@lumc.nl
* Correspondence: p.h.a.quax@lumc.nl; Tel.: +31-71-526-1584; Fax: +31-71-526-6570

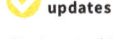

Citation: Aref, Z.; Quax, P.H.A. In Vivo Matrigel Plug Assay as a Potent Method to Investigate Specific Individual Contribution of Angiogenesis to Blood Flow Recovery in Mice. *Int. J. Mol. Sci.* **2021**, *22*, 8909. https://doi.org/10.3390/ijms22168909

Academic Editor: Giovanni Li Volti

Received: 26 May 2021
Accepted: 17 August 2021
Published: 18 August 2021

Publisher's Note: MDPI stays neutral with regard to jurisdictional claims in published maps and institutional affiliations.

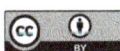

Copyright: © 2021 by the authors. Licensee MDPI, Basel, Switzerland. This article is an open access article distributed under the terms and conditions of the Creative Commons Attribution (CC BY) license (https://creativecommons.org/licenses/by/4.0/).

Abstract: Neovascularization restores blood flow recovery after ischemia in peripheral arterial disease. The main two components of neovascularization are angiogenesis and arteriogenesis. Both of these processes contribute to functional improvements of blood flow after occlusion. However, discriminating between the specific contribution of each process is difficult. A frequently used model for investigating neovascularization is the murine hind limb ischemia model (HLI). With this model, it is difficult to determine the role of angiogenesis, because usually the timing for the sacrifice of the mice is chosen to be optimal for the analysis of arteriogenesis. More importantly, the occurring angiogenesis in the distal calf muscles is probably affected by the proximally occurring arteriogenesis. Therefore, to understand and subsequently intervene in the process of angiogenesis, a model is needed which investigates angiogenesis without the influence of arteriogenesis. In this study we evaluated the in vivo Matrigel plug assay in genetic deficient mice to investigate angiogenesis. Mice deficient for *interferon regulatory factor (IRF)3, IRF7, RadioProtective 105 (RP105), Chemokine CC receptor CCR7,* and *p300/CBP-associated factor (PCAF)* underwent the in vivo Matrigel model. Histological analysis of the Matrigel plugs showed an increased angiogenesis in mice deficient of *IRF3, IRF7,* and *RP105,* and a decreased angiogenesis in *PCAF* deficient mice. Our results also suggest an involvement of *CCR7* in angiogenesis. Comparing our results with results of the HLI model found in the literature suggests that the in vivo Matrigel plug assay is superior in evaluating the angiogenic response after ischemia.

Keywords: angiogenesis; arteriogenesis; animal model; Matrigel plug assay

1. Introduction

The introduction of peripheral arterial disease (PAD) is a result of narrowing and frequently occlusion of the peripheral arteries by atherosclerotic plaque progression, which leads to impaired blood flow and subsequently ischemia in the tissue. The impaired blood flow leads to intermittent claudication and, in more severe stages when occlusion occurs, to critical limb ischemia (CLI). The prevalence of PAD increases with age to 20% in people over 70 years [1]. Current therapies for PAD are exercise rehabilitation and in severe cases endovascular revascularization or bypass surgery. Therapeutic neovascularization is a promising technique that has the potential to become an addition to conventional therapies [2].

Neovascularization is the natural mechanism that restores blood flow and recovers tissue perfusion after ischemia. The main two components of neovascularization are angiogenesis and arteriogenesis, both these mechanisms are essential for the restoration of blood flow after arterial occlusions. Identifying mediators that influence neovascularization may lead to discovering targets that can be utilized as therapeutic targets.

Angiogenesis is the process of sprouting of endothelial cells from pre-existing blood vessels resulting in a new capillary bed and is affected by several stimulators [3]. In PAD angiogenesis provides distribution of blood to ischemic distal tissue where gangrene occurs and is essential for protecting tissue from ischemia and for tissue repair. Angiogenesis is a complex process and different cascades are involved, among which are specific angiogenic growth factors, inflammation, and epigenetic factors [4].

The other component of neovascularization is arteriogenesis. Arteriogenesis is an inflammation driven process induced by shear stress and leads to the maturation of the pre-existing arterioles in functioning collateral arteries [5].

It is essential to consider that angiogenesis and arteriogenesis are different processes. Both of these processes occur in PAD and contribute to functional improvements of blood flow after occlusion, however, discriminating between the specific contribution of each process is difficult. A frequently used in vivo model for investigation of neovascularization is the mouse hind limb ischemia (HLI) model [6]. In this model the iliac or femoral artery is occluded by ligation, most commonly the femoral artery. In general, the occlusion of the femoral artery results in arteriogenesis, also referred to as collateral formation, proximally in the thigh, and angiogenesis in the distal part of the limb. However, ligation at different anatomical levels of the iliac and femoral artery triggers different pathways of neovascularization [6]. If the ligation of the femoral artery is distal to the origin of the collateral branches, arteriogenesis will occur, as it occurs after increasing shear stress in the pre-existing arterioles proximal to the collateral arteries.

Collateral formation as a result of arteriogenesis in the proximal thigh potentially influences the blood perfusion in the distal calf by resolving the ischemia that drives the angiogenesis. This impairs the reliability of angiogenesis determination in the distal calf muscles, which is usually determined in the soleus and gastrocnemius muscles by evaluating capillary formation via $CD31^+$ staining. Additionally, the timing of sacrificing the mice for histological analysis is complex, since usually this is done around two to four weeks after inducing limb ischemia. This is the optimal timing for analysis of arteriogenesis, but at this point the angiogenic response has passed its peak since the ischemia has been at least partly resolved. Therefore, to understand and subsequently intervene in the process of angiogenesis, a model is needed which investigates angiogenesis without the influence of arteriogenesis.

A suitable model to investigate angiogenesis is the in vivo Matrigel plug assay. In this assay, Matrigel is injected into the flank of mice inducing angiogenesis within the plug. The resulting angiogenesis can be evaluated after extracting the Matrigel plug. The Matrigel solution is a basement membrane preparation which is extracted from the Engelbreth–Holm–Swarm (EHS) mouse sarcoma, a tumor rich in extracellular matrix proteins [7]. It contains predominantly laminin, collagen IV, entactin, and small amounts of various growth factors. Matrigel is liquid at 4 °C and becomes a solid gel plug at 37 °C, the body temperature of mice. Matrigel mimics the physiological cell matrix and is the most frequently used substrate to investigate in vitro and in vivo angiogenesis [8]. Since the Matrigel plug is avascular at the beginning of the experiment, any vessel that is formed can be considered the result of angiogenesis. There are two main approaches in studying angiogenesis using the Matrigel plug assay. The first and most widely used approach is the use for evaluating of pro- or anti-angiogenic factors [9]. This is done by mixing a potential pro- or anti-angiogenic factor, cells, or exosomes with the Matrigel and thereafter injecting the mixture in (wild type) mice and subsequently analyzing, after the proper incubation period, the number of angiogenic vessels present in the plugs.

In the second approach, as used in our study, unmodified Matrigel is injected it in the flank of the (genetically modified) mice. Not manipulating the gel rules out the risk of influencing its functionality and warrants consistent results. This method analyzes the influence of the factors that are altered in the mice, e.g., by genetic modification, on angiogenesis.

The aim of this study is to demonstrate the potency of the in vivo Matrigel plug assay to investigate the role of different genetic factors in angiogenesis. To this end we performed the assay in mice genetically deficient for inflammatory factors like *interferon regulatory* factor (IRF)3, IRF7, RadioProtective 105 (RP105), Chemokine CC receptor CCR7, and p300/CBP-associated factor (PCAF). Similar mice were used previously by our group in studies on neovascularization by means of the HLI model [10–13]. Comparing the results of current and previous research in the aforementioned genetically deficient mice will give an insight into the additional value of the Matrigel plug over the HLI model and more specifically into the specific contribution of angiogenesis on blood flow recovery in vivo.

2. Results

2.1. Matrigel Ingrowth in Mice Deficient for Inflammation-Related Factors; $IRF3^{-/-}$, $IRF7^{-/-}$, and $RP105^{-/-}$ Mice

2.1.1. Increased Angiogenesis in the $IRF3^{-/-}$ Mice

The areas of the $CD31^+$ endothelial cells in the Matrigel sections of the $IRF3^{-/-}$ mice were 43% larger compared to the control wild type mice (1649 versus 1157 µm^2, p value < 0.0001) (Figure 1a). The depth of ingrowth of the $CD31^+$ endothelial cells into the subcutaneously injected Matrigel was 11% deeper in the $IRF3^{-/-}$ mice compared to the control wild type mice (162 versus 146 µm, p value 0.0049) (Figure 1b). This leads to the conclusion that angiogenesis was increased in the $IRF3$ deficient mice, thus $IRF3$ leads to decreasing angiogenesis.

These results support the predictions made in the literature, as $IRF3$ deficiency probably leads to increased angiogenesis through reduced production of type I IFNs. IRFs are transcription factors that form a dimer and translocate to the nucleus. In the nucleus, the IRFs bind to the promoter of the interferon (IFN) gene, resulting in the production of type I interferons. Type I interferons cause an increased production of several anti-angiogenic mediators such as TIMPs and a reduced production of proangiogenic factors such as VEGF, resulting in an anti-angiogenic effect. In addition, IFNs inhibit endothelial cell proliferation and migration, which are both required for angiogenesis.

In contrast to our observations, the angiogenic response in $IRF3^{-/-}$ mice which underwent HLI was decreased compared to control C57BL/6 mice [12]. We presume that the conflicting results in the HLI model are caused by the time point of evaluation. In HLI treated mice angiogenesis was assessed at sacrifice by determination of the number of $CD31^+$ capillaries in both the left ischemic and right non-ischemic soleus muscle of $IRF3^{-/-}$ and C57BL/6 mice. However, these data were obtained 28 days after inducing limb ischemia via surgical ligation of the femoral artery. The timing of 28 days after inducting of limb ischemia is probably not optimal for determination of the angiogenic response. At this time point angiogenesis has already passed its peak since the ischemia is partly or even totally is resolved due to concomitant arteriogenic response. In the Matrigel plug assay model analysis is performed at 7 days after injection, in a setting with full ischemia, stimulating the angiogenic activity.

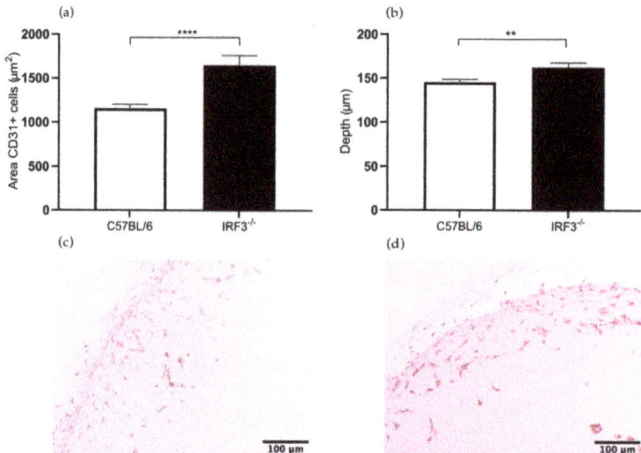

Figure 1. (**a**) Area of CD31$^+$ cells in the subcutaneously injected Matrigel, in interferon regulatory factor (IRF)3$^{-/-}$ and wild type C57BL/6 mice. (**b**) Quantification of the depth (μm) of ingrowth of CD31$^+$ cells into subcutaneously injected Matrigel, in IRF3$^{-/-}$ and wild type C57BL/6 mice. (**c**) Immunohistochemical staining of paraffin-embedded Matrigel plug of C57BL/6 7 days after Matrigel injection, using anti-CD31 antibodies. (**d**) Immunohistochemical staining of paraffin-embedded Matrigel plug of IRF3$^{-/-}$ mice 7 days after Matrigel injection, using anti-CD31 antibodies. N = 6 mice per group, 2 Matrigel plugs per mouse. Values are presented as the mean SEM. ** $p \leq 0.01$, **** $p \leq 0.0001$.

2.1.2. Increased Angiogenesis in IRF7$^{-/-}$ Mice

In the Matrigel sections of IRF7$^{-/-}$ mice the area of the CD31+ endothelial cells were 15% larger compared to the control C57BL/6 mice. However the difference was not significant (1326 versus 1157 μm^2, p value 0.07) (Figure 2a). Furthermore, the depth of ingrowth of these cells in the Matrigel plug was 56% deeper in the IRF7$^{-/-}$ mice compared to control wild type mice (228 versus 146 μm, p value < 0.0001) (Figure 2b). These results suggest that IRF7 is involved in the process of angiogenesis. Our experiment corroborates the hypothesis that an IRF3 and IRF7 deficiency leads to increased angiogenesis through reduced production of type I IFNs, as described above. In the HLI model the angiogenic response is decreased in the IRF7$^{-/-}$ mice compared to C57BL/6 mice [12]. Interesting to observe is that the results of Matrigel plug assay in IRF7$^{-/-}$ mice as in IRF3$^{-/-}$ mice do not match the results of the HLI mouse model. An explanation for the difference is the aforementioned limitations of performing the angiogenic response analysis at 28 days after inducing HLI, which is not an optimal timing for the determination of angiogenic response.

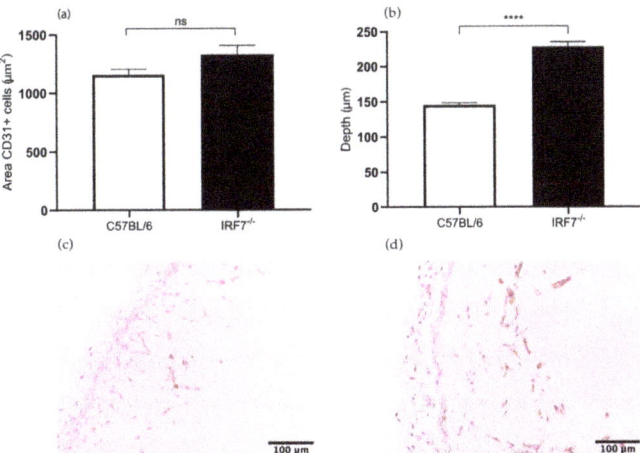

Figure 2. (a) Area of CD31$^+$ cells in the subcutaneously injected Matrigel, in $IRF7^{-/-}$ and wild type C57BL/6 mice. (b) Quantification of the depth (μm) of ingrowth of CD31$^+$ cells into subcutaneously injected Matrigel, in $IRF7^{-/-}$ and wild type C57BL/6 mice. (c) Immunohistochemical staining of paraffin-embedded Matrigel plug of C57BL/6 7 days after Matrigel injection, using anti-CD31 antibodies. (d) Immunohistochemical staining of paraffin-embedded Matrigel plug of $IRF7^{-/-}$ mice 7 days after Matrigel injection, using anti-CD31 antibodies. N = 6 mice per group, 2 Matrigel plugs per mouse. Values are presented as the mean SEM. ns not significant. **** $p \leq 0.0001$.

2.1.3. Increased Angiogenesis in the Matrigel Plug Assay in the $RP105^{-/-}$ Mice

In the Matrigel plug sections of *RadioProtective 105 (RP105)* deficient mice showed a 41% larger area of CD31+ endothelial cells within the Matrigel plug in comparison to the control wild type mice (1634 versus 1157 μm^2, *p* value < 0.0001) (Figure 3a). The depth of the cells in the Matrigel plug was 38% deeper in the $RP105^{-/-}$ mice compared to the control group (202 versus 146 μm, *p* value < 0.0001) (Figure 3b). These results confirm the hypothesis that RP105 is potentially an angiogenic inhibitor by inhibiting TLR4-signaling and thereby decreasing the production of several proangiogenic mediators. RP105 is a TLR4-signaling modulator and is a specific inhibitor of the TLR4-triggered response [14]. TLR4 may promote angiogenesis in pancreatic cancer tissues via activating the PI3K/AKT signaling pathway to induce VEGF expression [15]. TLR4-mediated responses also contribute to the oxygen-induced neovascularization in ischemic neural tissue [16]. However, the exact role of RP105 in angiogenesis in peripheral arterial disease remains unclear.

Previously, Bastiaansen et al. investigated angiogenesis in the HLI model by determination of capillary density in the ischemic calf muscle [11]. In their experiment the capillary density marginally increased in the gastrocnemius muscle in $RP105^{-/-}$ mice. However, the difference in angiogenic response measured by capillary density and size in the gastrocnemius muscle was not significant [11]. The results of the Matrigel plug assay is more evincive than the results of the HLI model, whereby *RP105* deficiency leads to increased angiogenic response 7 days after plug placement. This corresponds with our hypothesis that RP105 is potentially an angiogenic inhibitor.

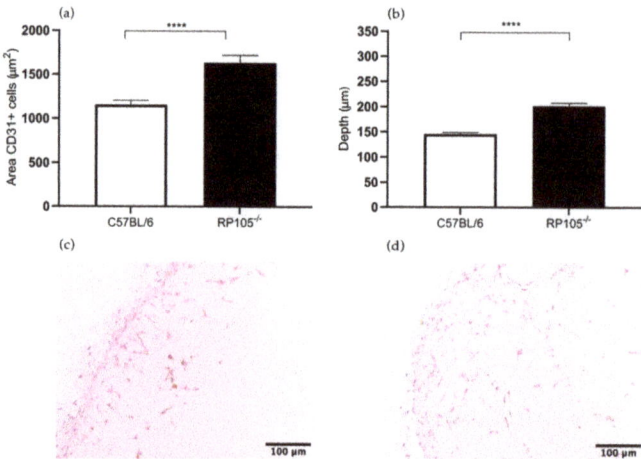

Figure 3. (**a**) Area of CD31$^+$ cells in the subcutaneously injected Matrigel, in *RadioProtective 105 (RP105)* $^{-/-}$ and wild type C57BL/6 mice. (**b**) Quantification of the depth (μm) of ingrowth of CD31$^+$ cells into subcutaneously injected Matrigel, in *RP105*$^{-/-}$ and wild type C57BL/6 mice. (**c**) Immunohistochemical staining of paraffin-embedded Matrigel plug of C57BL/6 7 days after Matrigel injection, using anti-CD31 antibodies. (**d**) Immunohistochemical staining of paraffin-embedded Matrigel plug of *RP105*$^{-/-}$ mice 7 days after Matrigel injection, using anti-CD31 antibodies. N = 6 mice per group, 2 Matrigel plugs per mouse. Values are presented as the mean SEM. **** $p \leq 0.0001$.

2.2. The Role of Chemokine CC Receptor CCR7 in Angiogenesis

Previously we studied the effects of CCR7 deficiency on blood flow recovery after HLI in *CCR7*$^{-/-}$ mice. These mice were bred on a *C57BL/6/LDLR*$^{-/-}$ background and, therefore, we used *C57BL/6/LDLR*$^{-/-}$ mice as controls [13]. Here we study the effects in angiogenesis in the Matrigel plugs in these mice.

The area of the CD31$^+$ cells was 25% larger in the *LDLR*$^{-/-}$/*CCR7*$^{-/-}$ mice compared to the control group (1984 versus 1583 μm^2, p value 0.0003) (Figure 4a). However, the *LDLR*$^{-/-}$/*CCR7*$^{-/-}$ and *LDLR*$^{-/-}$ mice showed the same depth of ingrowth of CD31$^+$ cells in the Matrigel plug (198 versus 200 μm) (Figure 4b). Both the total area of endothelial cells and the depth of the ingrowth are both parameters to assess the angiogenesis in the in vivo Matrigel plug assay. However, the area of cells is a more prominent parameter, the combination of these two parameters makes it possible to make a solid conclusion. This suggests that CCR7 is involved in angiogenesis.

CCR7 is expressed by various immune cells and is involved in homing of T cells and dendritic cells to lymph nodes [17]. Furthermore, in the literature it is demonstrated that CCR7 is overexpressed in different malignant cells, which leads to the suggestion that CCR7 induces angiogenesis. However the evidence for the latter is limited [18,19]. Regarding the neovascularization stimulatory effect, the chemokine contributes to arteriogenesis via inflammatory-mediated mechanisms [20]. On the contrary, in the HLI model in *LDLR*$^{-/-}$/*CCR7*$^{-/-}$ mice it was shown that the number of CD31$^+$ capillaries in the gastrocnemius muscles was not significantly different from the control *LDLR*$^{-/-}$ mice [13]. In this set-up of the HLI model, the evaluation was performed 10 days after HLI, which is a good time point to investigate angiogenesis, in contrast to 28 days.

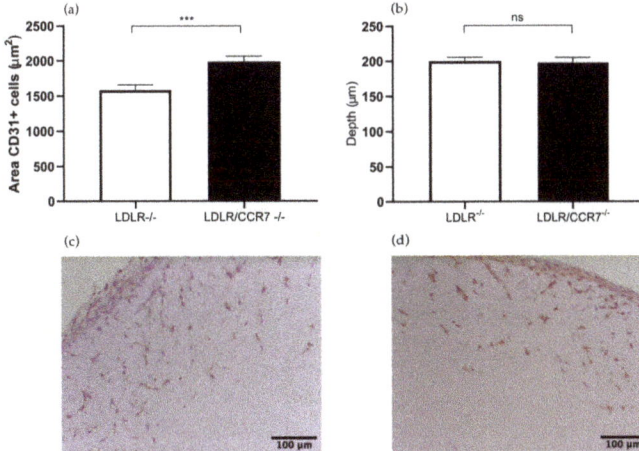

Figure 4. (**a**) Area of CD31$^+$ cells in the subcutaneously injected Matrigel, in $LDLR^{-/-}$ and $LDLR^{-/-}/CCR7^{-/-}$ mice. (**b**) Quantification of the depth (μm) of ingrowth of CD31$^+$ cells into subcutaneously injected Matrigel, in $LDLR^{-/-}$ and $LDLR^{-/-}/CCR7^{-/-}$ mice. (**c**) Immunohistochemical staining of paraffin-embedded Matrigel plug of $LDLR^{-/-}/CCR7^{-/-}$ mice using anti-CD31 antibodies. (**d**) Immunohistochemical staining of paraffin-embedded Matrigel plug of $LDLR^{-/-}$ mice using anti-CD31 antibodies. N = 7 mice per group, 2 Matrigel plugs per mouse. Values are presented as the mean SEM. *** $p \leq 0.001$. ns = not significant.

2.3. PCAF Deficiency Leads to Decrease in Angiogenesis

In the $PCAF^{-/-}$ Matrigel sections, the area of the CD31$^+$ endothelial cell area was 35% smaller compared to the control group (751 versus 1157 μm^2, p value < 0.0001) (Figure 5a). The depth of the CD31$^+$ endothelial cells in the Matrigel plug was 21% less deep in the $PCAF^{-/-}$ mice compared to the control group (116 versus 146 μm, p value < 0.0001) (Figure 5b). The results of the Matrigel plug assay in $PCAF^{-/-}$ mice demonstrate that PCAF has a role in angiogenesis. This result confirms the hypothesis that PCAF may have a role in angiogenesis considering the essential role of HIF-1 in angiogenesis. P300/CBP-associated factor (PCAF) acetylates histones H3 and H4 and this histone acetylating activity is crucial for NF-KB-mediated gene transcription and regulates inflammation-related genes [21]. PCAF also mediates the regulation of hypoxia-inducible factor-1α (HIF-1α), which increases lysyl-acetylted HIF-1α and delays the PHD-independent degradation of HIF-1α [22]. HIF-1 regulates the expression of proangiogenic factors and is even a master stimulator of vascular endothelial growth factor [23]. Previously, our group investigated the involvement of PCAF in arteriogenesis as is a key regulator of this process [10]. Additionally, our group showed that PCAF regulates vascular inflammation [24].

As to angiogenesis in hind limb ischemia, it has not yet been investigated in $PCAF^{-/-}$ mice. In consideration that PCAF mediates the regulation of hypoxia-inducible factor-1α (HIF-1α) and HIF-1 regulates the expression of proangiogenic factors, such as vascular endothelial growth factor, this is the result of this study that we expected.

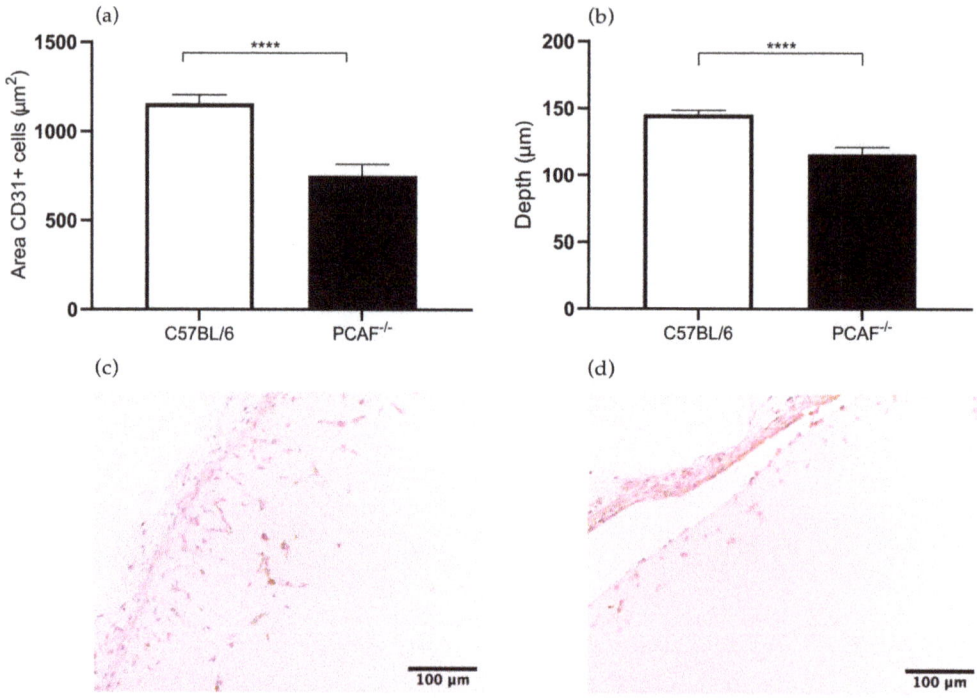

Figure 5. (a) Area of CD31+ cells in the subcutaneously injected Matrigel, in *p300/CBP-associated factor (PCAF)*$^{-/-}$ and wild type C57BL/6 mice. (b) Quantification of the depth (μm) of ingrowth of CD31$^+$ cells into subcutaneously injected Matrigel, in *PCAF*$^{-/-}$ and wild type C57BL/6 mice. (c) Immunohistochemical staining of paraffin-embedded Matrigel plug of C57BL/6 7 days after Matrigel injection, using anti-CD31 antibodies. (d) Immunohistochemical staining of paraffin-embedded Matrigel plug of *PCAF*$^{-/-}$ mice 7 days after Matrigel injection, using anti-CD31 antibodies. N = 6 mice per group, 2 Matrigel plugs per mouse. Values are presented as the mean SEM. **** $p \leq 0.000$.

3. Discussion

In this study we were able to quantify the angiogenic response in Matrigel plugs of various genetically modified mouse strains and compare these results with the results obtained in the HLI model. We found that the angiogenic response in the same genetic deficient mice determined through the Matrigel plug assay could be different from the angiogenic results found in the HLI model. The results showed that the in vivo Matrigel plus assay is more reliable than the HLI model to the determine the angiogenic response.

We performed the in vivo Matrigel plug assay in *IRF3*$^{-/-}$ and *IRF7*$^{-/-}$ mice because the exact role of these components is unknown and theoretically *IRF3* and *IRF7* may be anti-angiogenic and has a potential in therapeutic angiogenesis. The results of the Matrigel plug model in *IRF3*$^{-/-}$ and *IRF7*$^{-/-}$ mice were that angiogenesis is increased in *IRF3*$^{-/-}$ and *IRF7*$^{-/-}$ mice. These results are the opposite to the results of the HLI model, where it was demonstrated that the angiogenic response decreased in the *IRF3*$^{-/-}$ and *IRF7*$^{-/-}$ mice compared to C57BL/6 mice [12]. Since in the HLI model, the evaluation of angiogenesis was performed 28 days after surgery and the angiogenesis in the distal calf muscles is influenced by arteriogenesis proximal, we believe that the results in Matrigel plug assay are more reliable.

Mice deficient in *RP105* show a severely impaired blood flow recovery after HLI, where arteriogenesis was reduced [11], whereas the effects on angiogenesis were not studied. The Matrigel plug assay data from *RP105*$^{-/-}$ mice showed that *RP105* deficiency leads to increased angiogenesis. Previously we have shown that CCR7 expression is rapidly upregulated after induction of HLI in mice, and the neovascularization response after HLI in $LDLR^{-/-}/CCR7^{-/-}$ was reduced due to effects on arteriogenesis as well as angiogenesis [13]. Our data strongly support the involvement of CCR7 in the angiogenesis response, next to its role in arteriogenesis. Along the same line, we previously demonstrated a hampered blood flow recovery in $PCAF^{-/-}$ mice due to a decreased arteriogenesis [10] without analyzing the angiogenesis response. Here we show, using the Matrigel plug assay in $PCAF^{-/-}$ mice, that PCAF has a role in angiogenesis and more study to elucidate the role of PCAF in angiogenesis is needed.

In the in vivo Matrigel plug assay for accurate quantification through histological analysis, numerous tissue slides for each plug are needed. This makes it a time-consuming process. However, the histological analysis is still the preferred method to study angiogenesis in Matrigel plug assay as it provides information on morphology and localization of the endothelial cells, which cannot be obtained through other techniques. In histological analysis we used the area of endothelial cells and the depth of the ingrowth as a result parameter. It is challenging to interpret the results if both parameters do not show the same result. In our experiments we used a combination of both parameters and considered the area of the cells as a superior parameter.

Alternative quantitative techniques for the assessment of angiogenesis in the in vivo Matrigel plug model are hemoglobin content determination, injecting dextran, Matrigel cytometry, or using the qPCR technique [9,25–27]. The hemoglobin content assay is used to assess the blood content in the newly formed vessels. However this assay cannot differentiate between stagnant blood, blood in the capillaries, larger vessels, or in the vessels in the surrounding granulation tissue [28,29]. Strict separation of the surrounding tissue from the edge of the plug is challenging and can lead to damaging the edge where the most angiogenesis occurs. The other alternative method is injecting the dextran into the tail vein and extracting it from the plug for quantification. This approach can also not differentiate between the presence of stagnant blood due hemorrhage and blood in the vessels, also non-perfused vessels due to compression at the time of harvesting is not quantified. The new method is isolating RNA from the plugs and use qPCR of EC genes as a quantification technique [27]. However, the limited cellularity in the control plugs lead to a low yield of total RNA, making the comparison between two sets of samples unreliable.

4. Materials and Methods

4.1. Mice

All animal experiments were performed in compliance with Dutch government guidelines and the Directive 2010/63/EU of the European Parliament, all experiments were approved by the animal welfare committee of the LUMC under approval code 12173 (19-11-2012). In this study we used mice deficient for *IRF3*, *IRF7*, *RP105* and *PCAF* [10–12]. Also, $LDLR^{-/-}/CCR7^{-/-}$ and $LDLR^{-/-}$ mice were used [13]. All strains have a C57BL/6 background. In general, we used n= 6 mice per group. Wild type C57BL/6 were used as control. The mice were used at the age of 10–14 weeks.

4.2. The In Vivo Matrigel Plug Assay

A total of 500 μL of Matrigel Solution (BD Biosciences, Vianen, the Netherlands) was injected subcutaneously in the dorsal side of the mice, both the left and right flank. The solution had a temperature of 4 °C at time of injection, forming a plug as it warmed up to body temperature (37 °C) [8]. After seven days the mice were sacrificed and the Matrigel plug and the surrounding granulation tissue were removed. The color of the viscous plugs ranged from a (light) yellow (Figure 6), to a pink or red depending on the amount of blood vessel ingrowth. The Matrigel plugs were fixed in formaldehyde, embedded into paraffin blocks, and sectioned into slides of 5 μm.

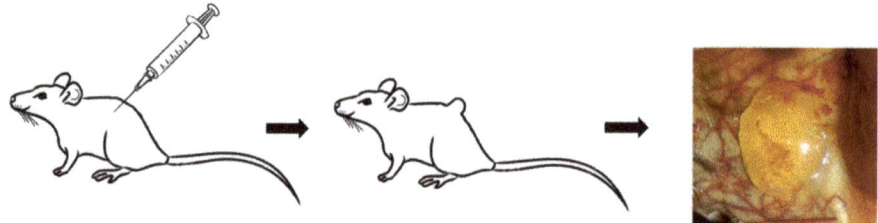

Figure 6. Matrigel plug in the flank of a mouse.

4.3. CD31-Immunohistochemistry Staining

The paraffin-embedded sections of the Matrigel plug (5 μm) were used for histological analysis. Sections were stained using anti-CD31 antibodies (BD Biosciences). The CD31-immunohistochemistry staining was performed to detect the CD31$^+$ endothelial cells in the Matrigel plugs. Most angiogenesis is observed at the edge of the plug, with ingrowth toward the center of the plug.

Photomicrographs of the CD31-stained sections were made and morphometric image analysis was performed (Figure 7). The Matrigel area (μm^2), endothelial cell areas (μm^2), endothelial cell ingrowth (%), and maximal endothelial cell depth (μm) were measured for quantification of angiogenesis using Image J software.

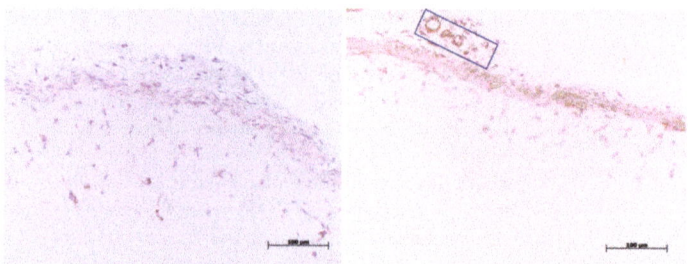

Figure 7. Representative images of the CD31 immunohistochemistry staining. CD31 positive cells (i.e., endothelial cells) are stained and visible as a brown staining. In the right figure, a blood vessel in the membrane surrounding the Matrigel plug is stained and serves as an internal positive control. In the box in the right panel some CD31 positive vessel structures in the surrounding granulation tissue around the plug can been seen, demonstrating the specificity of the endothelial cell staining. The left panel is representative of a section with a deeper ingrowth of endothelial cells. The maximal depth to the ingrowth as well as the CD31+ area in the plug were quantified using Image J software.

4.4. Statistical Analysis

Results are presented as mean ± SEM. Comparisons between groups were performed using Student *t*-test or Mann–Whitney U-test. Statistical analyses were performed using GraphPad Prism 7. A *p* value of <0.05 was considered statistically significant.

5. Conclusions

In conclusion, the Matrigel plug assay in mice should be the method of choice for the in vivo evaluation of angiogenesis and has an added value over HLI model in the research of neovascularization. The in vivo Matrigel plug assay can be used to identify factors that are involved in angiogenesis. This study indicates that RP105, IRF3, IRF7, CCR7, and PCAF are involved in angiogenesis.

Author Contributions: Z.A. and P.H.A.Q. both contributed to conceptualizing, formal analysis, investigation, writing, and editing the manuscript. All authors have read and agreed to the published version of the manuscript.

Funding: This research forms part of the Project P1.03 PENT of the research program of the Biomedical Materials institute, co-funded by the Dutch Ministry of Economic Affairs, Agriculture and Innovation.

Institutional Review Board Statement: All animal experiments were performed in compliance with Dutch government guidelines and the Directive 2010/63/EU of the European Parliament, all experiments were approved by the animal welfare committee of the LUMC under approval code 12173 (19-11-2012).

Informed Consent Statement: Not applicable.

Data Availability Statement: All relevant data will be made available upon request.

Conflicts of Interest: The authors declare no conflict of interest.

References

1. Norgren, L.; Hiatt, W.R.; Dormandy, J.A.; Nehler, M.R.; Harris, K.A.; Fowkes, F.G.; Rutherford, R.B. Inter-society consensus for the management of peripheral arterial disease. *Int. Angiol. J. Int. Union Angiol.* **2007**, *26*, 81–157.
2. Raval, Z.; Losordo, D.W. Cell therapy of peripheral arterial disease: From experimental findings to clinical trials. *Circ. Res.* **2013**, *112*, 1288–1302. [CrossRef] [PubMed]
3. Carmeliet, P. Angiogenesis in health and disease. *Nat. Med.* **2003**, *9*, 653–660. [CrossRef]
4. Potente, M.; Gerhardt, H.; Carmeliet, P. Basic and therapeutic aspects of angiogenesis. *Cell* **2011**, *146*, 873–887. [CrossRef]
5. Heil, M.; Eitenmuller, I.; Schmitz-Rixen, T.; Schaper, W. Arteriogenesis versus angiogenesis: Similarities and differences. *J. Cell Mol. Med.* **2006**, *10*, 45–55. [CrossRef] [PubMed]
6. Aref, Z.; de Vries, M.R.; Quax, P.H.A. Variations in Surgical Procedures for Inducing Hind Limb Ischemia in Mice and the Impact of These Variations on Neovascularization Assessment. *Int. J. Mol. Sci.* **2019**, *20*, 3704. [CrossRef] [PubMed]
7. Kleinman, H.K.; Martin, G.R. Matrigel: Basement membrane matrix with biological activity. *Semin. Cancer Biol.* **2005**, *15*, 378–386. [CrossRef]
8. Nowak-Sliwinska, P.; Alitalo, K.; Allen, E.; Anisimov, A.; Aplin, A.C.; Auerbach, R.; Augustin, H.G.; Bates, D.O.; van Beijnum, J.R.; Bender, R.H.F.; et al. Consensus guidelines for the use and interpretation of angiogenesis assays. *Angiogenesis* **2018**, *21*, 425–532. [CrossRef] [PubMed]
9. Passaniti, A.; Taylor, R.M.; Pili, R.; Guo, Y.; Long, P.V.; Haney, J.A.; Pauly, R.R.; Grant, D.S.; Martin, G.R. A simple, quantitative method for assessing angiogenesis and antiangiogenic agents using reconstituted basement membrane, heparin, and fibroblast growth factor. *Lab. Investig.* **1992**, *67*, 519–528.
10. Bastiaansen, A.J.; Ewing, M.M.; de Boer, H.C.; van der Pouw Kraan, T.C.; de Vries, M.R.; Peters, E.A.; Welten, S.M.; Arens, R.; Moore, S.M.; Faber, J.E.; et al. Lysine acetyltransferase PCAF is a key regulator of arteriogenesis. *Arterioscler. Thromb. Vasc. Biol.* **2013**, *33*, 1902–1910. [CrossRef]
11. Bastiaansen, A.J.; Karper, J.C.; Wezel, A.; de Boer, H.C.; Welten, S.M.; de Jong, R.C.; Peters, E.A.; de Vries, M.R.; van Oeveren-Rietdijk, A.M.; van Zonneveld, A.J.; et al. TLR4 accessory molecule RP105 (CD180) regulates monocyte-driven arteriogenesis in a murine hind limb ischemia model. *PLoS ONE* **2014**, *9*, e99882. [CrossRef]
12. Simons, K.H.; de Vries, M.R.; de Jong, R.C.M.; Peters, H.A.B.; Jukema, J.W.; Quax, P.H.A. IRF3 and IRF7 mediate neovascularization via inflammatory cytokines. *J. Cell. Mol. Med.* **2019**. [CrossRef] [PubMed]
13. Nossent, A.Y.; Bastiaansen, A.J.; Peters, E.A.; de Vries, M.R.; Aref, Z.; Welten, S.M.; de Jager, S.C.; van der Pouw Kraan, T.C.; Quax, P.H. CCR7-CCL19/CCL21 Axis is Essential for Effective Arteriogenesis in a Murine Model of Hindlimb Ischemia. *J. Am. Heart Assoc.* **2017**, *6*. [CrossRef]
14. Yildirim, C.; Nieuwenhuis, S.; Teunissen, P.F.; Horrevoets, A.J.; van Royen, N.; van der Pouw Kraan, T.C. Interferon-Beta, a Decisive Factor in Angiogenesis and Arteriogenesis. *J. Interferon Cytokine Res.* **2015**, *35*, 411–420. [CrossRef]
15. Sun, Y.; Wu, C.; Ma, J.; Yang, Y.; Man, X.; Wu, H.; Li, S. Toll-like receptor 4 promotes angiogenesis in pancreatic cancer via PI3K/AKT signaling. *Exp. Cell Res.* **2016**, *347*, 274–282. [CrossRef]
16. He, C.; Sun, Y.; Ren, X.; Lin, Q.; Hu, X.; Huang, X.; Su, S.-B.; Liu, Y.; Liu, X. Angiogenesis mediated by toll-like receptor 4 in ischemic neural tissue. *Arterioscler. Thromb. Vasc. Biol.* **2013**, *33*, 330–338. [CrossRef]
17. Forster, R.; Davalos-Misslitz, A.C.; Rot, A. CCR7 and its ligands: Balancing immunity and tolerance. *Nat. Rev. Immunol.* **2008**, *8*, 362–371. [CrossRef]
18. Chi, B.J.; Du, C.L.; Fu, Y.F.; Zhang, Y.N.; Wang, R.W. Silencing of CCR7 inhibits the growth, invasion and migration of prostate cancer cells induced by VEGFC. *Int. J. Clin. Exp. Pathol.* **2015**, *8*, 12533–12540.

19. Xiong, Y.; Huang, F.; Li, X.; Chen, Z.; Feng, D.; Jiang, H.; Chen, W.; Zhang, X. CCL21/CCR7 interaction promotes cellular migration and invasion via modulation of the MEK/ERK1/2 signaling pathway and correlates with lymphatic metastatic spread and poor prognosis in urinary bladder cancer. *Int. J. Oncol.* **2017**, *51*, 75–90. [CrossRef] [PubMed]
20. Shireman, P.K. The chemokine system in arteriogenesis and hind limb ischemia. *J. Vasc. Surg.* **2007**, *45* (Suppl. A), A48–A56. [CrossRef] [PubMed]
21. Sheppard, K.A.; Rose, D.W.; Haque, Z.K.; Kurokawa, R.; McInerney, E.; Westin, S.; Thanos, D.; Rosenfeld, M.G.; Glass, C.K.; Collins, T. Transcriptional activation by NF-kappaB requires multiple coactivators. *Mol. Cell. Biol.* **1999**, *19*, 6367–6378. [CrossRef] [PubMed]
22. Lim, J.H.; Lee, Y.M.; Chun, Y.S.; Chen, J.; Kim, J.E.; Park, J.W. Sirtuin 1 modulates cellular responses to hypoxia by deacetylating hypoxia-inducible factor 1alpha. *Mol. Cell* **2010**, *38*, 864–878. [CrossRef]
23. Zimna, A.; Kurpisz, M. Hypoxia-Inducible Factor-1 in Physiological and Pathophysiological Angiogenesis: Applications and Therapies. *BioMed Res. Int.* **2015**, *2015*, 549412. [CrossRef]
24. de Jong, R.C.M.; Ewing, M.M.; de Vries, M.R.; Karper, J.C.; Bastiaansen, A.; Peters, H.A.B.; Baghana, F.; van den Elsen, P.J.; Gongora, C.; Jukema, J.W.; et al. The epigenetic factor PCAF regulates vascular inflammation and is essential for intimal hyperplasia development. *PLoS ONE* **2017**, *12*, e0185820. [CrossRef] [PubMed]
25. Auerbach, R.; Lewis, R.; Shinners, B.; Kubai, L.; Akhtar, N. Angiogenesis assays: A critical overview. *Clin. Chem.* **2003**, *49*, 32–40. [CrossRef] [PubMed]
26. Adini, A.; Fainaru, O.; Udagawa, T.; Connor, K.M.; Folkman, J.; D'Amato, R.J. Matrigel cytometry: A novel method for quantifying angiogenesis in vivo. *J. Immunol. Methods* **2009**, *342*, 78–81. [CrossRef]
27. Coltrini, D.; Di Salle, E.; Ronca, R.; Belleri, M.; Testini, C.; Presta, M. Matrigel plug assay: Evaluation of the angiogenic response by reverse transcription-quantitative PCR. *Angiogenesis* **2013**, *16*, 469–477. [CrossRef] [PubMed]
28. Norrby, K. In vivo models of angiogenesis. *J. Cell. Mol. Med.* **2006**, *10*, 588–612. [CrossRef]
29. Auerbach, R.; Akhtar, N.; Lewis, R.L.; Shinners, B.L. Angiogenesis assays: Problems and pitfalls. *Cancer Metastasis Rev.* **2000**, *19*, 167–172. [CrossRef]

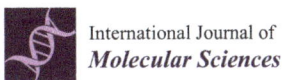

Article

Impact of *C57BL/6J* and *SV-129* Mouse Strain Differences on Ischemia-Induced Postnatal Angiogenesis and the Associated Leukocyte Infiltration in a Murine Hindlimb Model of Ischemia

Matthias Kübler [1,2,†], Philipp Götz [1,2,†], Anna Braumandl [1,2], Sebastian Beck [1,2], Hellen Ishikawa-Ankerhold [1,3] and Elisabeth Deindl [1,2,*]

1. Walter-Brendel-Centre of Experimental Medicine, University Hospital, Ludwig-Maximilians-Universität München, 81377 Munich, Germany; Matthias.Kuebler@med.uni-muenchen.de (M.K.); P.Goetz@med.uni-muenchen.de (P.G.); Anna.Braumandl@med.uni-muenchen.de (A.B.); sebastian.beck@med.uni-muenchen.de (S.B.); Hellen.Ishikawa-Ankerhold@med.uni-muenchen.de (H.I.-A.)
2. Biomedical Center, Institute of Cardiovascular Physiology and Pathophysiology, Ludwig-Maximilians-Universität München, 82152 Planegg-Martinsried, Germany
3. Department of Internal Medicine I, Faculty of Medicine, University Hospital, Ludwig-Maximilians-Universität München, 81377 Munich, Germany
* Correspondence: Elisabeth.Deindl@med.uni-muenchen.de; Tel.: +49-(0)-89-2180-76504
† These authors contributed equally to this work.

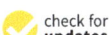

Citation: Kübler, M.; Götz, P.; Braumandl, A.; Beck, S.; Ishikawa-Ankerhold, H.; Deindl, E. Impact of *C57BL/6J* and *SV-129* Mouse Strain Differences on Ischemia-Induced Postnatal Angiogenesis and the Associated Leukocyte Infiltration in a Murine Hindlimb Model of Ischemia. *Int. J. Mol. Sci.* **2021**, *22*, 11795. https://doi.org/10.3390/ijms222111795

Academic Editor: Maria Luisa Balestrieri

Received: 21 September 2021
Accepted: 27 October 2021
Published: 30 October 2021

Publisher's Note: MDPI stays neutral with regard to jurisdictional claims in published maps and institutional affiliations.

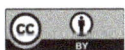

Copyright: © 2021 by the authors. Licensee MDPI, Basel, Switzerland. This article is an open access article distributed under the terms and conditions of the Creative Commons Attribution (CC BY) license (https://creativecommons.org/licenses/by/4.0/).

Abstract: Strain-related differences in arteriogenesis in inbred mouse strains have already been studied excessively. However, these analyses missed evaluating the mouse strain-related differences in ischemia-induced angiogenic capacities. With the present study, we wanted to shed light on the different angiogenic potentials and the associated leukocyte infiltration of *C57BL/6J* and *SV-129* mice to facilitate the comparison of angiogenesis-related analyses between these strains. For the induction of angiogenesis, we ligated the femoral artery in 8–12-week-old male *C57BL/6J* and *SV-129* mice and performed (immuno-) histological analyses on the ischemic gastrocnemius muscles collected 24 h or 7 days after ligation. As evidenced by hematoxylin and eosin staining, *C57BL/6J* mice showed reduced tissue damage but displayed an increased capillary-to-muscle fiber ratio and an elevated number of proliferating capillaries (CD31$^+$/BrdU$^+$ cells) compared to *SV-129* mice, thus showing improved angiogenesis. Regarding the associated leukocyte infiltration, we found increased numbers of neutrophils (MPO$^+$ cells), NETs (MPO$^+$/CitH3$^+$/DAPI$^+$), and macrophages (CD68$^+$ cells) in *SV-129* mice, whereas macrophage polarization (MRC1$^-$ vs. MRC1$^+$) and total leukocyte infiltration (CD45$^+$ cells) did not differ between the mouse strains. In summary, we show increased ischemia-induced angiogenic capacities in *C57BL/6J* mice compared to *SV-129* mice, with the latter showing aggravated tissue damage, inflammation, and impaired angiogenesis.

Keywords: angiogenesis; *C57BL/6J* mice; *SV-129* mice; leukocytes; macrophages; neutrophils; NETs; neutrophil extracellular traps; C57BL6; 129S1/Sv

1. Introduction

The terminal vessels of the vertebrate circulatory system are made up of arterioles, venules, and the capillary bed, with the latter being mandatory for maintaining the homeostasis of a living individual [1]. The anatomy and physiology of capillaries allow the direct exchange of gases, liquids, nutrients, signal molecules, and cells between blood and the adjacent tissue, thus ensuring proper tissue nourishment with oxygen and nutrients [1]. Furthermore, the regulation of capillary bed growth in the adult individual plays a vital role in physiological conditions as well as in many acute and chronic diseases, such as wound healing, cancer, and inflammation [2–4]. This process, denoted as angiogenesis, occurs either via capillary splitting or sprouting, leading to a more advanced capillary network structure accompanied by an amplification of the total capillary surface [5,6]. While, in cancer, uncontrolled capillary growth facilitates the nutrition and survival of tumor cells and their blood-dependent metastatic spread, in wound healing, impaired angiogenesis causes chronic stagnancy of the healing process. Thus, both promoting and inhibiting angiogenic processes are the object of different therapeutic approaches, dependent on the present pathology.

In vascular occlusive diseases, such as myocardial infarction and peripheral artery disease, the restoration of oxygen supply in the affected ischemic tissue downstream the occluded artery is only possible via the formation of natural bypasses, a process that is referred to as arteriogenesis [7,8]. Arteriogenesis describes the growth transformation of pre-existing collateral arteries, which is initially triggered by increasing fluid shear stress that leads to a local inflammatory process. This inflammation finally results in a caliber gain of the pre-existing interarterial anastomoses and therefore to a redirection of the blood flow, ensuring the appropriate re-supply of the ischemic tissue areas. Instead, angiogenesis does not occur to re-oxygenate the hypoxic tissue due to insufficient blood supply, but for cell debris removal and tissue reorganization in the ischemic muscle tissue areas [9–11].

The processes of angiogenesis are modified by a broad range of signaling molecules originating from a wide variety of cells. The most investigated pro-angiogenic factor is the vascular endothelial growth factor A (VEGFA) belonging to a family of strong pro-angiogenic regulators [1,12,13]. It is well described that VEGFA promotes endothelial cell differentiation, proliferation, and angiogenic remodeling via its binding to the receptor tyrosine kinase VEGF receptor 2 (VEGFR-2) [14,15]. VEGFA levels rise in an oxygen-dependent manner in hypoxic tissue [16]. However, VEGFA and other angiogenesis-modulating molecules, such as tissue modulating matrix metalloproteases (MMPs), are also distributed by leukocytes, such as neutrophils and macrophages [1,17,18]. Additionally, leukocytes directly affect angiogenesis by activating endothelial cells, remodeling the matrix, and stabilizing vessel anastomoses [17–19].

Thus, leukocytes play an essential role in controlling angiogenesis not only through the removal of cellular debris at the ischemic site but also through the remodeling of the surrounding matrix and tissue and the direct allocation of pro- and anti-angiogenic factors [1,19–24]. Consequently, the regulation of the inflammatory immune cell infiltration highlights a new therapeutic target to modulate the efficacy of the processes of angiogenesis.

In different experimental setups, different mouse strains are employed in murine hindlimb models of ischemia to evaluate the effects of different targets on arteriogenesis and angiogenesis. Following femoral artery ligation (FAL), collateral arteries in the adductor muscles in the upper leg grow to restore the hindlimb's blood supply (arteriogenesis), while the provoked ischemia in the gastrocnemius muscle of the lower leg leads to hypoxia-dependent muscle tissue destruction and accompanied angiogenesis [25–28]. In the past, astonishing differences regarding the arteriogenic capacities between different inbred mouse strains have been observed, yet without analyzing the strain-related differences in angiogenesis and the associated leukocyte recruitment [29,30].

Two extremes of arteriogenic capacity analysis were marked by the two inbred mouse strains of the *C57BL/6J* line and the *SV-129* line, both widely used and well-established experimental inbred mouse strains. Comparing their arteriogenic capacities upon FAL, *C57BL/6J* mice showed the highest reperfusion rate, while *SV-129* mice showed attenuated reperfusion recovery [29].

It is important to notice that in the model of femoral artery ligation, the extent of angiogenesis highly depends on the efficacy of arteriogenesis; impaired collateral artery growth in the adductor muscle of the upper leg leads to increased ischemia in the distal gastrocnemius muscle of the lower leg and thus to a stronger ischemic trigger for the processes of angiogenesis [31]. So, for comparing ischemia-dependent angiogenesis upon FAL between different mouse strains, the associated arteriogenic capacities of these inbred lines have to be taken into account when interpreting the acquired data.

Inbred mouse strains are commonly accepted in research. Their genetic uniformity facilitates genetic research as the use of fewer individuals may lead to a statistical significance level. Having their origin in genetics and cancer research, the *C57BL6* line became the standard for most research applications, especially in cardiovascular research, since C. C. Little, the founder of Jackson Laboratory, established the line with mice from Abbie Lathrop about 100 years ago [32]. Due to the well-established embryonic stem cell line, *SV-129* mice are often used for targeted mutations, thus being the preferable mouse line concerning transgenic mouse strain design.

In the past, the yet unknown differences in ischemia-induced angiogenic efficacy between the two different inbred mouse strains of *C57BL/6J* and *SV-129* made it challenging to evaluate and compare findings in experiments conducted with these two strains. As *SV-129* mice show a decreased arteriogenic capacity, we hypothesized that a higher ischemic force might lead to a higher level of angiogenesis. The present study aimed to investigate whether this was the case and how the strains react pathophysiologically to femoral artery occlusion. Thus, with the present study, we shed light on the differences in ischemia-provoked angiogenic capacities and the accompanied leukocyte infiltration in a murine hindlimb model between the *C57BL/6J* and *SV-129* inbred mouse strains.

2. Results

To compare the angiogenic potential of the two different mouse strains, we followed a well-established model of hindlimb ischemia: the right femoral artery of *C57BL/6J* and *SV-129* mice was occluded (FAL), leading to collateral growth (arteriogenesis) in the upper leg and angiogenesis in the lower leg on the occluded side, while the left leg underwent a sham operation [25]. At 24 h or 7 days after FAL, mice were sacrificed and the gastrocnemius muscles of the lower leg were collected for (immuno-) histological studies.

Monitoring the animal's health in the experiment, we could not observe any strain-related differences concerning wound healing. No grave necrosis of the foot could be observed. As known, both strains regain their hindlimb function within 7 days after surgery [29]. A systemic assessment of the foot active use score was not performed in this study.

The area of ischemic damage in gastrocnemius muscles 7 days after FAL was analyzed using a hematoxylin and eosin (H&E) staining. *C57BL/6J* mice showed a decreased ischemic damage area compared to *SV-129* mice (Figure 1). Neither gastrocnemius muscles isolated from *C57BL/6J* nor *SV-129* mice showed any ischemic damage after sham operation (Figure S1).

To measure the angiogenic capacity of the mouse strains under ischemic conditions, we stained gastrocnemius muscles for CD31/BrdU/DAPI and calculated the capillary-to-muscle fiber ratio from muscle tissue isolated 7 days after FAL. CD31 served as a capillary marker and bromodeoxyuridine (BrdU) served as a proliferation marker. As platelets also express CD31, only $CD31^+/DAPI^+$ signals were counted as capillary signals and quantified. In addition, $CD31^+/BrdU^+/DAPI^+$ signals were quantified to investigate the number of proliferating capillaries. Compared to *SV-129* mice, *C57BL/6J* mice showed a higher number of capillaries and a higher number of proliferating capillaries per muscle fiber, indicating the increased angiogenic capacity of *C57BL/6J* mice (Figure 2a,b,d). To exclude any a priori differences in capillarity between the mouse strains, we analyzed non-ischemic gastrocnemius muscles, finding no significant differences in capillary-to-muscle fiber ratio (Figure 2c).

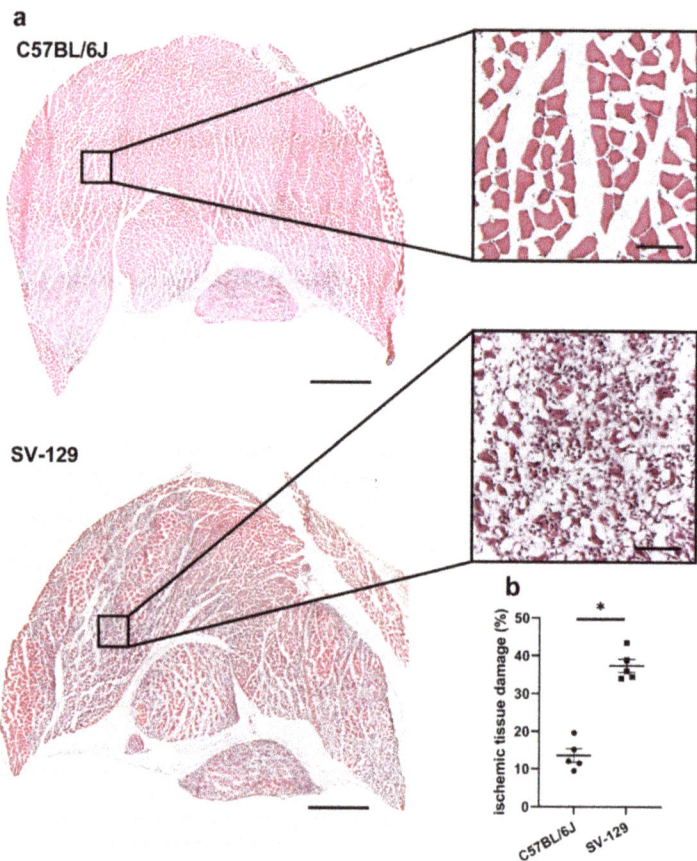

Figure 1. *C57BL/6J* mice show a smaller cross-sectional area of ischemic tissue damage in comparison to *SV-129* mice. (**a**) Representative pictures of hematoxylin and eosin (H&E)-stained gastrocnemius muscles of *C57BL/6J* (top) and *SV-129* mice (bottom) collected 7 days after femoral artery ligation (FAL). Skeletal muscle cells that show centralized nuclei are a sign of regenerating muscle cells and hence ischemic damage. Scale bars: 1000 µm (overview), 100 µm (detail). (**b**) The scatter plot displays the relative area of ischemic tissue damage (%) in gastrocnemius muscles of *C57BL/6J* and *SV-129* mice isolated 7 days after FAL. One complete sectional area was analyzed per mouse per group. Data are means ± S.E.M., $n = 5$ per group. * $p < 0.05$ (*C57BL/6J* vs. *SV-129*) by unpaired, two-sided Student's *t*-test.

Leukocytes are known as regulators as well as enhancers of ischemia-induced inflammation, including cell debris removal and tissue regeneration, and directly influence vascular cell proliferation by their supply of growth factors. Consequently, we focused on changes in leukocyte accumulation related to the different mouse strains. Using CD45 as a pan-leukocyte marker, we quantified $CD45^+/DAPI^+$ signals in gastrocnemius muscles 7 days after surgery. Comparing both mouse strains, we did not find a significant difference between the *SV-129* and the *C57BL/6J* line (Figure 3a,c) in ischemic tissue samples. In addition, we observed no significant difference in the number of leukocytes in sham-operated muscles (Figure 3b).

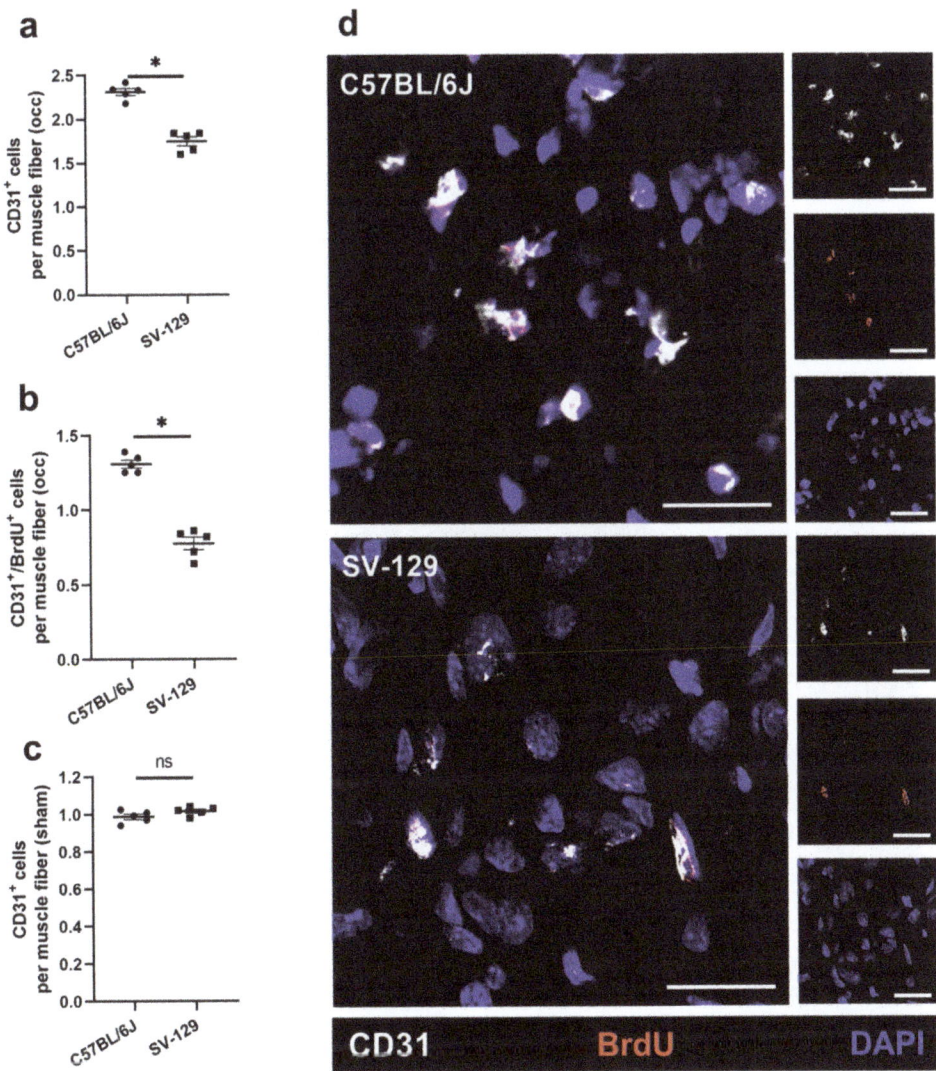

Figure 2. *C57BL/6J* mice show a higher capillarity under ischemic conditions than *SV-129* mice. The scatter plots display (**a**) endothelial cells (CD31$^+$/DAPI$^+$) per muscle fiber as well as (**b**) proliferating endothelial cells (CD31$^+$/BrdU$^+$ (bromodeoxyuridine)/DAPI$^+$) per muscle fiber of *C57BL/6J* and *SV-129* mice in occluded (occ) ischemic gastrocnemius muscles isolated 7 days after femoral artery ligation (FAL). Scatter plot (**c**) displays the capillary-to-muscle fiber ratio of sham-operated (sham) non-ischemic gastrocnemius muscles isolated from *C57BL/6J* and *SV-129* mice 7 days after FAL. A defined ischemic area (1.5 mm^2) of muscle tissue was analyzed per mouse. Data are means ± S.E.M., n = 5 per group. $^{n.s.}$ $p \geq 0.05$, * $p < 0.05$ (*C57BL/6J* vs. *SV-129*) by unpaired, two-sided Student's *t*-test. (**d**) Representative immunofluorescence staining of ischemic gastrocnemius muscles of *C57BL/6J* (top) and *SV-129* mice (bottom) collected 7 days after FAL. Cells were stained with an antibody labeling CD31 (white), BrdU (red), and DAPI (blue) to label nucleic DNA. Scale bars: 20 µm.

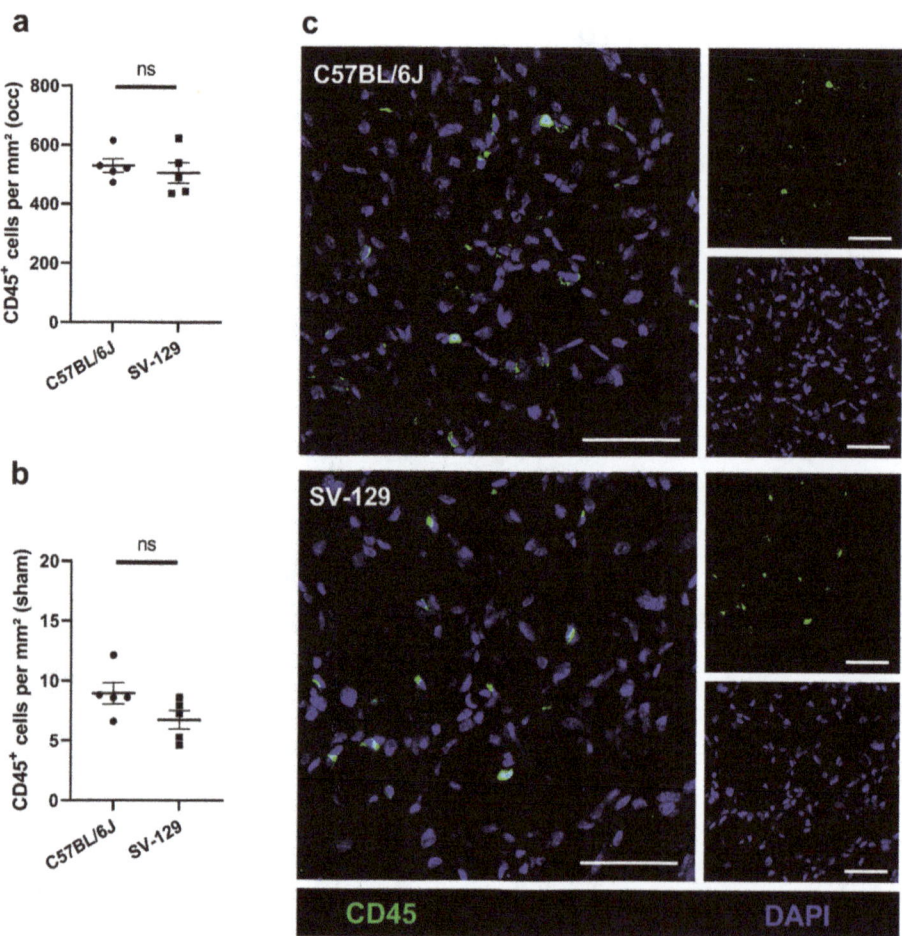

Figure 3. *C57BL/6J* and *SV-129* mouse strains show comparable leukocyte accumulation under ischemic conditions. The scatter plots display (**a**) the number of infiltrating leukocytes (CD45$^+$/DAPI$^+$) per mm^2 in occluded (occ) ischemic gastrocnemius muscles of *C57BL/6J* and *SV-129* mice as well as (**b**) the number of leukocytes per mm^2 in sham-operated (sham) non-ischemic tissue, all collected 7 days after femoral artery ligation (FAL). A defined ischemic area (1.5 mm^2) of muscle tissue was analyzed per mouse. Data are means ± S.E.M., n = 5 per group. $^{n.s.}$ $p \geq 0.05$, (*C57BL/6J* vs. *SV-129*) by unpaired, two-sided Student's *t*-test. (**c**) Representative immunofluorescence staining of ischemic gastrocnemius muscles of *C57BL/6J* (top) and *SV-129* mice (bottom) isolated 7 days after FAL. Cells were stained with an antibody against CD45 (green) and DAPI (blue) to label nucleic DNA. Scale bars: 50 µm.

To gain further information concerning leukocyte subpopulations with a focus on neutrophils and macrophages, we detected neutrophils and their formation of neutrophil extracellular traps (NETs) using a combined staining for myeloperoxidase (MPO) as a neutrophil marker and citrullinated histone H3 (CitH3) as a NET marker on tissue isolated 24 h after FAL. We found a significantly reduced number of neutrophils (MPO$^+$/DAPI$^+$), NETs (MPO$^+$/CitH3$^+$/DAPI$^+$), and neutrophils, which are in the process of NET formation, in mice of the *C57BL/6J* strain in comparison to the *SV-129* line in ischemic tissue (Figure 4). Under non-ischemic conditions after sham operation, we could not observe differences in the number of neutrophils in tissue samples of both mouse strains (data not shown), while NETs were completely absent.

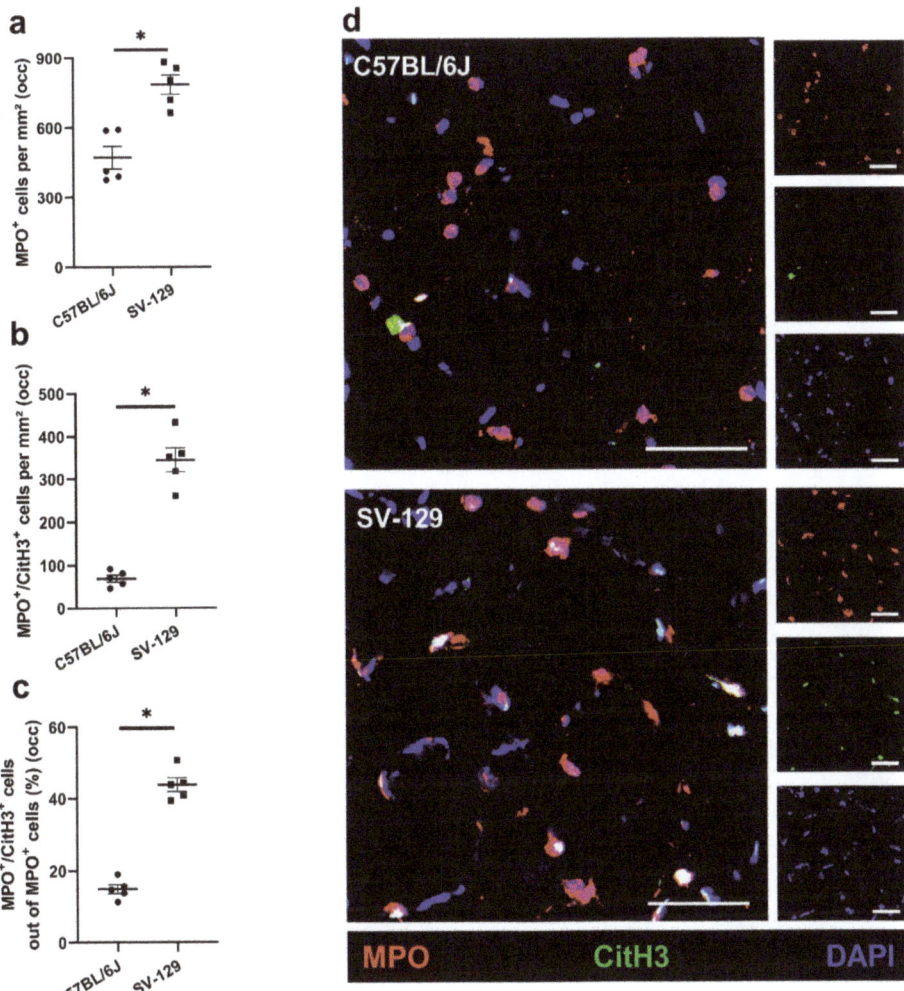

Figure 4. Compared to *SV-129* mice, accumulation of neutrophils and neutrophil extracellular trap (NET) formation is diminished in *C57BL/6J* mice under ischemic conditions. Scatter plots display the number of (**a**) neutrophils (MPO$^+$ (myeloperoxidase)/DAPI$^+$) per mm^2, (**b**) neutrophil extracellular traps (MPO$^+$/CitH3$^+$ (citrullinated histone H3)/DAPI$^+$) per mm^2, and (**c**) the percentage of NETs/neutrophils in occluded (occ) ischemic gastrocnemius muscles isolated from *C57BL/6J* and *SV-129* mice 24 h after femoral artery ligation (FAL). A defined ischemic area (0.86 mm^2) of muscle tissue was analyzed per mouse. Data are means ± S.E.M., n = 5 per group. * $p < 0.05$ (*C57BL/6J* vs. *SV-129*) by unpaired, two-sided Student's *t*-test. (**d**) Representative immunofluorescence staining of ischemic gastrocnemius muscles of *C57BL/6J* (top) and *SV-129* mice (bottom) collected 24 h after FAL. Cells were stained with an antibody against MPO (red), CitH3 (green), and DAPI (blue) to label nucleic DNA. Scale bars: 50 µm.

Analyzing strain-dependent changes in macrophage accumulation and polarization in ischemic tissue 7 days after FAL, we used CD68 as a macrophage and mannose receptor C-type 1 (MRC1) as a macrophage polarization marker. CD68$^+$/MRC1$^-$ cells were counted as pro-inflammatory M1-like polarized macrophages and CD68$^+$/MRC1$^+$ cells as anti-inflammatory M2-like polarized macrophages accordingly. *C57BL/6J* mice displayed a lower infiltration of macrophages in ischemic tissue than *SV-129* mice, but no change in macrophage polarization was observed (Figure 5). In non-ischemic tissue, both mouse strains differed neither in macrophage accumulation nor macrophage polarization (data not shown).

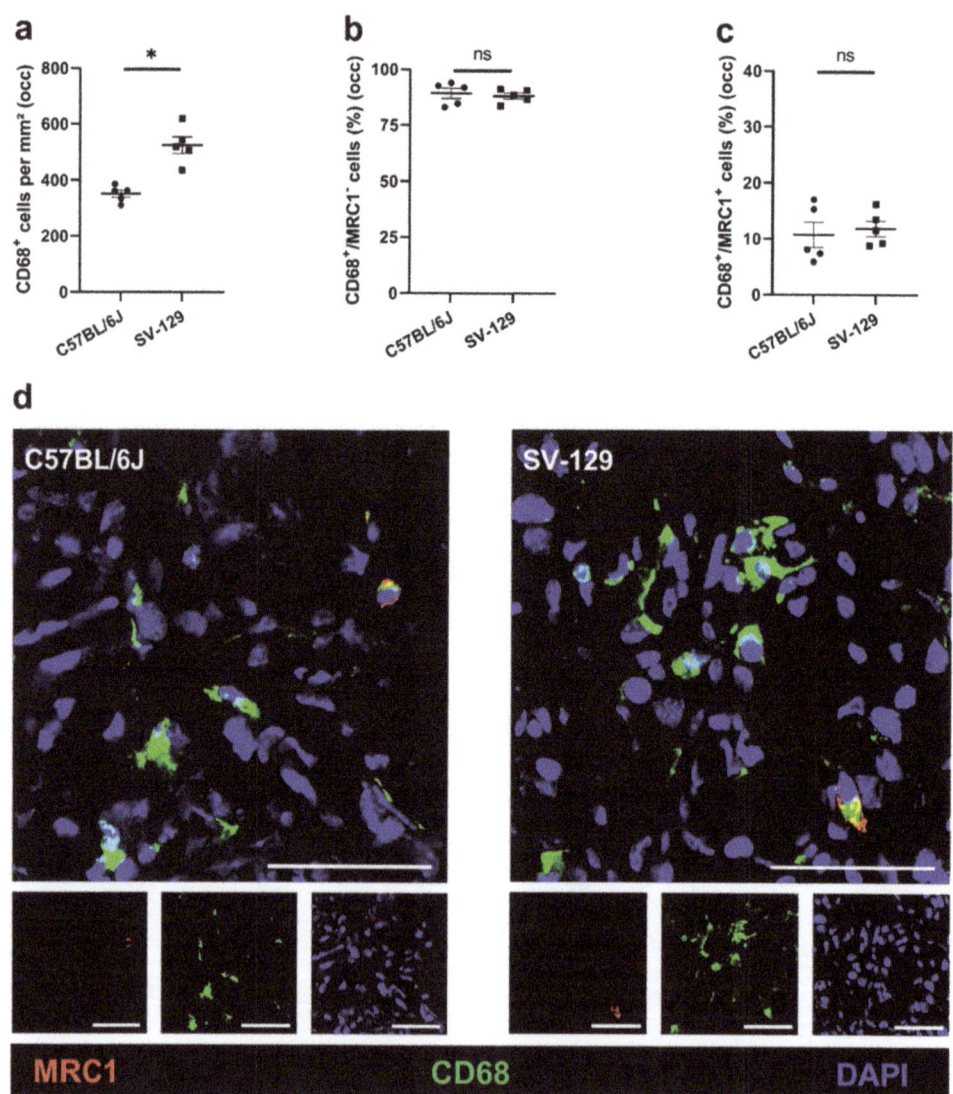

Figure 5. *C57BL/6J* mice show a lower number of macrophages than *SV-129* mice at the side of sterile, ischemic inflammation, while macrophage polarization is unaffected. Scatter plots display (**a**) the number of macrophages (CD68$^+$/DAPI$^+$) per mm^2, (**b**) the percentage of M1-like polarized macrophages (CD68$^+$/MRC1$^-$ (mannose receptor C-type 1)/DAPI$^+$), and (**c**) the percentage of M2-like polarized macrophages (CD68$^+$/MRC1$^+$/DAPI$^+$) in occluded (occ) ischemic gastrocnemius muscles isolated from *C57BL/6J* and *SV-129* mice 7 days after femoral artery ligation (FAL). A defined ischemic area (1.5 mm^2) of muscle tissue was analyzed per mouse. Data are means ± S.E.M., *nüber* = 5 per group. $^{n.s.}$ $p \geq 0.05$, * $p < 0.05$ (*C57BL/6J* vs. *SV-129*) by unpaired, two-sided Student's *t*-test. (**d**) Representative immunofluorescence staining of ischemic gastrocnemius muscles of *C57BL/6J* (left) and *SV-129* mice (right) collected 7 days after FAL. Cells were stained with an antibody against MRC1 (red), CD68 (green), and DAPI (blue) to label nucleic DNA. Scale bars: 50 µm.

3. Discussion

Researchers working with mouse models are often not aware of differences in the pathophysiological reactions of inbred mouse strains to experimental manipulations. In the case of experimental setups using FAL, the differences in the degree and the underlying molecular pathways of angiogenesis between inbred mouse strains have never been taken into account. Over the last few years, numerous studies on ischemia-induced angiogenesis using the well-established and important murine hindlimb model of FAL have been conducted using both the *C57BL/6J* and *SV-129* mouse strains. Yet, the angiogenic capacities of both inbred strains have never been compared, complicating the retrospective comparison and evaluation of already collected data [28,31,33,34]. With the present study, we performed a detailed investigation of *C57BL/6J* and *SV-129* mouse strains known for their different pathological reactions towards FAL, focusing on postnatal ischemia-induced angiogenesis and the associated leukocyte recruitment in the gastrocnemius muscle.

Our results demonstrate that *C57BL/6J* mice show an increased capillary-to-muscle fiber ratio 7 days after FAL with an elevated number of proliferating capillaries and a reduced area of ischemia-induced tissue damage compared to *SV-129* mice. These findings were accompanied by a total reduction in infiltrating neutrophils (MPO^+ cells), NETs ($MPO^+/CitH3^+/DAPI^+$), and macrophages ($CD68^+$ cells) in ischemic muscle tissue of *C57BL/6J* mice, while no significant differences in macrophage polarization and the total number of infiltrative immune cells ($CD45^+$ cells) were observed. Altogether, our data suggest that *C57BL/6J* mice possessed better angiogenic capacities resulting in minor ischemic muscle tissue damage, probably caused by a milder, more pro-angiogenic inflammatory environment in *C57BL/6J* mice than in *SV-129* mice.

Compared to *SV-129* mice, *C57BL/6J* mice showed a decreased area of ischemic tissue damage. In the mouse model of hindlimb ischemia, FAL results in the arteriogenic growth of collateral arteries in the upper leg and in ischemia-induced angiogenesis in the lower leg [25]. It was found that improved arteriogenesis in the upper leg results in a reduction in the ischemic tissue damage in the distal gastrocnemius muscle [31]. However, it is well described that the *C57BL/6J* strain has higher arteriogenic capacities than the *SV-129* strain, attributable to an improved increase in luminal diameter upon ligation [29]. Our results confirm these findings, as we found a decreased ischemic tissue damage area in *C57BL/6J* mice compared to *SV-129* mice, which is partly attributable to *C57BL/6J*'s improved arteriogenesis and the resulting higher perfusion of the lower limb.

Due to increased ischemia as the main angiogenic trigger, increased ischemic tissue damage is expected to be associated with enhanced angiogenesis. However, we found that despite the reduced tissue damage, *C57BL/6J* mice show a higher capillary-to-muscle fiber ratio and a higher number of proliferating capillaries per muscle fiber than *SV-129* mice. Accordingly, our results demonstrate that mice of the *C57BL/6J* strain show a more effective ischemia-induced angiogenesis than *SV-129* mice. Therefore, the observed decrease in ischemic tissue damage in *C57BL/6J* mice could also be a result of improved arteriogenesis, angiogenesis, and accompanied tissue reorganization.

In ischemic tissue damage, leukocytes migrate from the vasculature into the perivascular space to phagocyte damaged cells and initiate tissue reorganization comprising new capillary bed formation. Part of this tissue reorganization is creating local inflammation, leading to the release of other leukocyte-originating pro-inflammatory cytokines and chemokines. The allocation of these messenger substances results in further leukocyte recruitment at the damaged tissue area [17,18,35,36]. Additionally, this leukocyte migration is facilitated through a cytokine-dependent leakage of the endothelial cell barrier. After clearing the cellular debris and reorganizing the tissue, pro-inflammatory leukocytes leave the affected area, giving space for an anti-inflammatory and regenerating environment leading to tissue remodeling of the affected muscle tissue. While leukocytes, especially macrophages and neutrophils, are described to promote angiogenesis through the release of pro-angiogenic and tissue remodeling factors, excessive leukocyte accumulation is associated with the prolongation of infiltration and therefore decelerated healing processes [18,35,37]. However, we could not show a significant difference in the number of infiltrating leukocytes between both mouse strains.

In the earliest stages after the induction of FAL, neutrophils are recruited to the site of ischemic tissue damage, playing a pivotal role in initiating and modulating the local inflammatory and angiogenic processes [17]. By releasing potent forms of VEGFA, MMP-9, and other angiogenic factors, neutrophils are essential to promote the induction of angiogenesis as neutropenic mice failed to revascularize transplanted pancreatic island tissue [21,38–40]. Through their ability of phagocytosis, neutrophils participate in tissue repair and cell debris removal. Moreover, it was found that neutrophils form tunnels for vessel sprouts, supporting their growth and development in a model of thermal hepatic injury [37,41]. Nevertheless, neutrophils also release cytotoxic factors and excessive neutrophil accumulation is known to cause the aggravation of tissue damage [35,37,42].

Apart from that, neutrophil extracellular traps (NETs) are shown to promote angiogenesis in vivo and in vitro directly [43]. NETs are neutrophil-originated chromatin filaments with citrullinated histone H3 (CitH3) that are released into the extracellular space accompanied by various enzymes such as myeloperoxidase (MPO) as a reaction towards different inflammatory stimuli [44,45]. It was recently found that NETs promote angiogenesis through the modulation of intercellular adhesion molecule 1 (ICAM-1) expression on endothelial cells, thus affecting leukocyte migration out of the vasculature into the perivascular space and the modulation of VEGF signaling leading to changes in progenitor cell recruitment and endothelial cell migration [43]. Moreover, NETs are also described to participate in tissue remodeling by promoting apoptosis in senescent vasculature in retinopathy [46]. However, excessive NET accumulation at the inflammatory site is associated with the aggravation and general prolongation of inflammation [47,48].

We observed an increased number of neutrophils, NETs, and neutrophils forming NETs in the ischemic muscle tissue of mice belonging to the *SV-129* inbred strain. Thus, mice from the *C57BL/6J* strain show a milder, more pro-angiogenic inflammatory picture, whereas *SV-129* mice display aggravated inflammation in their ischemic muscle tissue one day after FAL.

In ischemic tissue, macrophages play a crucial role in supporting angiogenic tissue remodeling [18]. Hereby, their role depends on their plastic and changeable polarization state [49]. The shift in the macrophage polarization phenotype mirrors the shift from the pro- to the anti-inflammatory environment. The M1-like polarization (CD68$^+$MRC1$^-$) indicates a pro-inflammatory state of the macrophages, which shifts to an M2-like polarization (CD68$^+$MRC1$^+$), designating the change towards the subsequent regenerative anti-inflammatory phase of tissue restitution [18,50]. However, macrophages' M1- and M2-like polarization states only reflect the extremes in a wide spectrum of macrophage polarization [49].

In the beginning, pro-inflammatory M1-like polarized macrophages are mainly responsible for clearing cellular debris through phagocytosis and promoting further local leukocyte recruitment via the allocation of pro-inflammatory chemoattractants [18]. Apart from that, M1-like polarized macrophages are described to support endothelial tip cell sprouting and to guide the growth of the newly formed vessels [51]. Furthermore, M1-like polarized macrophages are potent distributors of pro-angiogenic factors such as VEGFA and tumor necrosis factor-alpha (TNF-α) and are described to play an important role in angiogenesis as their depletion showed impaired angiogenic processes in zebrafish [51]. However, their impact on angiogenesis and tissue restitution is limited due to their restrained ability for matrix remodeling [18].

Afterward, the macrophages change their polarization towards an alternatively activated regenerative anti-inflammatory M2-like polarized phenotype [49]. The M2-like polarization state is mainly associated with tissue repair and the resolution of the previous inflammation [52–55]. In contrast to M1-like polarized macrophages, the M2-like polarized phenotype is essential for matrix remodeling. While in M1-like polarized macrophages, matrix remodeling proteases like matrix metalloproteinase 9 (MMP-9) are complexed and thus downregulated and inactive, in M2-like polarized macrophages, the complexation of these proteases is abolished and thus the enzymes can easily be released in their potent active form [56]. Thus, the M2-like polarized phenotype is denoted as the classic pro-angiogenic macrophage polarization state [18,57–59].

We found an increased number of infiltrating macrophages in the ischemic tissue of *SV-129* mice compared to *C57BL/6J* mice, while no differences in the ratio of M1- or M2-like proliferation state were detected. Nevertheless, the total number of M1- as well as M2-like polarized macrophages was higher in the ischemic muscle tissue of *SV-129* mice. Thus, the difference between the inbred mouse strains had no impact on macrophage polarization but on the number of infiltrating macrophages. Even though we found more pro-angiogenic M2-like polarized macrophages in the ischemic muscle tissue of *SV-129* mice, they did not show ameliorated angiogenesis compared to *C57BL/6J* mice. Accordingly, the increased number of infiltrative macrophages, especially the M1-like polarized phenotype, in *SV-129* mice could mirror an aggravated and prolonged inflammatory state associated with the increased ischemic tissue damage found in this mouse strain.

Moreover, we want to mention that the spatial distribution of macrophage subpopulation is well investigated in the process of arteriogenesis. C. Troidl et al. have observed a rising number of both M1- and M2-like polarized macrophages in the perivascular space until 28 days after ligation [60]. Interestingly, M1-like polarized macrophages were most likely found in the media, while M2-like polarized macrophages were found in the adventitia of the vessels, leading to the conclusion that they might fulfill different distinct roles in arteriogenesis. In contrast to the findings in collateral growth, in angiogenesis we could observe a predominantly pro-inflammatory M1-like polarized phenotype at 7 days after surgery with a spatial distribution throughout all the affected ischemic muscle tissue.

Altogether, we could show that *C57BL/6J* mice show improved angiogenesis after the onset of ischemia compared to mice from the *SV-129* strain. This difference in increased angiogenic growth capacity in *C57BL/6J* mice might be partly attributable to a milder, more pro-angiogenic inflammation based on reduced numbers of infiltrative macrophages, neutrophils, and NETs as compared to *SV-129* mice.

Concerning their specific impact, angiogenic factors and receptors have been extensively studied in various in vitro and in vivo experimental settings and reviewed [1]. The quantitative amounts of individual angiogenic factors alone are not exclusively responsible for modulating angiogenesis. Instead, the activation state of receptors, the number of co-receptors, and the activation status of co-receptors are as important as the number of angiogenic factors alone [61]. To gain a better overall understanding of the angiogenic capacities and their mediation in *C57BL/6J* and *SV-129* mice, we representatively analyzed the present immune microenvironmental conditions. However, further in-depth studies are necessary to evaluate the possible differences of other angiogenesis-modulating factors in *C57BL/6J* and *SV-129* mice.

With the present study, we aimed to advance the field of angiogenesis research by allowing a retrospective comparison and evaluation of already conducted studies on angiogenesis that used either *C57BL/6J* or *SV-129* mice. Furthermore, as researchers are often unaware of the importance of the appropriate mouse strain choice for their experimental setups, disregarding the differences in the pathophysiological reactions of inbred mouse strains to experimental manipulations, we also tried to point out the importance of mouse strain choice for experimental setup design. In synopsis with the presented immunological analysis concerning leukocyte infiltration and inflammation, we could show the detrimental differences between *C57BL/6J* and *SV-129* mouse strains for FAL-induced angiogenesis. Thus, evaluating the applicability of mouse strain choice regarding the research's question for the planned experimental setup before conducting the experiments is still a very important and crucial part in experimental design.

4. Materials and Methods

4.1. Animals and Treatments

Experimental setups and animal care were permitted by the Bavarian Animal Care and Use Committee (ethical approval code: ROB-55.2Vet-2532.Vet_02-17-99, approved on the 8 December 2017) and were performed in strict accordance with the German animal legislation guidelines. Mice were housed in a temperature-controlled room on a 12-h light-dark cycle and received a standard laboratory diet. For all investigations, adult male C57BL/6J and 129S1/Sv (SV-129) (both Charles River Laboratories, Sulzfeld, Germany) mice, aged 8–12 weeks, were sacrificed at 24 h or 7 days (per timepoint $n = 5$ per group) after FAL. For determining the proliferation rate of endothelial cells in the gastrocnemius muscle 7 days after surgery, mice received a daily injection of 100 µL BrdU (Sigma-Aldrich, St. Louis, MO, USA) (12.5 mg/mL BrdU in PBS (PAN Biotech)) i.p., starting directly after the surgical intervention.

4.2. Femoral Artery Ligation and Tissue Processing

To initiate the processes of angiogenesis in the gastrocnemius muscle of the lower hindlimb, the right femoral artery was unilaterally ligated while the left hindlimb was sham-operated and served as an internal control, as previously described [25]. Before the ligation, mice were anesthetized with a s.c. injection of fentanyl (0.05 mg/kg, CuraMED Pharma, Karlsruhe, Germany), midazolam (5.0 mg/kg, Ratiopharm GmbH, Ulm, Germany), and medetomidine (0.5 mg/kg, Pfister Pharma, Berlin, Germany). Before tissue collection 24 h or 7 days after FAL, mice were again anesthetized as described above. After sacrificing, the hindlimbs were perfused with a combination of adenosine buffer (1% adenosine (Sigma-Aldrich, St. Louis, MO, USA), 5% bovine serum albumin (BSA, Sigma-Aldrich, St. Louis, MO, USA, dissolved in PBS) and 3% (for cryopreservation) paraformaldehyde (PFA, Merck, Darmstadt, Germany, dissolved in PBS). For immunohistology, the ligated and the sham-operated hindlimbs of each mouse were collected after the perfusion, then embedded in Tissue-Tek compound (Sakura Finetek Germany GmbH, Staufen, Germany), and finally cryopreserved at $-80\ °C$ for further analysis.

4.3. Histology and Immunohistology

For (immuno-) histological staining, the cryopreserved gastrocnemius muscles were cut in 10-µm-thick slices. Tissue collected 7 days after FAL was used for immunohistological staining of endothelial cells, leukocytes, and macrophages as well as H&E staining, whereas neutrophils and NETs were analyzed on gastrocnemius muscles collected 1 day after ligation.

For the labeling of proliferating cells, the BrdU-treated tissue was incubated with 1 N HCl in a humidified chamber at 37 °C for 30 min, then permeabilized with a 0.2% Triton X-100 solution (AppliChem GmbH, Darmstadt, Germany) in $1 \times$ PBS/0.1% Tween-20 (AppliChem GmbH, Darmstadt, Germany)/0.5% BSA for 2 min, followed by blocking with 10% goat serum (Abcam, ab7481, Cambridge, UK) in $1 \times$ PBS/0.1% Tween-20/0.5% BSA for 1 h at room temperature (RT). Subsequently, the BrdU-treated muscle tissues were incubated with the primary anti-BrdU-antibody (Abcam, ab6326, dilution 1:50 in 10% goat serum, Cambridge, UK) at 4 °C overnight. Following the next day, the cryosections were labeled with a secondary goat anti-rat Alexa Fluor®-546 antibody (Invitrogen, Thermo Fischer Scientific, A-11081, Carlsbad, CA, USA, dilution 1:100) for 1 h at RT. After secondary blocking with $1 \times$ PBS/0.1% Tween-20/4% BSA for 30 min at RT, we applied an anti-CD31-Alexa Fluor® 647 antibody (Biolegend, 102516, San Diego, CA, USA, dilution 1:50 in $1 \times$ PBS/0.1% Tween-20) for labeling endothelial cells for 2 h at RT.

For macrophage labeling, we used an anti-CD68-Alexa Fluor® 488 antibody (Abcam, ab201844, dilution 1:200 in PBS, Cambridge, UK) together with a primary anti-MRC1 antibody (Abcam, ab64693, dilution 1:200 in PBS, Cambridge, UK) to ascertain macrophage polarization and incubated both at 4 °C overnight. Secondary antibody staining was conducted with a donkey-anti-rabbit Alexa Fluor® 546 antibody (Invitrogen, A-10040) for 1 h at RT.

For NETs staining, cryosections collected 24 h after FAL were initially permeabilized with 0.2% Triton X-100 solution in 1 × PBS/0.1% Tween-20/0.5% BSA for 2 min, then blocked with 10% donkey serum (Abcam, ab7475, Cambridge, UK) in 1 × PBS/0.1% Tween-20/0.5% BSA for 1 h at RT followed by incubation with the primary antibodies anti-myeloperoxidase (MPO; R&D Systems, AF3667, Minneapolis, MN, USA, dilution 1:20 in 10% donkey serum in 1 × PBS/0.1% Tween-20/0.5% BSA) and anti-CitH3 antibody (polyclonal rabbit anti-Histone H3 (citrulline R2+R8+R17), Abcam (Cambridge, UK), ab5103, dilution 1:100 in 10% donkey serum in 1 × PBS/0.1% Tween-20/0.5% BSA) at 4 °C overnight. A donkey anti-goat Alexa Fluor® 594 (Invitrogen, A-11058, dilution 1:100 in 1 × PBS/0.1% Tween-20) and a donkey anti-rabbit Alexa Fluor® 488 antibody (Invitrogen, A-21206, dilution 1:200 in 1 × PBS/0.1% Tween-20) were used for secondary antibody staining for 1 h at RT.

Additionally, DAPI (Thermo Fisher Scientific, Waltham, MA, 62248, dilution 1:1000 in PBS) was co-incubated on all cryosections for nucleic DNA labeling for 10 min at RT. The stained tissue sections were finally mounted with an antifade mounting medium (Dako, Agilent, Santa Clara, CA, USA). H&E staining was conducted according to the manufacturer's instruction (Carl Roth GmbH, Karlsruhe, Germany).

For microscopic imaging, we employed a confocal laser scanning microscope LSM 880 (Carl-Zeiss Jena GmbH, Jena, Germany) with a 20× objective (415 µm × 415 µm) as well as an epifluorescence microscope (Leica DM6 B, Leica microsystems, Wetzlar, Germany) with a 20× objective (630 µm × 475µm). For each muscle section, we imaged 5 defined fields to quantify cells, muscle fibers, and NETs. To ascertain the areas of damaged tissue (%), the total gastrocnemius muscle area was analyzed. Gastrocnemius sections stained with H&E, CD45/DAPI, and CD31/BrdU/DAPI were analyzed with the epifluorescence microscope. CD68/MRC1/DAPI and MPO/CitH3/DAPI labeled muscle sections were investigated with the confocal laser scanning microscope. Cell quantification and analysis of the damaged muscle area were conducted using ImageJ software. We calculated the capillary-to-muscle fiber ratio (CD31$^+$/DAPI$^+$ cells were counted as endothelial cells) as described before to assess the processes of angiogenesis [62].

4.4. Statistical Analysis

Statistical analyses were performed and graphically outlined with GraphPad Prism 8 (GraphPad Software, La Jolla, CA, USA). Data are means ± standard error of the mean (S.E.M.). Statistical analyses were calculated as described in the figure legends. Results were considered as statistically significant at $p < 0.05$.

Supplementary Materials: The following are available online at https://www.mdpi.com/article/10.3390/ijms222111795/s1.

Author Contributions: Surgeries, A.B., S.B., P.G. and M.K.; histology, M.K. and P.G.; conceptualization, M.K., P.G. and E.D.; methodology, P.G., M.K., S.B., A.B., H.I.-A. and E.D.; software, M.K. and P.G.; validation, P.G., M.K. and E.D.; formal analysis, M.K. and P.G.; investigation, P.G., M.K. and E.D.; resources, P.G., M.K., A.B., S.B., H.I.-A. and E.D.; data curation, M.K. and P.G.; writing—original draft preparation, M.K. and P.G.; writing—review and editing, M.K., P.G., H.I.-A. and E.D.; visualization, M.K. and P.G.; supervision, E.D.; project administration and funding acquisition, E.D. All authors have read and agreed to the published version of the manuscript.

Funding: This research was funded by Förderprogramm für Forschung und Lehre (FöFoLe) (S.B., P.G.), the Lehre@LMU program, both from the Ludwig-Maximilians-Universität, Munich, Germany and by the DFG-SFB 914 (Project Z01 to H.I.-A.).

Institutional Review Board Statement: The study was approved by the Institutional Review Board of Walter-Brendel-Centre of Experimental Medicine and the Bavarian Animal Care and Use Committee (ethical approval code: ROB-55.2Vet-2532.Vet_02-17-99, approved on the 8 December 2017).

Informed Consent Statement: Not applicable.

Data Availability Statement: The data presented in this study are available on request from the first authors.

Acknowledgments: The authors thank C. Eder and D. van den Heuvel for technical support.

Conflicts of Interest: The authors declare no conflict of interest.

References

1. Adams, R.H.; Alitalo, K. Molecular regulation of angiogenesis and lymphangiogenesis. *Nat. Rev. Mol. Cell Biol.* **2007**, *8*, 464–478. [CrossRef] [PubMed]
2. Folkman, J. Angiogenesis in cancer, vascular, rheumatoid and other disease. *Nat. Med.* **1995**, *1*, 27–31. [CrossRef]
3. Tonnesen, M.G.; Feng, X.; Clark, R.A. Angiogenesis in wound healing. *J. Investig. Dermatol. Symp. Proc.* **2000**, *5*, 40–46. [CrossRef] [PubMed]
4. Carmeliet, P. Angiogenesis in health and disease. *Nat. Med.* **2003**, *9*, 653–660. [CrossRef] [PubMed]
5. Carmeliet, P. Mechanisms of angiogenesis and arteriogenesis. *Nat. Med.* **2000**, *6*, 389–395. [CrossRef]
6. Egginton, S.; Zhou, A.-L.; Brown, M.D.; Hudlická, O. Unorthodox angiogenesis in skeletal muscle. *Cardiovasc. Res.* **2001**, *49*, 634–646. [CrossRef]
7. Pipp, F.; Boehm, S.; Cai, W.J.; Adili, F.; Ziegler, B.; Karanovic, G.; Ritter, R.; Balzer, J.; Scheler, C.; Schaper, W.; et al. Elevated fluid shear stress enhances postocclusive collateral artery growth and gene expression in the pig hind limb. *Arterioscler. Thromb. Vasc. Biol.* **2004**, *24*, 1664–1668. [CrossRef]
8. Deindl, E.; Schaper, W. The art of arteriogenesis. *Cell Biochem. Biophys.* **2005**, *43*, 1–15. [CrossRef]
9. Deindl, E.; Zaruba, M.M.; Brunner, S.; Huber, B.; Mehl, U.; Assmann, G.; Hoefer, I.E.; Mueller-Hoecker, J.; Franz, W.M. G-CSF administration after myocardial infarction in mice attenuates late ischemic cardiomyopathy by enhanced arteriogenesis. *FASEB J.* **2006**, *20*, 956–958. [CrossRef]
10. Heil, M.I.; Eitenmüller, T. Arteriogenesis versus angiogenesis: Similarities and differences. *J. Cell. Mol. Med.* **2006**, *10*, 45–55. [CrossRef]
11. Rizzi, A.; Benagiano, V.; Ribatti, D. Angiogenesis versus arteriogenesis. *Rom. J. Morphol. Embryol.* **2017**, *58*, 15–19.
12. Ferrara, N.; Henzel, W.J. Pituitary follicular cells secrete a novel heparin-binding growth factor specific for vascular endothelial cells. *Biochem. Biophys. Res. Commun.* **1989**, *161*, 851–858. [CrossRef]
13. Gerhardt, H.; Golding, M.; Fruttiger, M.; Ruhrberg, C.; Lundkvist, A.; Abramsson, A.; Jeltsch, M.; Mitchell, C.; Alitalo, K.; Shima, D.; et al. VEGF guides angiogenic sprouting utilizing endothelial tip cell filopodia. *J. Cell Biol.* **2003**, *161*, 1163–1177. [CrossRef] [PubMed]
14. Schwarz, E.R.; Speakman, M.T.; Patterson, M.; Hale, S.S.; Isner, J.M.; Kedes, L.H.; Kloner, R.A. Evaluation of the effects of intramyocardial injection of DNA expressing vascular endothelial growth factor (VEGF) in a myocardial infarction model in the rat—Angiogenesis and angioma formation. *J. Am. Coll. Cardiol.* **2000**, *35*, 1323–1330. [CrossRef]
15. Fukumura, D.; Xu, L.; Chen, Y.; Gohongi, T.; Seed, B.; Jain, R.K. Hypoxia and acidosis independently up-regulate vascular endothelial growth factor transcription in brain tumors in vivo. *Cancer Res.* **2001**, *61*, 6020–6024. [PubMed]
16. Shima, D.T.; Adamis, A.P.; Ferrara, N.; Yeo, K.T.; Yeo, T.K.; Allende, R.; Folkman, J.; D'Amore, P.A. Hypoxic induction of endothelial cell growth factors in retinal cells: Identification and characterization of vascular endothelial growth factor (VEGF) as the mitogen. *Mol. Med.* **1995**, *1*, 182–193. [CrossRef] [PubMed]
17. Wang, J. Neutrophils in tissue injury and repair. *Cell Tissue Res.* **2018**, *371*, 531–539. [CrossRef]
18. Du Cheyne, C.; Tay, H.; De Spiegelaere, W. The complex TIE between macrophages and angiogenesis. *Anat. Histol. Embryol.* **2020**, *49*, 585–596. [CrossRef]
19. Scapini, P.; Morini, M.; Tecchio, C.; Minghelli, S.; Di Carlo, E.; Tanghetti, E.; Albini, A.; Lowell, C.; Berton, G.; Noonan, D.M.; et al. CXCL1/macrophage inflammatory protein-2-induced angiogenesis in vivo is mediated by neutrophil-derived vascular endothelial growth factor-A. *J. Immunol.* **2004**, *172*, 5034–5040. [CrossRef]
20. Scapini, P.; Calzetti, F.; Cassatella, M.A. On the detection of neutrophil-derived vascular endothelial growth factor (VEGF). *J. Immunol. Methods* **1999**, *232*, 121–129. [CrossRef]
21. Gaudry, M.; Brégerie, O.; Andrieu, V.; El Benna, J.; Pocidalo, M.A.; Hakim, J. Intracellular pool of vascular endothelial growth factor in human neutrophils. *Blood* **1997**, *90*, 4153–4161. [CrossRef]
22. Stockmann, C.; Kirmse, S.; Helfrich, I.; Weidemann, A.; Takeda, N.; Doedens, A.; Johnson, R.S. A wound size-dependent effect of myeloid cell-derived vascular endothelial growth factor on wound healing. *J. Investig. Dermatol.* **2011**, *131*, 797–801. [CrossRef]
23. Nissen, N.N.; Polverini, P.J.; Koch, A.E.; Volin, M.V.; Gamelli, R.L.; DiPietro, L.A. Vascular endothelial growth factor mediates angiogenic activity during the proliferative phase of wound healing. *Am. J. Pathol.* **1998**, *152*, 1445–1452.
24. Berse, B.; Brown, L.F.; Van de Water, L.; Dvorak, H.F.; Senger, D.R. Vascular permeability factor (vascular endothelial growth factor) gene is expressed differentially in normal tissues, macrophages, and tumors. *Mol. Biol. Cell* **1992**, *3*, 211–220. [CrossRef] [PubMed]
25. Limbourg, A.; Korff, T.; Napp, L.C.; Schaper, W.; Drexler, H.; Limbourg, F.P. Evaluation of postnatal arteriogenesis and angiogenesis in a mouse model of hind-limb ischemia. *Nat. Protoc.* **2009**, *4*, 1737–1746. [CrossRef]

26. Kübler, M.; Beck, S.; Fischer, S.; Götz, P.; Kumaraswami, K.; Ishikawa-Ankerhold, H.; Lasch, M.; Deindl, E. Absence of Cold-Inducible RNA-Binding Protein (CIRP) Promotes Angiogenesis and Regeneration of Ischemic Tissue by Inducing M2-Like Macrophage Polarization. *Biomedicines* **2021**, *9*, 395. [CrossRef] [PubMed]
27. Götz, P.; Braumandl, A.; Kübler, M.; Kumaraswami, K.; Ishikawa-Ankerhold, H.; Lasch, M.; Deindl, E. C3 Deficiency Leads to Increased Angiogenesis and Elevated Pro-Angiogenic Leukocyte Recruitment in Ischemic Muscle Tissue. *Int. J. Mol. Sci.* **2021**, *22*, 5800. [CrossRef]
28. Kübler, M.; Beck, S.; Peffenköver, L.L.; Götz, P.; Ishikawa-Ankerhold, H.; Preissner, K.T.; Fischer, S.; Lasch, M.; Deindl, E. The Absence of Extracellular Cold-Inducible RNA-Binding Protein (eCIRP) Promotes Pro-Angiogenic Microenvironmental Conditions and Angiogenesis in Muscle Tissue Ischemia. *Int. J. Mol. Sci.* **2021**, *22*, 9484. [CrossRef]
29. Helisch, A.; Wagner, S.; Khan, N.; Drinane, M.; Wolfram, S.; Heil, M.; Ziegelhoeffer, T.; Brandt, U.; Pearlman, J.D.; Swartz, H.M.; et al. Impact of mouse strain differences in innate hindlimb collateral vasculature. *Arterioscler. Thromb. Vasc. Biol.* **2006**, *26*, 520–526. [CrossRef]
30. Scholz, D.; Ziegelhoeffer, T.; Helisch, A.; Wagner, S.; Friedrich, C.; Podzuweit, T.; Schaper, W. Contribution of arteriogenesis and angiogenesis to postocclusive hindlimb perfusion in mice. *J. Mol. Cell Cardiol.* **2002**, *34*, 775–787. [CrossRef] [PubMed]
31. Chillo, O.; Kleinert, E.C.; Lautz, T.; Lasch, M.; Pagel, J.-I.; Heun, Y.; Troidl, K.; Fischer, S.; Caballero-Martinez, A.; Mauer, A.; et al. Perivascular Mast Cells Govern Shear Stress-Induced Arteriogenesis by Orchestrating Leukocyte Function. *Cell Rep.* **2016**, *16*, 2197–2207. [CrossRef] [PubMed]
32. Morse, H.C. *Origins of Inbred Mice*; Academic Press: Cambridge, MA, USA, 1978.
33. Lee, J.J.; Arpino, J.M.; Yin, H.; Nong, Z.; Szpakowski, A.; Hashi, A.A.; Chevalier, J.; O'Neil, C.; Pickering, J.G. Systematic In-terrogation of Angiogenesis in the Ischemic Mouse Hind Limb: Vulnerabilities and Quality Assurance. *Arterioscler. Thromb. Vasc. Biol.* **2020**, *40*, 2454–2467. [CrossRef] [PubMed]
34. Bot, I.; Velden, D.V.; Bouwman, M.; Kröner, M.J.; Kuiper, J.; Quax, P.H.A.; de Vries, M.R. Local Mast Cell Activation Pro-motes Neovascularization. *Cells* **2020**, *9*, 701. [CrossRef]
35. Seignez, C.; Phillipson, M. The multitasking neutrophils and their involvement in angiogenesis. *Curr. Opin. Hematol.* **2017**, *24*, 3–8. [CrossRef]
36. Castanheira, F.V.S.; Kubes, P. Neutrophils and NETs in modulating acute and chronic inflammation. *Blood* **2019**, *133*, 2178–2185. [CrossRef] [PubMed]
37. Wang, J.; Hossain, M.; Thanabalasuriar, A.; Gunzer, M.; Meininger, C.; Kubes, P. Visualizing the function and fate of neutro-phils in sterile injury and repair. *Science* **2017**, *358*, 111–116. [CrossRef]
38. Ardi, V.C.; Kupriyanova, T.A.; Deryugina, E.I.; Quigley, J.P. Human neutrophils uniquely release TIMP-free MMP-9 to pro-vide a potent catalytic stimulator of angiogenesis. *Proc. Natl. Acad. Sci. USA* **2007**, *104*, 20262–20267. [CrossRef] [PubMed]
39. Gong, Y.; Koh, D.-R. Neutrophils promote inflammatory angiogenesis via release of preformed VEGF in an in vivo corneal model. *Cell Tissue Res.* **2009**, *339*, 437–448. [CrossRef]
40. Christoffersson, G.; Vågesjö, E.; Vandooren, J.; Lidén, M.; Massena, S.; Reinert, R.B.; Brissova, M.; Powers, A.C.; Opdenakker, G.; Phillipson, M. VEGF-A recruits a proangiogenic MMP-9-delivering neutrophil subset that induces angiogenesis in trans-planted hypoxic tissue. *Blood* **2012**, *120*, 4653–4662. [CrossRef]
41. Kolaczkowska, E.; Kubes, P. Neutrophil recruitment and function in health and inflammation. *Nat. Rev. Immunol.* **2013**, *13*, 159–175. [CrossRef]
42. Mittal, M.; Siddiqui, M.R.; Tran, K.; Reddy, S.P.; Malik, A.B. Reactive Oxygen Species in Inflammation and Tissue Injury. *Antioxid. Redox Signal.* **2014**, *20*, 1126–1167. [CrossRef]
43. Aldabbous, L.; Abdul-Salam, V.; McKinnon, T.; Duluc, L.; Pepke-Zaba, J.; Southwood, M.; Ainscough, A.J.; Hadinnapola, C.; Wilkins, M.R.; Toshner, M.; et al. Neutrophil Extracellular Traps Promote Angiogenesis: Evidence From Vascular Pathology in Pul-monary Hypertension. *Arterioscler. Thromb. Vasc. Biol.* **2016**, *36*, 2078–2087. [CrossRef] [PubMed]
44. Rohrbach, A.S.; Slade, D.J.; Thompson, P.R.; Mowen, K.A. Activation of PAD4 in NET formation. *Front. Immunol.* **2012**, *3*, 360. [CrossRef] [PubMed]
45. Zawrotniak, M.; Rapala-Kozik, M. Neutrophil extracellular traps (NETs)—Formation and implications. *Acta Biochim. Pol.* **2013**, *60*, 277–284. [CrossRef]
46. Binet, F.; Cagnone, G.; Crespo-Garcia, S.; Hata, M.; Neault, M.; Dejda, A.; Wilson, A.M.; Buscarlet, M.; Mawambo, G.T.; Howard, J.P.; et al. Neutrophil extracellular traps target senescent vasculature for tissue remodeling in retinopathy. *Science* **2020**, *369*, eaay5356. [CrossRef]
47. Lefrançais, E.; Mallavia, B.; Zhuo, H.; Calfee, C.S.; Looney, M.R. Maladaptive role of neutrophil extracellular traps in patho-gen-induced lung injury. *JCI Insight* **2018**, *3*, e98178. [CrossRef]
48. Wong, S.L.; Demers, M.; Martinod, K.; Gallant, M.; Wang, Y.; Goldfine, A.B.; Kahn, C.R.; Wagner, D.D. Diabetes primes neu-trophils to undergo NETosis, which impairs wound healing. *Nat. Med.* **2015**, *21*, 815–819. [CrossRef]
49. Murray, P.J. Macrophage Polarization. *Annu. Rev. Physiol.* **2017**, *79*, 541–566. [CrossRef] [PubMed]
50. Wynn, T.A.; Vannella, K.M. Macrophages in Tissue Repair, Regeneration, and Fibrosis. *Immunity* **2016**, *44*, 450–462. [CrossRef] [PubMed]
51. Gurevich, D.; Severn, C.; Twomey, C.; Greenhough, A.; Cash, J.; Toye, A.M.; Mellor, H.; Martin, P. Live imaging of wound angiogenesis reveals macrophage orchestrated vessel sprouting and regression. *EMBO J.* **2018**, *37*, e97786. [CrossRef]

52. Zhang, J.; Muri, J.; Fitzgerald, G.; Gorski, T.; Gianni-Barrera, R.; Masschelein, E.; D'Hulst, G.; Gilardoni, P.; Turiel, G.; Fan, Z.; et al. Endothelial Lactate Controls Muscle Regeneration from Ischemia by Inducing M2-like Macrophage Polarization. *Cell Metab.* **2020**, *31*, 1136.e7–1153.e7. [CrossRef]
53. Willenborg, S.; Lucas, T.; Van Loo, G.; Knipper, J.; Krieg, T.; Haase, I.; Brachvogel, B.; Hammerschmidt, M.; Nagy, A.; Ferrara, N.; et al. CCR2 recruits an inflammatory macrophage subpopulation critical for angiogenesis in tissue repair. *Blood* **2012**, *120*, 613–625. [CrossRef]
54. Dort, J.; Fabre, P.; Molina, T.; Dumont, N.A. Macrophages Are Key Regulators of Stem Cells during Skeletal Muscle Re-generation and Diseases. *Stem Cells Int.* **2019**, *2019*, 4761427. [CrossRef] [PubMed]
55. Gordon, S.; Martinez, F.O. Alternative Activation of Macrophages: Mechanism and Functions. *Immunity* **2010**, *32*, 593–604. [CrossRef] [PubMed]
56. Zajac, E.; Schweighofer, B.; Kupriyanova, T.A.; Juncker-Jensen, A.; Minder, P.; Quigley, J.P.; Deryugina, E.I. Angiogenic capacity of M1- and M2-polarized macrophages is determined by the levels of TIMP-1 complexed with their secreted proMMP-9. *Blood* **2013**, *122*, 4054–4067. [CrossRef]
57. Moore, E.M.; West, J.L. Harnessing Macrophages for Vascularization in Tissue Engineering. *Ann. Biomed. Eng.* **2018**, *47*, 354–365. [CrossRef]
58. Gordon, S.; Taylor, P. Monocyte and macrophage heterogeneity. *Nat. Rev. Immunol.* **2005**, *5*, 953–964. [CrossRef]
59. Pollard, J.W. Trophic macrophages in development and disease. *Nat. Rev. Immunol.* **2009**, *9*, 259–270. [CrossRef]
60. Troidl, C.; Jung, G.; Troidl, K.; Hoffmann, J.; Mollmann, H.; Nef, H.; Schaper, W.; Hamm, C.W.; Schmitz-Rixen, T. The tem-poral and spatial distribution of macrophage subpopulations during arteriogenesis. *Curr. Vasc. Pharmacol.* **2013**, *11*, 5–12. [CrossRef] [PubMed]
61. Lasch, M.; Kleinert, E.C.; Meister, S.; Kumaraswami, K.; Buchheim, J.-I.; Grantzow, T.; Lautz, T.; Salpisti, S.; Fischer, S.; Troidl, K.; et al. Extracellular RNA released due to shear stress controls natural bypass growth by mediating mechanotransduction in mice. *Blood* **2019**, *134*, 1469–1479. [CrossRef]
62. Olfert, I.M.; Baum, O.; Hellsten, Y.; Egginton, S. Advances and challenges in skeletal muscle angiogenesis. *Am. J. Physiol. Heart Circ. Physiol.* **2016**, *310*, H326–H336. [CrossRef] [PubMed]

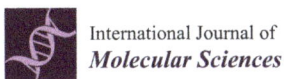

Article

The Absence of Extracellular Cold-Inducible RNA-Binding Protein (eCIRP) Promotes Pro-Angiogenic Microenvironmental Conditions and Angiogenesis in Muscle Tissue Ischemia

Matthias Kübler [1,2], Sebastian Beck [1,2], Lisa Lilian Peffenköver [3], Philipp Götz [1,2], Hellen Ishikawa-Ankerhold [1,4], Klaus T. Preissner [3], Silvia Fischer [3], Manuel Lasch [1,2,5] and Elisabeth Deindl [1,2,*]

1. Walter-Brendel-Centre of Experimental Medicine, University Hospital, Ludwig-Maximilians-Universität München, 81377 Munich, Germany; Matthias.Kuebler@med.uni-muenchen.de (M.K.); sebastian.beck@med.uni-muenchen.de (S.B.); P.Goetz@med.uni-muenchen.de (P.G.); Hellen.Ishikawa-Ankerhold@med.uni-muenchen.de (H.I.-A.); manuel_lasch@gmx.de (M.L.)
2. Biomedical Center, Institute of Cardiovascular Physiology and Pathophysiology, Ludwig-Maximilians-Universität München, 82152 Planegg-Martinsried, Germany
3. Department of Biochemistry, Faculty of Medicine, Justus Liebig University, 35392 Giessen, Germany; Lilli.Peffenkoever@gmail.com (L.L.P.); Klaus.T.Preissner@biochemie.med.uni-giessen.de (K.T.P.); Silvia.Fischer@biochemie.med.uni-giessen.de (S.F.)
4. Department of Internal Medicine I, Faculty of Medicine, University Hospital, Ludwig-Maximilians-Universität München, 81377 Munich, Germany
5. Department of Otorhinolaryngology, Head and Neck Surgery, University Hospital, Ludwig-Maximilians-Universität München, 81377 Munich, Germany
* Correspondence: Elisabeth.Deindl@med.uni-muenchen.de; Tel.: +49-(0)89-2180-76504

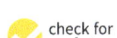

Abstract: Extracellular Cold-inducible RNA-binding protein (eCIRP), a damage-associated molecular pattern, is released from cells upon hypoxia and cold-stress. The overall absence of extra- and intracellular CIRP is associated with increased angiogenesis, most likely induced through influencing leukocyte accumulation. The aim of the present study was to specifically characterize the role of eCIRP in ischemia-induced angiogenesis together with the associated leukocyte recruitment. For analyzing eCIRPs impact, we induced muscle ischemia via femoral artery ligation (FAL) in mice in the presence or absence of an anti-CIRP antibody and isolated the gastrocnemius muscle for immunohistological analyses. Upon eCIRP-depletion, mice showed increased capillary/muscle fiber ratio and numbers of proliferating endothelial cells (CD31$^+$/CD45$^-$/BrdU$^+$). This was accompanied by a reduction of total leukocyte count (CD45$^+$), neutrophils (MPO$^+$), neutrophil extracellular traps (NETs) (MPO$^+$CitH3$^+$), apoptotic area (ascertained via TUNEL assay), and pro-inflammatory M1-like polarized macrophages (CD68$^+$/MRC1$^-$) in ischemic muscle tissue. Conversely, the number of regenerative M2-like polarized macrophages (CD68$^+$/MRC1$^+$) was elevated. Altogether, we observed that eCIRP depletion similarly affected angiogenesis and leukocyte recruitment as described for the overall absence of CIRP. Thus, we propose that eCIRP is mainly responsible for modulating angiogenesis via promoting pro-angiogenic microenvironmental conditions in muscle ischemia.

Keywords: angiogenesis; cold-inducible RNA-binding protein; extracellular cold-inducible RNA-binding protein; CIRP; eCIRP; neutrophil extracellular traps; NETs; macrophage polarization; inflammation; apoptosis; ischemia

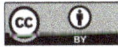

1. Introduction

The cold-inducible RNA binding protein (CIRP) is a member of the glycine-rich RNA-binding protein family, including several proteins which regulate nucleic acid interactions through their RNA-binding sites [1,2]. The expression of intracellular CIRP (iCIRP) in various cell types, particularly in immune cells, is induced in response to diverse cellular stresses such as mild hypothermia, hypoxia, or oxidative stress, and in response, the intracellular protein can be translocated from the nucleus to the cytoplasm [1,3–7]. In particular, as a reaction to hypoxia, in hemorrhagic shock and other ischemia-related pathologies, iCIRP translocates from the cytoplasm towards the extracellular space (possibly via lysosomal secretion) [8–12]. Once secreted, extracellular CIRP (eCIRP) acts as a damage-associated molecular pattern (DAMP) molecule, leading to tissue damage and aggravation of inflammation [8]. eCIRP activates a wide range of immune cells, such as neutrophils and macrophages, via the "Toll-like receptor 4" (TLR4)-myeloid differentiation factor 2 (MD2)-complex as well as via the "Triggering receptor expressed on myeloid cells 1" (TREM-1). These interactions result in amplified inflammatory processes through the release of pro-inflammatory cytokines and chemokines [8,13,14].

The absence of eCIRP in most of the studied ischemic disease-related animal models was correlated with a significant mitigation of the investigated inflammatory reaction, while the injection of recombinant CIRP led to liver and lung injury [10,15–19]. Furthermore, patients brought to the intensive care unit due to hemorrhagic shock or sepsis presented with a significantly higher survival chance when serum levels of CIRP were low [8,20]. Hence, the modulation of eCIRP's bioavailability may provide a novel approach in therapeutic drug treatment in the immune regulation of different inflammatory-dependent pathologies.

Several RNA-binding proteins (RBP) have been implicated in the post-transcriptional regulation of mRNAs involved in the processes of angiogenesis [21–23]. Angiogenesis describes the generation of new capillaries from a pre-existing capillary network, particularly in response to ischemia, necessary for embryonic development as well as for wound healing, menstruation, or pregnancy in healthy adults [24–27]. The predominant pro-angiogenic cytokine involved in these processes is vascular endothelial growth factor A (VEGF-A) [24,28,29], whose expression is induced in ischemic tissues under the control of a molecular oxygen-sensor, present in virtually all cell types [30,31]. Following endothelial cell activation, extracellular matrix remodeling by proteases and anastomosis formation of capillary beds, regulatory humoral factors, as well as immune cells (particularly macrophages) contribute to the orchestration and control of angiogenesis [24].

To increase the capillarity of an ischemic tissue, there are two different mechanisms through which angiogenesis can proceed: (a) splitting the capillaries of a pre-existing microvasculature network, a process which is denoted as intussusceptive angiogenesis; (b) de novo formation of new capillary branches by migration and proliferation of endothelial cells, a mechanism that is referred to as sprouting angiogenesis [25,32,33]. Besides physiological angiogenesis, uncontrolled pathological angiogenesis drives solid tumor growth, psoriasis, or diabetic retinopathy [24,26,27,34–36], where the indicated factors appear to operate in an uncontrolled manner. Concerning vascular diseases, like myocardial infarction or peripheral artery disease, the process of angiogenesis alone is not sufficient to restore the blood supply in the affected ischemic areas [37]. In this case, capillary growth is promoted to clear the cell debris congregated at the site of ischemia. Instead, only the process of arteriogenesis, the growth transformation of pre-existing vessels acting as natural bypasses in response to increased shear-stress, can compensate for the occlusion of a nutrient supplying artery [38–42].

Particularly myeloid cells, such as neutrophils and macrophages, but also blood platelets, are major sources of VEGF-A and other vascular remodeling factors like matrix metalloproteinases (MMPs) that regulate the bioavailability of VEGF-A and participating in vessel formation and the clearance of cell debris at the ischemic tissue site [43–47]. As a consequence, the accumulation and activation of different leukocyte subpopulations in certain vascular regions may directly influence the outcome of angiogenic vessel formation.

Neutrophil extracellular traps (NETs), comprised of the decondensed extracellular chromatin network of activated neutrophils, and necessary for catching and killing of microbes in innate immunity, were found to positively affect angiogenesis in a preclinical model of pulmonary hypertension through the upregulation of intercellular adhesion molecule 1 (ICAM-1) expression, affecting VEGF-signaling and endothelial cell migration [48].

Recently, a new subset of pro-inflammatory neutrophils that could be triggered by eCIRP under septic conditions were shown to express high levels of C-X-X chemokine receptor type 4 (CXCR4), ICAM-1, inducible nitric oxide synthase (iNOS), reactive oxygen species (ROS), and NETs [49]. Furthermore, eCIRP was described to excessively induce NET formation by activating the "Triggering receptor expressed on myeloid cells 1" (TREM-1) in a Rho-GTPase-dependent manner and via the upregulated expression of "Peptidylarginine deiminase 4" (PAD4), which catalyzes the citrullination of histones as an essential step in NET formation to decondense the cellular chromatin [50–53].

Idrovo et al. (2016) found a significant improvement of wound healing of skin lesions in CIRP-deficient mice as compared to wild-type mice. The elevated inflammatory state (such as changes in tumor necrosis factor-α (TNF-α) dynamics, reduced numbers of Gr1$^+$ leukocytes) was accompanied by an elevated number of CD31$^+$ cells, resulting in the hypothesis that the absence of CIRP could improve tissue regeneration and angiogenesis [54]. Moreover, iCIRP was suggested to regulate the post-transcriptional processing of specific microRNAs of the 14q32 locus, which are known to be involved in regulating ischemia-induced angiogenesis [55,56]. It was shown that the blocking of miR-329, a microRNA belonging to the 14q32 cluster and a possible target of post-transcriptional processing of CIRP, enhanced the expression of CD146, a co-receptor of VEGF receptor 2 (VEGFR-2) on endothelial cells, also to ameliorate angiogenic processes [56–58].

Recently, we showed in a murine hindlimb model that the genetic ablation of CIRP (including eCIRP and iCIRP) improves angiogenesis and the regeneration of ischemic tissue damage, most likely through the predominance of regenerative anti-inflammatory M2-like polarized macrophages and the reduced accumulation of neutrophils and NETs [59]. Whether these changes in leukocyte recruitment, macrophage polarization, and ameliorated angiogenesis are attributed to the lack of intra- or extracellular CIRP remains unclear so far. In the present study, we have analyzed the ramifications of blocking eCIRP on ischemia-induced angiogenesis and cell apoptosis together with the accompanied leukocyte infiltration and macrophage polarization in order to demonstrate that eCIRP appears to be sufficient to modulate the efficacy of angiogenesis in vivo.

2. Results

To analyze the impact of the lack of eCIRP on the process of angiogenesis in ischemic muscle tissue, a well-established murine hindlimb model was used. Following femoral artery ligation (FAL), the formation of collateral blood vessels (arteriogenesis) is initiated in the adductor muscle of the upper leg, and in ischemia-induced angiogenesis in the gastrocnemius muscle of the lower leg, due to the reduced blood flow [60]. After intravenous injection of mice with a neutralizing anti-CIRP antibody prior to and following FAL (every second day) [9], gastrocnemius muscles were collected for immunohistological analyses at day 1 and day 7 after FAL. An isotype antibody or phosphate-buffered saline (PBS), respectively, was used in the control groups.

In order to investigate whether the depletion of eCIRP affects angiogenesis, a CD31/CD45/BrdU/DAPI quadruple immunofluorescence staining on tissue sections collected 7 days after FAL was performed. CD31 was implemented as an endothelial cell marker, CD45 was used as a pan-leukocyte marker to exclude CD31$^+$ leukocytes. To exclude platelets from the quantification (which also express CD31), only CD31$^+$ cells that colocalized with a signal for nuclear DNA (DAPI) were counted. Hence, CD31$^+$/CD45$^-$/DAPI$^+$ cells were defined as capillary endothelial cells. Bromodeoxyuridine (BrdU) was used as a proliferation marker. To quantitate the extent of angiogenesis, the number of capillaries per muscle fiber ratio was determined [61]. Compared to both control groups (isotype antibody-and PBS-treated mice), the anti-CIRP antibody-treated group showed a significant increase in capillary/muscle fiber ratio (Figure 1a,b). Furthermore, an elevated ratio of proliferating capillaries (CD31$^+$/CD45$^-$/BrdU$^+$/DAPI$^+$) per muscle fiber was found in anti-CIRP antibody-treated mice compared to both control groups (Figure 1a,c). Isotype antibody- and PBS-treated mice did not show any statistically significant difference between their capillarity and proliferating endothelial cells per muscle fiber. In tissue samples of non-ischemic (sham-operated) gastrocnemius muscles no significant difference in capillary per muscle fiber ratio between all treatment groups was noted (data not shown).

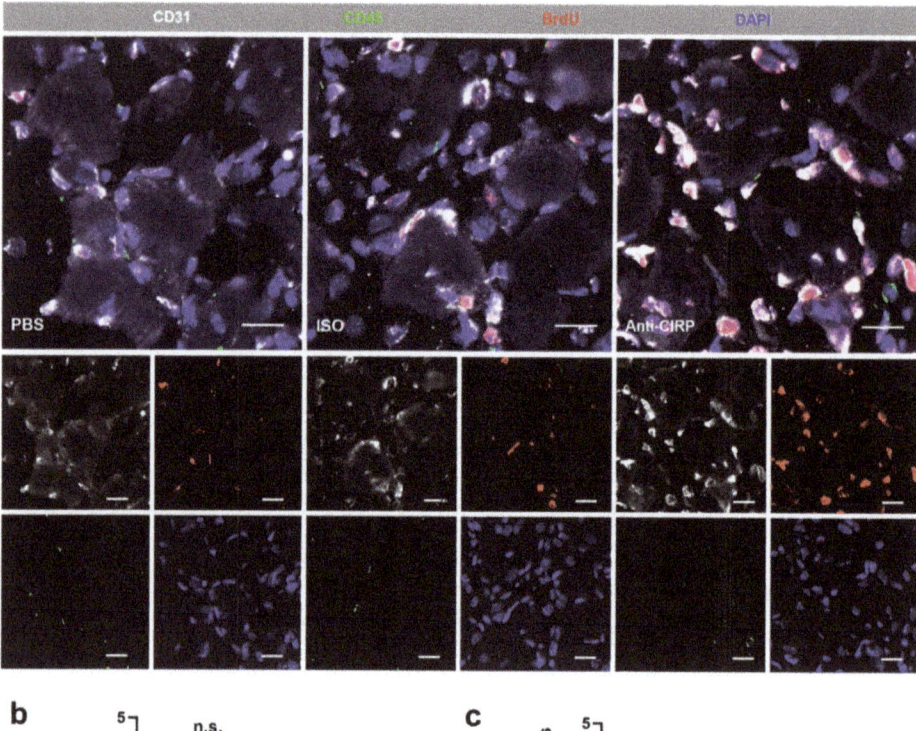

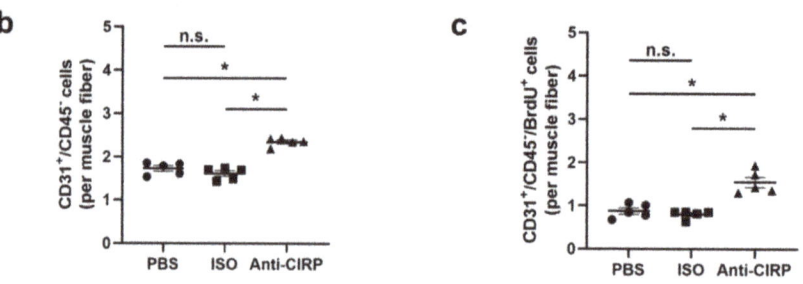

Figure 1. Lack of extracellular "Cold-inducible RNA-binding protein" (eCIRP) enhances capillary growth. (**a**) Representative immunofluorescence stains of ischemic gastrocnemius muscle slices from control mice (treated with phosphate-buffeCDred saline (PBS) or isotype antibody (ISO)), and mice which received anti-CIRP antibody (Anti-CIRP) 7 days after femoral artery ligation (FAL). Smaller images show single channels, large images show all merged channels of endothelial cells (anti-CD31, white), proliferating cells (anti-BrdU (bromodeoxyuridine), red), leukocytes (anti-CD45, green), and nucleic acid (DAPI, blue). Scale bars represent 20 µm. Scatter plots displaying (**b**) $CD31^+/CD45^-$ (endothelial) cells and (**c**) $CD31^+/CD45^-/BrdU^+$ (proliferating endothelial) cells per muscle fiber of ischemic gastrocnemius muscles of PBS-, ISO- (both control groups), and anti-CIRP antibody-treated mice 7 days after FAL. Data are means ± S.E.M., n.s. $p > 0.05$, * $p < 0.05$ (PBS vs. ISO vs. anti-CIRP) by one-way ANOVA with the Tukey's multiple comparisons test, a defined ischemic area (1.5 mm^2) of muscle tissue was analyzed per mouse.

Upon treatment of microvascular endothelial cells in vitro with recombinant murine CIRP (rmCIRP), a significant reduction in fetal calf serum (FCS)-initiated cell proliferation was seen (Figure S1). Moreover, after rmCIRP treatment of cells, the mRNA levels of the inflammatory genes interleukin 6 (IL-6) and monocyte chemoattractant protein-1 (MCP-1) were significantly elevated, whereas the expression level of CIRP did not change (Figure S2).

Leukocytes, such as neutrophils and macrophages, play a regulatory role in ischemia-induced inflammation through the removal of cellular debris, the promotion of tissue repair, and their direct influence on vascular proliferation by supplying a broad range of growth factors. In response to the neutralization of eCIRP in the anti-CIRP antibody-treated mice on day 7 after FAL, the number of infiltrated CD45$^+$ cells in ischemic areas was significantly decreased as compared to both control groups (Figure 2a,b). In all non-ischemic (sham-operated) muscle tissues of each group, no difference in the numbers of infiltrated CD45$^+$ cells was found (data not shown).

In order to assess the influence of eCIRP neutralization on the accumulation of different neutrophil subpopulations and their specific products (such as NETs) in ischemic muscle tissue sections, double immuno-staining at day 1 after FAL for myeloperoxidase (MPO) (to detect neutrophils) and for citrullinated histone H3 (CitH3) (to detect NETs) was performed. MPO$^+$/DAPI$^+$ cells were classified as neutrophils and MPO$^+$/CitH3$^+$/DAPI$^+$ cells were considered as NETs. A significantly reduced number of both, neutrophils and NETs, was seen in tissue samples of mice treated with anti-CIRP antibody compared to the two control groups (Figure 3a,b,d). Also, the portion of neutrophils forming NETs in comparison to the total neutrophil count was significantly reduced in anti-CIRP antibody-treated mice (Figure 3c,d). No differences were observed between all control groups in non-ischemic (sham-operated) muscle tissue sections (data not shown).

Based on the observation that eCIRP-induced NETs have an impact on efferocytotic clearance of apoptotic cells by macrophages [62], the extent of apoptotosis in ischemic muscle tissue sections 7 days after FAL was assessed by using a TdT-mediated dUTP-biotin neck end labeling (TUNEL) assay. A significant reduction of the apoptotic area in gastrocnemius muscle sections from the anti-CIRP antibody-treated group was found compared to the isotype antibody-treated and PBS-treated control groups, respectively (Figure 4a–c). There was no sign of apoptosis in the isolated non-ischemic (sham-operated) gastrocnemius muscles from all groups (data not shown).

The influence of the neutralization of eCIRP on macrophage accumulation and polarization was analyzed by using anti-CD68 antibody staining to label macrophages as well as anti-MRC1 (mannose receptor C-type 1) antibody to identify M2-like polarized macrophages. Consequently, CD68$^+$/MRC1$^-$/DAPI$^+$ cells were counted as M1-like polarized macrophages, while CD68$^+$/MRC1$^+$/DAPI$^+$ cells were assessed as M2-like polarized macrophages. No significant differences in macrophage accumulation at the site of ischemia of gastrocnemius muscles, collected 7 days after FAL, were observed between all three different treatment groups (Figure 5a,d). However, a significantly higher portion of M2-like polarized macrophages and a significant reduction in the portion of M1-like polarized macrophages in the ischemic muscle tissue in anti-CIRP antibody-treated mice was found (Figure 5b–d). Gastrocnemius muscles of all experimental groups isolated from the contralateral sham-operated (non-ischemic) site did not show any significant difference in macrophage accumulation and polarization (data not shown).

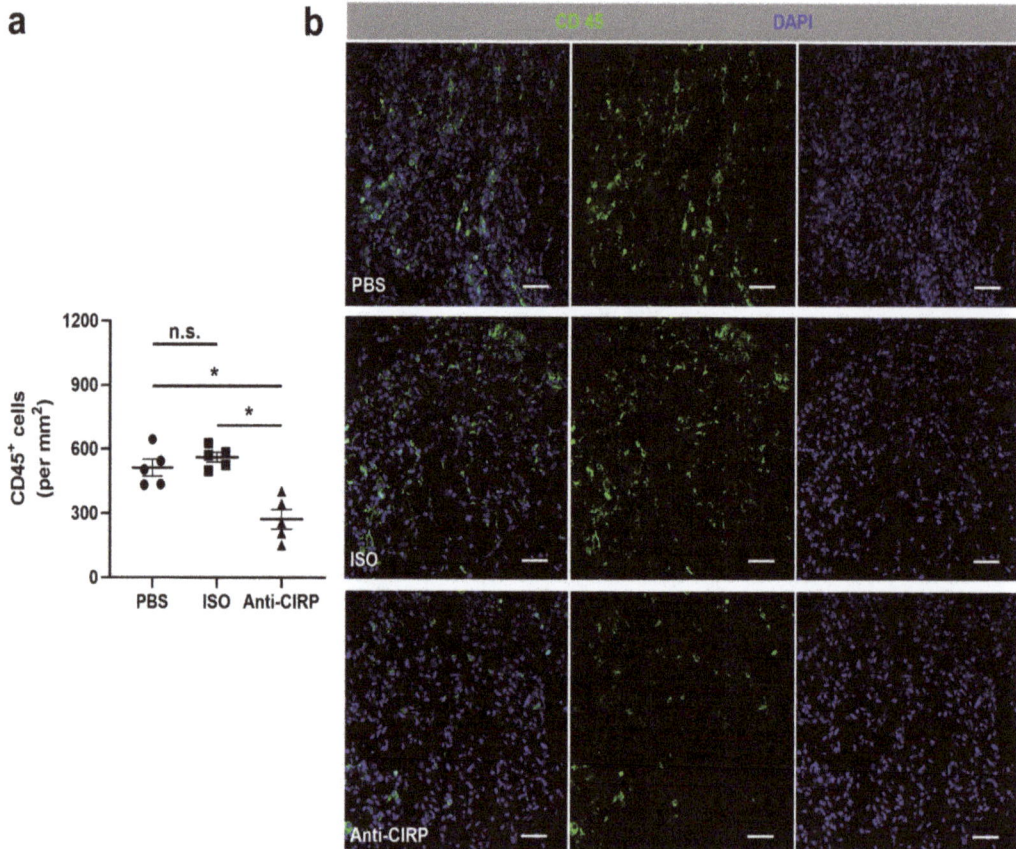

Figure 2. Neutralization of extracellular "Cold-inducible RNA-binding protein" (eCIRP) decreases leukocyte accumulation in ischemic tissue. (**a**) The scatter plot displays the relative number of CD45$^+$ (pan-leukocyte marker) cells (per mm^2) in the ischemic gastrocnemius muscles of mice that received phosphate-buffered saline (PBS), isotype antibody (ISO) (control groups), or the anti-CIRP antibody (Anti-CIRP) and were sacrificed 7 days after femoral artery ligation (FAL). Data are means ± S.E.M., n = 5 per group. n.s. p > 0.05, * p < 0.05 (PBS vs. ISO vs. Anti-CIRP) by one-way ANOVA with the Tukey's multiple comparisons test, a defined ischemic area (1.5 mm^2) of muscle tissue was analyzed per mouse. (**b**) Representative immunofluorescence staining of ischemic gastrocnemius muscles of mice treated with PBS (top), isotype antibody (middle), or anti-CIRP antibody (bottom) 7 days after FAL. Cells were stained with an antibody against CD45 (green) and DAPI (blue) to label nucleic DNA. Scale bars represent 50 μm.

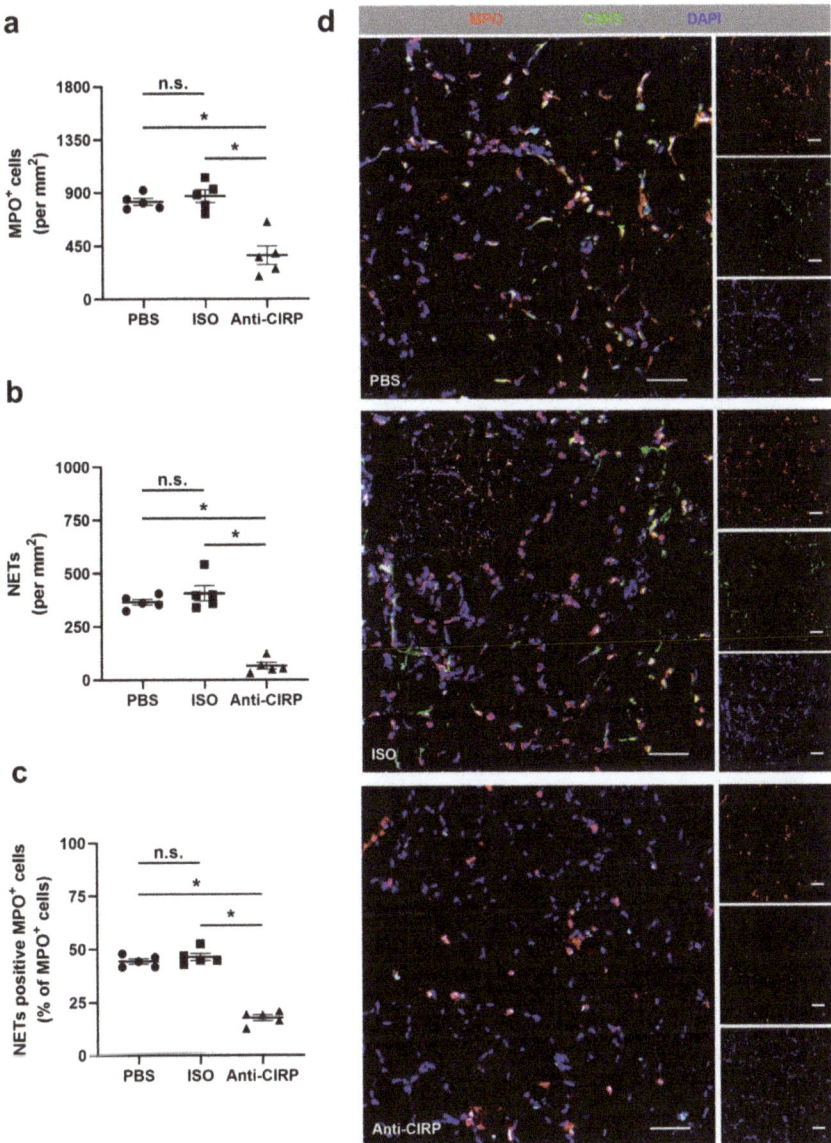

Figure 3. Depletion of extracellular "Cold-inducible RNA-binding protein" (eCIRP) interferes with neutrophil recruitment and neutrophil extracellular trap (NET) formation in ischemic muscle tissue. The scatter plots display the number of (**a**) MPO$^+$ (myeloperoxidase, marker for neutrophils) cells, (**b**) NETs (MPO$^+$/CitH3$^+$ (citrullinated histone 3)/DAPI$^+$) (both per mm^2), and (**c**) NET positive MPO$^+$ cells per total MPO$^+$ cells in ischemic gastrocnemius muscles isolated from phosphate-buffered saline- (PBS), isotype antibody- (ISO) (control groups) and anti-CIRP antibody- (Anti-CIRP) treated mice, isolated on day 1 after femoral artery ligation (FAL). Data are means ± S.E.M., n = 5 per group. n.s. $p > 0.05$, * $p < 0.05$ (PBS vs. ISO vs. Anti-CIRP) by one-way ANOVA with the Tukey's multiple comparisons test, a defined ischemic area (1.5 mm^2) of muscle tissue was analyzed per mouse. (**d**) Representative immunofluorescence staining of ischemic gastrocnemius muscle slices of PBS- (top), isotype antibody- (middle), and anti-CIRP antibody-treated mice (bottom) collected 1 day after FAL. Images display single and merged channels of neutrophils (MPO$^+$/DAPI$^+$) and NETs (MPO$^+$/CitH3$^+$/DAPI$^+$) labeled with anti-MPO (red), anti-CitH3 (green), and DAPI (nucleic acid, blue). Scale bars represent 50 µm.

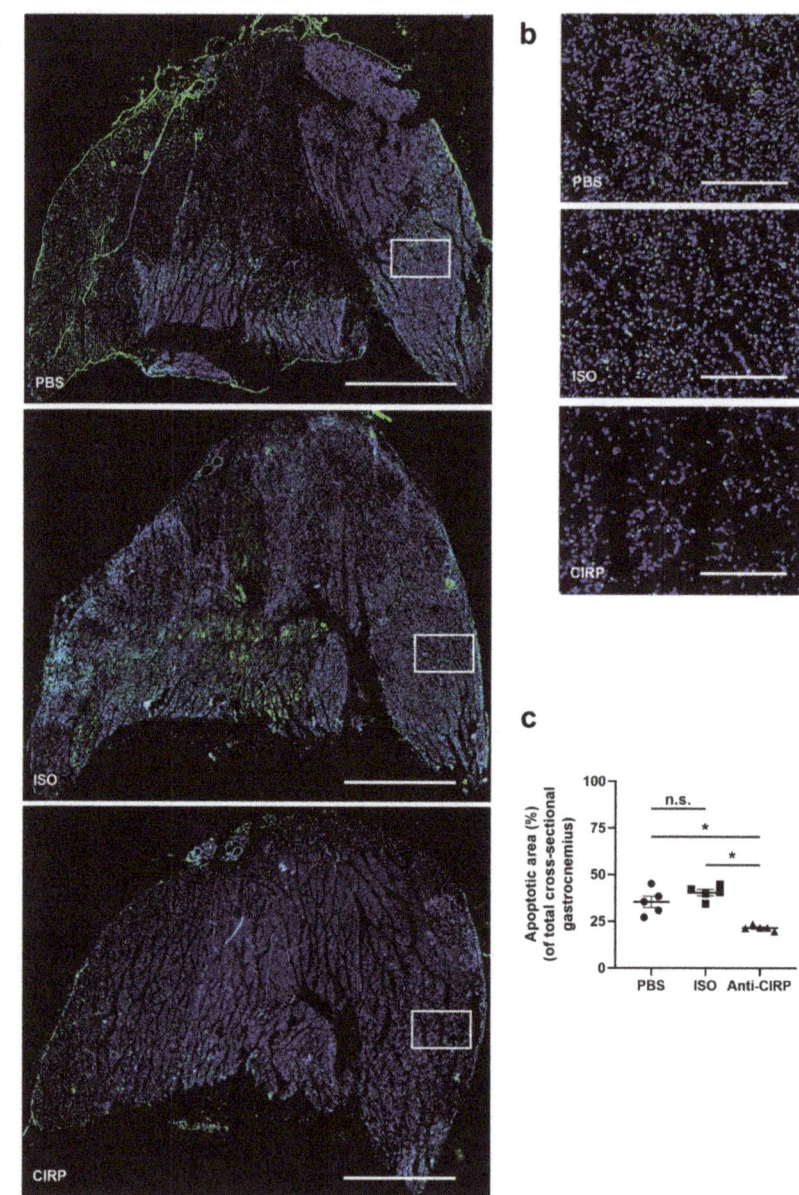

Figure 4. Depletion of extracellular "Cold-inducible RNA-binding protein" (eCIRP) mitigates apoptosis. (**a**) Representative pictures of TUNEL-stained gastrocnemius muscle slices of mice, treated with phosphate-buffered saline (PBS) (top), isotype antibody (ISO) (middle) (both control groups), and anti-CIRP antibody (Anti-CIRP) (bottom) 7 days after femoral artery ligation (FAL). Scale bars represent 50 μm. (**b**) Magnification of white boxes in (**a**), showing TUNEL-stained apoptotic cells (green). Scale bars represent 7 μm. (**c**) The scatter plot displays the extent of the apoptotic areas in relation to the whole gastrocnemius muscle of PBS-, ISO-, and anti-CIRP antibody-treated mice 7 days after FAL. The total gastrocnemius cross-sectional area (about 20 mm^2) was analyzed. Data are means ± S.E.M., n = 5 per group. n.s. $p > 0.05$, * $p < 0.05$ (PBS vs. ISO vs. Anti-CIRP) by one-way ANOVA with the Tukey's multiple comparisons test.

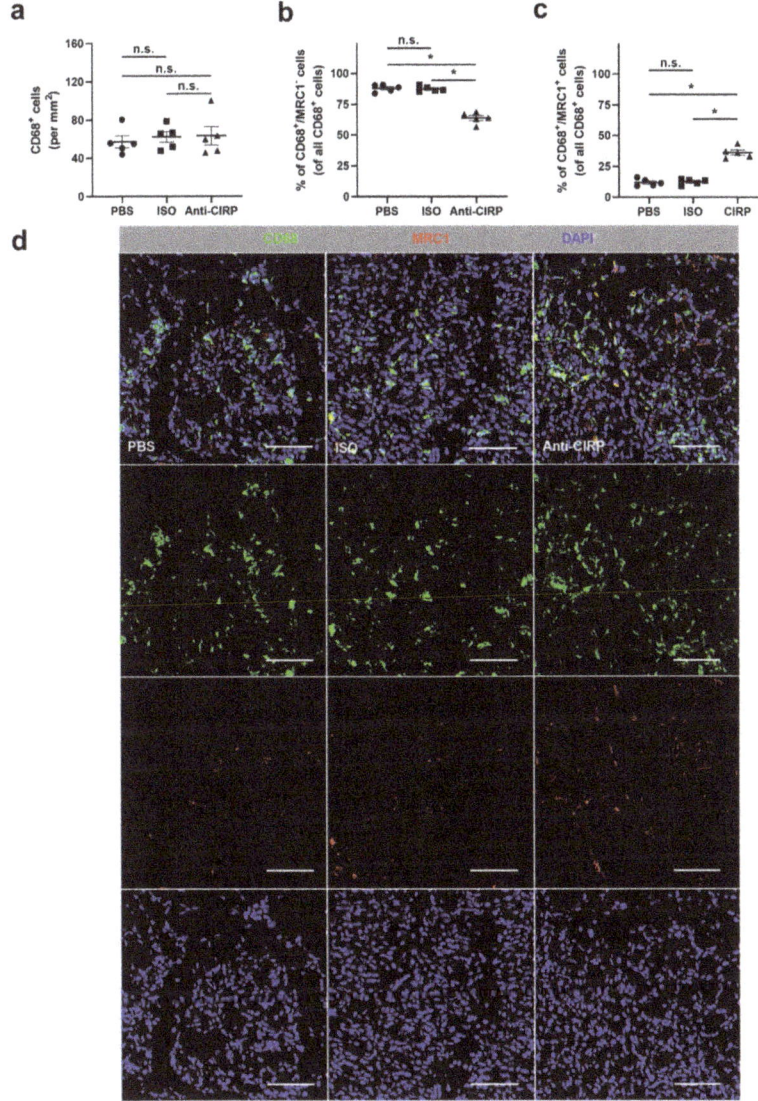

Figure 5. Neutralization of extracellular "Cold-inducible RNA-binding protein" (eCIRP) affects macrophage polarization. The scatter plots display (**a**) the relative amount of CD68$^+$ cells (macrophages) (per mm^2), (**b**) CD68$^+$/MRC1$^-$ (mannose receptor c-type 1) cells (M1-like polarized macrophages), and (**c**) CD68$^+$/MRC1$^+$ cells (M2-like polarized macrophages) in relation to all CD68$^+$ cells (in percent) in ischemic gastrocnemius muscles of phosphate-buffered saline- (PBS), isotype antibody- (ISO) (both control groups), or anti-CIRP antibody-treated mice (Anti-CIRP) 7 days after femoral artery ligation (FAL). Data are means ± S.E.M., n = 5 per group. n.s. $p > 0.05$, * $p < 0.05$ (PBS vs. ISO vs. Anti-CIRP) by one-way ANOVA with the Tukey's multiple comparisons test, a defined ischemic area (1.5 mm^2) of muscle tissue was analyzed per mouse. (**d**) Representative immunofluorescence staining of ischemic gastrocnemius muscle slices of PBS- (left), isotype antibody- (middle), and anti-CIRP-antibody-treated mice (right) 7 days after FAL. Images show single and merged channels of CD68 and MRC1 labeled macrophages (anti-CD68, green; anti-MRC1, red) and nucleic acid (DAPI, blue). Scale bars represent 50 μm.

3. Discussion

In the current study, the impact of the neutralization of extracellular CIRP (eCIRP) on angiogenesis and the associated leukocyte accumulation in a murine hindlimb model of muscle ischemia was investigated. The depletion of eCIRP resulted in ameliorated angiogenesis, evidenced by an increased capillary to muscle fiber ratio, as well as a reduction of the total apoptotic area in gastrocnemius muscle of mice treated with an anti-CIRP antibody. These responses might be due to a significant reduction in leukocyte accumulation, particularly neutrophil infiltration and NET formation, and a pronounced influence on macrophage polarization, although the number of infiltrated macrophages was not altered in ischemic gastrocnemius. In anti-CIRP antibody-treated mice a predominance of the anti-inflammatory M2-like polarized macrophages at the ischemic muscle tissue site was observed, as compared to control mice (for an overview see Figure 6). Overall, the blockade of eCIRP enhanced angiogenesis in vivo, reminiscent of results obtained in CIRP-deficient mice [59], to indicate that eCIRP is mainly responsible for modulating angiogenesis.

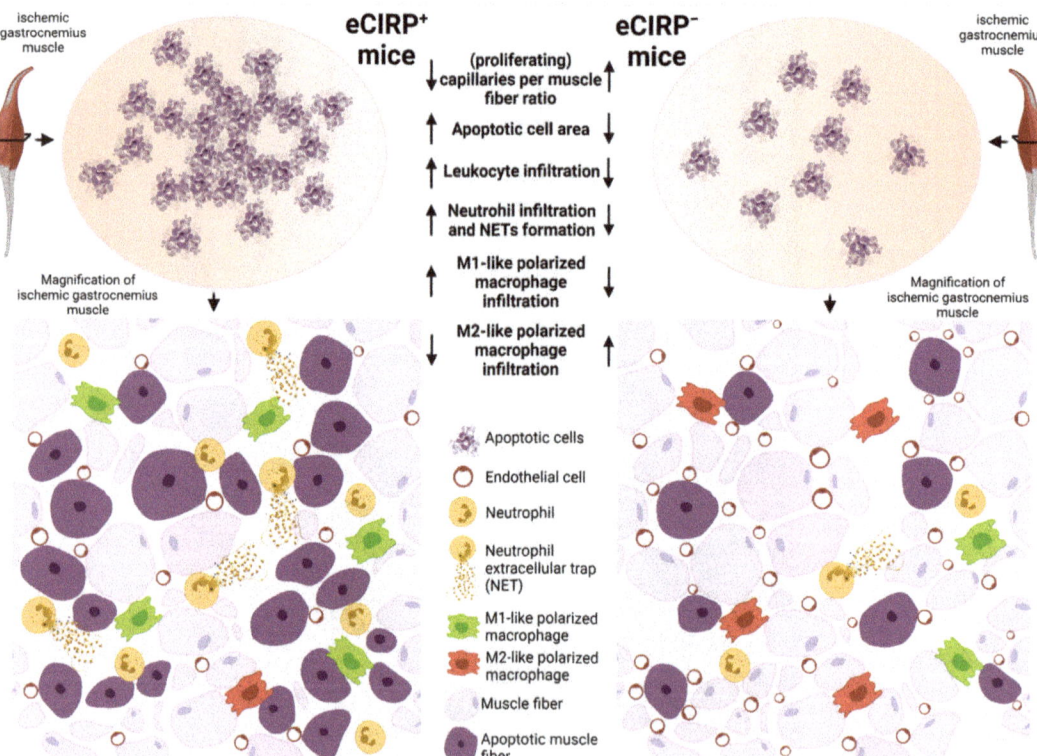

Figure 6. Depletion of extracellular "Cold-inducible RNA-binding protein" (eCIRP) promotes ischemia-induced angiogenesis and affects the associated leukocyte infiltration. In comparison to control mice, which still harbor eCIRP, mice with neutralized eCIRP showed an increased (proliferating) capillaries per muscle fiber ratio, reduced areas of apoptotic cells, reduced leukocyte infiltration with lower numbers of neutrophils, neutrophils that produce neutrophil extracellular traps (NETs), and pro-inflammatory M1-like polarized macrophages, whereas the number of infiltrative anti-inflammatory regenerative M2-like polarized macrophages was elevated. Thus, eCIRP-depleted mice show an ameliorated angiogenic capacity upon ischemia, mediated through a more pro-angiogenic inflammatory environment.

It has been described that the deficiency of CIRP in mice did affect angiogenesis in association with different pathologies [54,56]. We recently demonstrated that the overall absence of CIRP, intra- and extracellularly, resulted in ameliorated angiogenesis in muscle ischemia [59]. As evidenced by immunohistological analysis, the present study now shows that the blockade of eCIRP resulted in an elevated capillary to muscle fiber ratio and a raised proliferating capillary to muscle fiber ratio, thus improving angiogenesis. Furthermore, we confirmed our in vivo findings, as the administration of rmCIRP on microvascular endothelial cells abolished their FCS-induced proliferation in vitro. Consequently, for the first time it is shown that the neutralization of eCIRP by the administration of a specific antibody in the indicated mouse model resulted in ameliorated angiogenesis. Hence, the improved angiogenesis in CIRP-deficient mice is largely attributable to their lack of eCIRP.

Since connections between eCIRP as DAMP and immune cells are well described [63,64], we evaluated the influence of eCIRP depletion on leukocyte accumulation at the site of the ischemic gastrocnemius muscle tissue. In fact, a significant reduction in leukocyte accumulation, particularly neutrophils, at the site of muscle ischemia was observed when eCIRP was blocked.

In the context of angiogenesis and tissue reorganization, infiltrative leukocytes, predominantly neutrophils and macrophages, are known to be essential sources of pro-angiogenic growth factors, including VEGF-A, and several proteases, such as matrix metalloproteinase 9 (MMP9) which are important modulators of the extracellular matrix remodeling [43,47,65–67]. The diminished numbers of leukocytes are likely attributable to the lack of eCIRP as an inflammatory DAMP. eCIRP activates both macrophages and neutrophils via its direct binding to the pattern recognition receptor (PRR) TLR4-MD2-complex, resulting in nuclear factor 'kappa-light-chain-enhancer' of activated B-cells (NF-κB) activation and nuclear translocation, or to the TREM-1, thereby activating the tyrosine kinase Syk to ultimately catalyze the release of pro-inflammatory chemokines and cytokines, relevant for the exacerbation of inflammation and the enhancement of leukocyte recruitment [8,13,14,68]. Leukocyte accumulation and transmigration into the damaged tissue might be further facilitated by eCIRP´s propensity to increase vascular permeability and to activate endothelial cells, causing additional pro-inflammatory chemoattractant release and an upregulation of cell-surface adhesion molecules like endothelial-selectin (E-selectin) and ICAM-1 [19]. In addition, the administration of rmCIRP was shown to strongly induce the expression of inflammatory genes in microvascular endothelial cells in vitro. Consequently, the blocking of eCIRP could be responsible for a reduced accumulation of leukocytes at the site of the ischemic muscle tissue due to the absence of eCIRP´s pro-inflammatory properties as a DAMP and an attenuated extravasation induced by a more stable endothelial cell barrier and a decreased upregulation of cell-surface adhesion molecules.

It is important to mention that an excessive and prolonged accumulation of leukocytes at the site of inflammation can lead to aggravated tissue damage and thus may interfere with ischemic tissue restitution [47,65,69]. The blockade of eCIRP in many other pathologies had an attenuating influence on the inflammation in animal models, while low eCIRP levels in septic patients correlated with improved survival chances. By comparing the ischemic muscle tissue of CIRP-deficient and wild-type mice, we found a significant reduction in leukocyte accumulation in the CIRP knockout mice [59]. Accordingly, we propose that the decreased leukocyte infiltration in CIRP-deficient mice is mainly attributed to the lack of eCIRP. Whether iCIRP plays a role in leukocyte accumulation and its affection on immune cells in general, possibly through miRNA interactions or via binding of intracellular PRRs like nucleotide-binding, oligomerization domain (NOD)-like receptors (NLRs) or the RIG-like helicases (RLHs), must be elucidated in further in-depth immunology studies.

In the early phase of tissue damage, neutrophils infiltrate the ischemic tissue as one of the first innate immune cell types, playing an essential role in orchestrating angiogenesis and inflammation [66]. Comparable to macrophages, they are also capable of phagocyting apoptotic cells, thus clearing cell debris from the damaged tissue areas and consequently participating in tissue homeostasis restitution. Particularly important, neutrophils significantly influence the initiation of angiogenesis, since neutropenic mice showed impaired induction of angiogenesis [70]. Most likely, neutrophils participate in angiogenesis initiation through their direct allocation of preformed VEGF-A and other growth factors [44,45]. Their supply of active MMP9 and the protease-associated deconstruction of the extracellular matrix leads to further release of former matrix-bound VEGF-A and consequently to angiogenic sprouting [46,71]. Besides delivering VEGF-A to the ischemic site, activated neutrophils release a wide range of pro-inflammatory cytokines and chemokines, leading to the disruption of the endothelial cell barrier and further leukocyte recruitment, ultimately exacerbating the inflammation in damaged tissue [72]. For a long time, neutrophils were thought to be the major cause for aggravated and prolonged muscle injury [73]. Recent studies discounted this by proving that the blockade of neutrophils interfered with tissue restoration processes in muscle injury [74,75]. Hence, neutrophil-associated damage in muscle tissue could be substantial for recovery processes. After clearing cell debris, modulating inflammation, and initiating angiogenesis, neutrophils do not get phagocyted by macrophages but may reenter the vasculature by a process declared as reverse transendothelial migration [76].

Although neutrophils are important players in initiating angiogenesis, in our study, we found reduced numbers of neutrophils in eCIRP-depleted mice which, however, exhibited increased capillarity. We made similar observations in CIRP-knockout mice [59]. Furthermore, decreased neutrophil recruitment in anti-CIRP antibody-treated mice was also observed in a model of hepatic ischemia and reperfusion injury [9]. In our study, the diminished number of accumulated neutrophils observed 24 h after FAL in eCIRP-depleted mice might not be related to an overall reduction of neutrophil infiltration at all. It could reflect an augmented reverse transendothelial migration after phagocytosis of cell debris, initiation of angiogenesis, culminating in the orchestration of inflammation. Interestingly, under septic conditions, eCIRP was found to induce reverse transendothelial migration [77]. Yet, in contrast to sterile inflammation, reverse transendothelial migration of neutrophils in sepsis does not contribute to tissue reconstitution. Instead, neutrophils reentering the circulation in sepsis may further fuel inflammatory reactions and lead to dissemination of a local towards a systemic inflammation [77]. Whether the increased number of neutrophils in control mice that harbor eCIRP rather reflects an unrestrained inflammation as opposed to the effective induction of angiogenesis and whether the lack of eCIRP possibly ameliorates neutrophil reverse transendothelial migration in ischemia-dependent tissue damage are two possible processes that deserve further analysis.

In the present study, we found a significant reduction of NETs and NET-forming neutrophils in mice treated with the anti-CIRP antibody compared to the control groups. These observations are in line with previous findings, showing that DAMPs in general and eCIRP in particular are potent inducers of NET formation [50–52,78]. Interestingly, eCIRP promotes the induction of a specific pro-inflammatory subtype of neutrophils, expressing ICAM-1, and are characterized among others through their increased formation of NETs [52]. Moreover, we found decreased NET formation in ischemic muscle tissue of CIRP-deficient mice as well [59]. Whether NETs released by pro-inflammatory ICAM-1$^+$ neutrophils have the same effect on angiogenesis needs to be addressed in further investigations. Here, it is important to mention that NETs have been described not only to be associated with ongoing inflammation, angiogenesis, and vascular regeneration but are also causative for aggravated inflammation and thus evoke exacerbated tissue damage and delayed tissue restitution [79–83]. Therefore, we propose that the depletion of eCIRP may promote a more pro-angiogenic type of NET formation, contributing to tissue remodeling in the ischemic mice muscle.

A recent study on sepsis showed that NET formation, caused by eCIRP, limited efferocytosis [62]. Efferocytosis describes the process by which apoptotic cells are cleared by phagocytic cells, such as macrophages, and provides a prerequisite for resolving inflammation [84]. Efferocytotic clearance of apoptotic cells stimulates anti-inflammatory and pro-regenerating signals, marking the start of the tissue remodeling phase [84]. To ascertain whether abated efferocytosis also affected apoptotic processes in our study, we implemented a TUNEL assay to measure the area of apoptotic cells throughout the entire sections of the gastrocnemius muscle. The observation that reduced apoptotic areas in eCIRP-depleted mice were found may reflect an improved efferocytosis in these animals. Accordingly, excessive NET formation in control mice would not promote angiogenesis but would prolong the inflammatory phase leading to enhanced leukocyte recruitment. In contrast, apoptotic areas in eCIRP-depleted mice would be cleared much faster and could lead to an earlier start of the subsequent tissue remodeling phase. Whether the diminished areas of apoptotic cell death in the ischemic muscles of eCIRP-depleted mice are a direct consequence of eCIRP's effect on efferocytosis or are caused by another independent mechanism needs to be elucidated.

After the initial inflammatory phase, mainly characterized by the infiltration of neutrophils, macrophages accumulate at the site of ischemic muscle tissue damage, and have a significant impact on angiogenesis [24,47,85–87]. It is important to note that macrophages are a heterogeneous cell population, presenting high plasticity, reflected by their variable polarization states [88,89]. Therefore, the M1- and M2-like polarization status classification only marks extremes in a broad spectrum of possible differentiations.

Initially, M0-like polarized monocytes infiltrate the damaged tissue and locally mature to classically activated pro-inflammatory M1-like ($CD68^+$/$MRC1^-$) polarized macrophages. Macrophages showing this pro-inflammatory polarization state are responsible for phagocytosis and further leukocyte recruitment. In terms of angiogenesis, macrophages representing the M1-like polarized phenotype are associated with the supply of pro-angiogenic factors, such as VEGF-A and TNF-α, thus being relevant for the induction of angiogenesis [90]. It has been shown that M1-like polarized macrophages cumulate around endothelial tip cells, guiding the new sprouts, whereas the absence of pro-inflammatory macrophages resulted in the thwarted instigation of angiogenesis [91].

Following this, the pro-inflammatory M1-like polarization state changes towards an alternatively activated regenerative anti-inflammatory M2-like polarized phenotype, marking the beginning of the subsequent tissue restoration phase to resolve the inflammatory process [92–94]. In contrast to M1-like polarized macrophages, M2-like polarized macrophages play a crucial role in initiating matrix remodeling; while the M1-like polarized phenotype can only release an inactive complexed form of the matrix protease MMP9, M2-like polarized macrophages release an active form of MMP9 [95]. Consequently, the anti-inflammatory M2-like polarized phenotype mirrors the classical pro-angiogenic polarization state correlating with matrix remodeling, resolution of inflammation, and tissue repair [47,96].

Previous studies of our own group showed that administration of recombinant CIRP induced the expression of M1-like but not M2-like polarization markers on macrophages in vitro. Moreover, we found a predominance of M2-like polarized macrophages in ischemic muscle tissue in CIRP-deficient mice without any altered general macrophage accumulation compared to wild-type control mice [59]. In the present study, we observed similar findings, i.e., a significant increase in M2-like and a significant reduction in M1-like polarized macrophages with no changes in the total number of macrophages accumulated in ischemic muscle tissue of eCIRP-depleted mice compared to control mice. The increased number of M2-like polarized macrophages in mice that underwent eCIRP depletion possibly indicates that these mice—in contrast to control mice that still show a high number of infiltrating M1-like polarized macrophages—have already moved from the initial inflammatory phase towards the tissue regenerating phase.

In accordance with our in vitro results along with published information, the high number of M1-like polarized macrophages in control mice may be related to three different responses, triggered by eCIRP: (a) eCIRP promotes the expression of pro-inflammatory M1-like polarization markers in macrophages; (b) eCIRP strongly induces the expression of the pro-inflammatory genes IL-6 and MCP-1 in microvascular endothelial cells. The latter reaction will result in increased immune cell migration and infiltration, especially for monocytes, to the site of inflammation [97]. Moreover, since a deficiency of MCP-1 was described to enhance M2-like polarization in macrophages [98], a reduced expression of MCP-1 in mice lacking eCIRP could lead to a reduced induction of pro-inflammatory M1-like polarized macrophages in eCIRP-deficient mice. Also, an eCIRP-dependent release of pro-inflammatory chemokines and cytokines from a wide range of cells has been described [63]. Thus, a pro-inflammatory environment, induced by eCIRP´s propensity as a DAMP, is likely to promote the pro-inflammatory M1-like polarization status in macrophages and could lead to the observed high number of neutrophils, NETs, and the leukocyte infiltration at the site of ischemic muscle tissue. (c) As already mentioned above, eCIRP induces a particular subtype of NETs that are described to impair macrophage efferocytosis and thus may prolong the inflammatory phase. Therefore, the decreased amount of phagocyting M1-like polarized macrophages in combination with decreased apoptotic areas in eCIRP-blocked mice could reflect an improved macrophage efferocytosis and consequently an enhanced transition from the inflammatory to the tissue restitution phase.

Recently, a protective effect in ischemic stroke was reported for an eCIRP-derived peptide, which interferes with eCIRP´s binding ability to the MD2 receptor, resulting in a significant reduction of the ischemic infarct area as well as the inhibition of apoptosis and necroptosis in murine and rhesus monkey models [99]. This experimental approach highlights an important milestone in designing CIRP-related therapeutic treatments for ischemia-related pathologies.

With the present study, we demonstrated that several observations regarding angiogenesis and the associated leukocyte recruitment in CIRP-deficient mice also hold true for eCIRP-blocked mice. Thus, we propose that the lack of CIRP´s extracellular properties, especially as an inflammatory DAMP, are mainly responsible for the increased angiogenic process we have found in CIRP-deficient mice. Taken together, the administration of eCIRP-depleting drugs may be a valuable approach to modulate inflammatory processes and to improve angiogenesis in ischemic muscle tissue via the induction of M2-like macrophage polarization.

4. Materials and Methods

4.1. Animals and Treatments

All experimental setups were permitted by the Bavarian Animal Care and Use Committee (ethical approval code: ROB-55.2Vet-2532.Vet_02-17-99, approved on 8 December 2017) and were conducted in strict accordance with the German animal legislation guidelines. Mice were fed a standard laboratory diet and were housed in a temperature-controlled room on a 12 h light–dark cycle. For all experiments, adult male SV-129 (Charles River Laboratories, Sulzfeld, Germany) mice, aged 8–12 weeks, were sacrificed at 24 h or 7 days ($n = 5$ per group) after the surgical procedure. 30 minutes prior to surgical intervention, mice were either treated i.v. with a neutralizing anti-CIRP antibody (Abcam, ab106230, Cambridge, UK, 1 mg/kg), an isotype antibody (Abcam, ab37373, 1 mg/kg), or phosphate-buffered saline (PBS, PAN Biotech, Aidenbach, Germany, pH 7.4, 1 mL/kg) and then two, four and six days after surgery. To ascertain the proliferation rate of endothelial cells in the lower hindlimb 7 days after surgery, SV-129 mice were daily injected with 100 µL BrdU (bromodeoxyuridine) (Sigma-Aldrich, St. Louis, MO, USA) (12.5 mg/mL BrdU in PBS) i.p., starting directly after the surgical intervention.

4.2. Femoral Artery Ligation and Tissue Processing

To promote angiogenesis in the gastrocnemius muscle of the lower hindlimb, unilateral femoral artery ligation (FAL) was performed on the right femoral artery while the left artery was sham-operated and served as an internal control, as previously described [60]. Twenty minutes in advance of the surgical procedure, mice were anesthetized with a combination of fentanyl (0.05 mg/kg, CuraMED Pharma, Karlsruhe, Germany), midazolam (5.0 mg/kg, Ratiopharm GmbH, Ulm, Germany), and medetomidine (0.5 mg/kg, Pfister Pharma, Berlin, Germany). Prior to tissue sampling, 24 h or 7 days after FAL, mice were again anesthetized as described above. For tissue collection, the hindlimbs were perfused with adenosine buffer (1% adenosine (Sigma-Aldrich), 5% bovine serum albumin (BSA, Sigma-Aldrich), dissolved in PBS) and 3% paraformaldehyde (PFA, Merck, Darmstadt, Germany, dissolved in PBS). For immunohistology, both gastrocnemius muscles of each mouse were collected subsequently to perfusion, embedded in Tissue-Tek compound (Sakura Finetek Germany GmbH, Staufen, Germany), and cryopreserved at −80 °C.

4.3. Immunohistology

The cryopreserved gastrocnemius muscles from 24 h and 7 days after FAL were cut in 10 μm thick slices. For BrdU-staining, 1 N HCl was added to the cryosections in a humidified chamber at 37 °C for 30 min, followed by permeabilization with 0.2% Triton X-100 solution (AppliChem GmbH, Darmstadt, Germany) in 1 × PBS/0.1% Tween-20 (AppliChem GmbH)/0.5% BSA for 2 min, then blocked with 10% goat serum (Abcam, ab7481, Cambridge, UK) in 1 × PBS/0.1% Tween-20/0.5% BSA) for 1 h at room temperature (RT), and subsequently incubated with the primary anti-BrdU-antibody (Abcam, ab6326, dilution 1:50 in 10% goat serum) at 4 °C overnight. For secondary staining, the cryosections were treated with a goat anti-rat Alexa Fluor®-546 antibody (Invitrogen, Thermo Fischer Scientific, A-11081, Carlsbad, CA, USA, dilution 1:100) for 1 h at RT. Following secondary blocking with 1 × PBS/0.1% Tween-20/4% BSA for 30 min at RT, the sections were incubated with an anti-CD31-Alexa Fluor® 647 antibody (Biolegend, 102516, San Diego, CA, USA, dilution 1:50 in 1 × PBS/0.1% Tween-20) applied to label endothelial cells, together with an anti-CD45-Alexa Fluor® 488 antibody anti-CD45-Alexa Fluor® 488 antibody (BioLegend, 11-0451-85, dilution 1:100 in 1 × PBS/0.1% Tween-20) implemented as a pan-leukocyte marker for 2 h at RT.

Macrophages were stained with an anti-CD68-Alexa Fluor® 488 antibody (Abcam, ab201844, dilution 1:200 in PBS), which was co-incubated with an anti-MRC1 antibody (Abcam, ab64693, dilution 1:200 in PBS) as a macrophage polarization marker, at 4 °C overnight. Secondary antibody staining was performed with a donkey-anti-rabbit Alexa Fluor® 546 (Invitrogen, A-10040) for 1 h at RT.

To label NETs in tissue collected 24 h after FAL, cryosections were firstly permeabilized with 0.2% Triton X-100 solution in 1 × PBS/0.1% Tween-20/0.5% BSA for 2 min, followed by blocking with 10% donkey serum (Abcam, ab7475) in 1 × PBS/0.1% Tween-20/0.5% BSA for 1 h at RT and then incubated with the primary antibodies anti-myeloperoxidase (MPO; R&D Systems, AF3667, Minneapolis, MN, USA, dilution 1:20 in 10% donkey serum in 1 × PBS/0.1% Tween-20/0.5% BSA) and anti-citrullinated histone H3 antibody (Cit-H3; polyclonal rabbit anti-Histone H3 (citrulline R2 + R8 + R17), Abcam, ab5103, dilution 1:100 in 10% donkey serum in 1 × PBS/0.1% Tween-20/0.5% BSA) at 4 °C overnight. Secondary antibody staining was performed with a donkey anti-goat Alexa Fluor® 594 (Invitrogen, A-11058, dilution 1:100 in 1 × PBS/0.1% Tween-20) and a donkey anti-rabbit Alexa Fluor® 488 antibody (Invitrogen, A-21206, dilution 1:200 in 1 × PBS/0.1% Tween-20) for 1 h at RT.

To quantify apoptotic cells throughout the gastrocnemius muscle sections, we used an ApopTag® Plus Fluorescein in Situ Apoptosis Detection Kit (EMD Millipore Corp., Burlington, MA, USA) according to the manufacturers' instruction. Additionally, all cryosections were counter-stained with DAPI (Thermo Fisher Scientific, 62248, dilution 1:1000 in PBS) for labeling of nucleic DNA for 10 min at RT.

An antifade mounting medium (Dako, Agilent, Santa Clara, CA, USA) was applied to mount the stained tissue samples. Gastrocnemius cryosections from ischemic (occluded) and non-ischemic (sham-operated) side harvested 24 h after FAL was used for neutrophil and NETs labeling, while tissue collected 7 days after FAL were stained for capillaries, leukocytes, macrophages, and apoptotic cells.

For microscopic analysis, we used a confocal laser scanning microscope LSM 880 (Carl-Zeiss Jena GmbH, Jena, Germany) with a 20× objective (415 μm × 415 μm) as well as an epifluorescence microscope (Leica DM6 B, Leica microsystems, Wetzlar, Germany) with a 20× objective (630 μm × 475μm). For each muscle section, we analyzed 5 defined fields of view to count cells, muscle fibers, and NETs. To ascertain the areas of apoptotic cells (%), the total gastrocnemius muscle area and the apoptotic cell areas were measured and compared. CD31/CD45/BrdU/DAPI and apoptosis staining were investigated with the epifluorescence microscope. CD68/MRC1/DAPI and MPO/CitH3/DAPI stains were analyzed with the confocal laser scanning microscope. Cell counting, as well as analysis of the apoptotic muscle area, were conducted using ImageJ software with the Cell Counting and Region of Interest plugins. We calculated the capillary ($CD31^+$/$CD45^-$ cells were considered endothelial cells) per muscle fiber ratio as described before to evaluate the processes of angiogenesis [61].

4.4. Cell Culture and Proliferation Assays

The myocardial endothelial MyEnd cell line was grown in Dulbecco's modified Eagle medium (DMEM, Gibco, Darmstadt, Germany) with 10% fetal calf serum (FCS) and 1% penicillin/streptomycin (100 U/mL and 100 mg/mL, Sigma-Aldrich). The MyEnd cells showed typical endothelial properties and, as they grew to complete confluence, were highly positive for the endothelial marker CD31 [100].

The viability of cells was determined using the CellTiter 96™ non-radioactive cell proliferation assay from Promega (Mannheim, Germany). The cells were seeded on 96-well culture plates and cultured for 4 h. Prior to stimulation, cells were washed once with phosphate-buffered saline (PBS) and incubated in serum-free cell culture medium containing different concentrations of recombinant murine CIRP (Hölzel Diagnostika, Köln, Germany). After 24 h, one solution reagent from Promega was added and the amount of the formazan product was measured by its absorbance at 500 nm, which corresponds to the number of viable cells. Absorbance measured in the absence of rmCIRP was set to 100%.

4.5. Quantitative Real-Time PCR (qPCR)

Following treatment of MyEND with different concentrations of rmCIRP as indicated in the legends of the corresponding figure, cells were washed twice with PBS, lysed, and RNA was isolated with the total RNA extraction kit (Peqlab). For qPCR analysis, 1 µg of RNA was reverse-transcribed using the High-Capacity cDNA Reverse Transcription Kit (Applied Biosystems, Carlsbad, CA, USA) and DNA amplification was performed with a StepOne Plus cycler (Applied Biosystems) in a reaction volume of 10 µL using the SensiMix Sybr Kit (Bioline, Luckenwalde, Germany) with 50 pmol of each primer. To avoid the amplification of genomic DNA, primers were designed to span exon-exon junctions. The qPCR was performed under the following conditions: an initial denaturation step at 95 °C for 8.5 min followed by 45 cycles, consisting of denaturation (95 °C, 30 s), annealing (60 °C, 30 s) and elongation (72 °C, 30 s). Melt curve analysis was performed to control specific amplification. Results were normalized to the expression levels (E) of actin and expressed as the ratio of E(target)/E(Actin). The following mouse primers were used: IL-6 forward 5′-CTCTGCAAGAGACTTCCATCCA-3′; IL-6 reverse 5′-TTGGAAGTAGGGAAGGCCG-3′; MCP-1 forward 5′-AAGCTGTAGTTTTTGTCA CCAAGC-3′; MCP-1 reverse 5′-GACCTTAGGGCAGATGCAGTT-3′; CIRP forward 5′-CTACTATGCCAGCCGGAGTC; CIRP reverse 5′-GCTCTGAGGACACAAGGGTT-3′; ß-actin forward 5′-CGCGAGCACAGCTTCTTTG-3′; ß-actin reverse 5′-CGTCATCCAT GGCGAACTGG-3′.

4.6. Statistical Analysis

Statistical analyses were carried out and graphically plotted with GraphPad Prism 8 (GraphPad Software, La Jolla, CA, USA). Data are means ± standard error of the mean (S.E.M.). Statistical analyses were performed by using the one-way analysis of variance (ANOVA) with the Tukey's multiple comparisons test. The findings were considered statistically significant at $p < 0.05$.

4.7. Illustration

The illustration from Figure 6 was designed and rendered with BioRender.com.

Supplementary Materials: The following are available online at https://www.mdpi.com/article/10.3390/ijms22179484/s1.

Author Contributions: Conceptualization, M.K., S.F., M.L. and E.D.; Data curation, M.K., L.L.P. and S.F.; Formal analysis, M.K., L.L.P. and S.F.; Funding acquisition, E.D.; Investigation, M.K., L.L.P., S.F., M.L. and E.D.; Methodology, M.K., S.B., L.L.P., P.G., H.I.-A., S.F., M.L. and E.D.; Project administration, E.D.; Resources, M.K., S.B., P.G., H.I.-A., S.F. and E.D.; Software, M.K. and H.I.-A.; Supervision, M.K., L.L.P., K.T.P., S.F., M.L. and E.D.; Validation, M.K., L.L.P., S.F., M.L. and E.D.; Visualization, M.K.; Writing—original draft, M.K.; Writing—review & editing, M.K., H.I.-A., K.T.P., S.F., M.L. and E.D. All authors have read and agreed to the published version of the manuscript.

Funding: This research was funded by the Lehre@LMU program (M.K.), and the Förderprogramm für Forschung und Lehre (FöFoLe) (S.B., P.G.), both from the Ludwig-Maximilians-Universität, Munich, Germany and by the DFG- SFB 914 (Project Z01 to H.I.-A.).

Institutional Review Board Statement: The study was approved by the Institutional Review Board of Walter-Brendel-Centre of Experimental Medicine and the Bavarian Animal Care and Use Committee (ethical approval code: ROB-55.2Vet-2532.Vet_02-17-99).

Data Availability Statement: The data presented in this study is available on request from the first author.

Acknowledgments: The authors thank C. Eder and D. van den Heuvel for their technical assistance and A. Kübler, M. F. Frutos Marquez, J. Böhlhoff-Martin, and G. Di Todaro for their support in text editing.

Conflicts of Interest: The authors declare no conflict of interest.

References

1. Nishiyama, H.; Itoh, K.; Kaneko, Y.; Kishishita, M.; Yoshida, O.; Fujita, J. A Glycine-rich RNA-binding Protein Mediating Cold-inducible Suppression of Mammalian Cell Growth. *J. Cell Biol.* **1997**, *137*, 899–908. [CrossRef] [PubMed]
2. Thandapani, P.; O'Connor, T.R.; Bailey, T.L.; Richard, S. Defining the RGG/RG Motif. *Mol. Cell* **2013**, *50*, 613–623. [CrossRef]
3. De Leeuw, F.; Zhang, T.; Wauquier, C.; Huez, G.; Kruys, V.; Gueydan, C. The cold-inducible RNA-binding protein migrates from the nucleus to cytoplasmic stress granules by a methylation-dependent mechanism and acts as a translational repressor. *Exp. Cell Res.* **2007**, *313*, 4130–4144. [CrossRef]
4. Yang, R.; Zhan, M.; Nalabothula, N.R.; Yang, Q.; Indig, F.E.; Carrier, F. Functional Significance for a Heterogenous Ribonucleoprotein A18 Signature RNA Motif in the 3′-Untranslated Region of Ataxia Telangiectasia Mutated and Rad3-related (ATR) Transcript. *J. Biol. Chem.* **2010**, *285*, 8887–8893. [CrossRef]
5. Chen, X.; Liu, X.; Li, B.; Zhang, Q.; Wang, J.; Zhang, W.; Luo, W.; Chen, J. Cold Inducible RNA Binding Protein Is Involved in Chronic Hypoxia Induced Neuron Apoptosis by Down-Regulating HIF-1α Expression and Regulated By microRNA-23a. *Int. J. Biol. Sci.* **2017**, *13*, 518–531. [CrossRef]
6. Sumitomo, Y.; Higashitsuji, H.; Higashitsuji, H.; Liu, Y.; Fujita, T.; Sakurai, T.; Candeias, M.M.; Itoh, K.; Chiba, T.; Fujita, J. Identification of a novel enhancer that binds Sp1 and contributes to induction of cold-inducible RNA-binding protein (cirp) expression in mammalian cells. *BMC Biotechnol.* **2012**, *12*, 72. [CrossRef] [PubMed]
7. Yang, R.; Weber, D.J.; Carrier, F. Post-transcriptional regulation of thioredoxin by the stress inducible heterogenous ribonucleoprotein A18. *Nucleic Acids Res.* **2006**, *34*, 1224–1236. [CrossRef]
8. Qiang, X.; Yang, W.L.; Wu, R.; Zhou, M.; Jacob, A.; Dong, W.; Kuncewitch, M.; Ji, Y.; Yang, H.; Wang, H.; et al. Cold-inducible RNA-binding protein (CIRP) triggers inflammatory responses in hemorrhagic shock and sepsis. *Nat. Med.* **2013**, *19*, 1489–1495. [CrossRef]
9. Godwin, A.; Yang, W.-L.; Sharma, A.; Khader, A.; Wang, Z.; Zhang, F.; Nicastro, J.; Coppa, G.F.; Wang, P. Blocking Cold-Inducible RNA-Binding Protein Protects Liver From Ischemia-Reperfusion Injury. *Shock* **2015**, *43*, 24–30. [CrossRef] [PubMed]
10. McGinn, J.T.; Aziz, M.; Zhang, F.; Yang, W.-L.; Nicastro, J.M.; Coppa, G.F.; Wang, P. Cold-inducible RNA-binding protein-derived peptide C23 attenuates inflammation and tissue injury in a murine model of intestinal ischemia-reperfusion. *Surgery* **2018**, *164*, 1191–1197. [CrossRef]
11. Cen, C.; Yang, W.-L.; Yen, H.-T.; Nicastro, J.M.; Coppa, G.F.; Wang, P. Deficiency of cold-inducible ribonucleic acid-binding protein reduces renal injury after ischemia-reperfusion. *Surgery* **2016**, *160*, 473–483. [CrossRef] [PubMed]
12. Zhou, M.; Yang, W.-L.; Ji, Y.; Qiang, X.; Wang, P. Cold-inducible RNA-binding protein mediates neuroinflammation in cerebral ischemia. *Biochim. Biophys. Acta* **2014**, *1840*, 2253–2261. [CrossRef]
13. Pittman, K.; Kubes, P. Damage-Associated Molecular Patterns Control Neutrophil Recruitment. *J. Innate Immun.* **2013**, *5*, 315–323. [CrossRef]
14. Denning, N.-L.; Aziz, M.; Murao, A.; Gurien, S.D.; Ochani, M.; Prince, J.M.; Wang, P. Extracellular CIRP as an endogenous TREM-1 ligand to fuel inflammation in sepsis. *JCI Insight* **2020**, *5*. [CrossRef] [PubMed]

15. Sakurai, T.; Kashida, H.; Watanabe, T.; Hagiwara, S.; Mizushima, T.; Iijima, H.; Nishida, N.; Higashitsuji, H.; Fujita, J.; Kudo, M. Stress Response Protein Cirp Links Inflammation and Tumorigenesis in Colitis-Associated Cancer. *Cancer Res.* **2014**, *74*, 6119–6128. [CrossRef] [PubMed]
16. Sakurai, T.; Kashida, H.; Komeda, Y.; Nagai, T.; Hagiwara, S.; Watanabe, T.; Kitano, M.; Nishida, N.; Fujita, J.; Kudo, M. Stress Response Protein RBM3 Promotes the Development of Colitis-associated Cancer. *Inflamm. Bowel Dis.* **2017**, *23*, 57–65. [CrossRef]
17. McGinn, J.; Zhang, F.; Aziz, M.; Yang, W.L.; Nicastro, J.; Coppa, G.F.; Wang, P. The Protective Effect of a Short Peptide Derived from Cold-Inducible RNA-Binding Protein in Renal Ischemia-Reperfusion Injury. *Shock* **2018**, *49*, 269–276. [CrossRef]
18. Zhang, F.; Brenner, M.; Yang, W.-L.; Wang, P. A cold-inducible RNA-binding protein (CIRP)-derived peptide attenuates inflammation and organ injury in septic mice. *Sci. Rep.* **2018**, *8*, 3052. [CrossRef]
19. Yang, W.-L.; Sharma, A.; Wang, Z.; Li, Z.; Fan, J.; Wang, P. Cold-inducible RNA-binding protein causes endothelial dysfunction via activation of Nlrp3 inflammasome. *Sci. Rep.* **2016**, *6*, 26571. [CrossRef]
20. Zhou, Y.; Dong, H.; Zhong, Y.; Huang, J.; Lv, J.; Li, J. The Cold-Inducible RNA-Binding Protein (CIRP) Level in Peripheral Blood Predicts Sepsis Outcome. *PLoS ONE* **2015**, *10*, e0137721. [CrossRef]
21. Chang, S.-H.; Hla, T. Gene regulation by RNA binding proteins and microRNAs in angiogenesis. *Trends Mol. Med.* **2011**, *17*, 650–658. [CrossRef] [PubMed]
22. Gerstberger, S.; Hafner, M.; Tuschl, T. A census of human RNA-binding proteins. *Nat. Rev. Genet.* **2014**, *15*, 829–845. [CrossRef] [PubMed]
23. Lukong, K.E.; Chang, K.-W.; Khandjian, E.W.; Richard, S. RNA-binding proteins in human genetic disease. *Trends Genet.* **2008**, *24*, 416–425. [CrossRef]
24. Adams, R.H.; Alitalo, K. Molecular regulation of angiogenesis and lymphangiogenesis. *Nat. Rev. Mol. Cell Biol.* **2007**, *8*, 464–478. [CrossRef]
25. Egginton, S.; Zhou, A.-L.; Brown, M.D.; Hudlická, O. Unorthodox angiogenesis in skeletal muscle. *Cardiovasc. Res.* **2001**, *49*, 634–646. [CrossRef]
26. Tonnesen, M.G.; Feng, X.; Clark, R.A. Angiogenesis in wound healing. *J. Investig. Dermatol. Symp. Proc.* **2000**, *5*, 40–46. [CrossRef]
27. Karizbodagh, M.P.; Rashidi, B.; Sahebkar, A.; Masoudifar, A.; Mirzaei, H. Implantation Window and Angiogenesis. *J. Cell. Biochem.* **2017**, *118*, 4141–4151. [CrossRef]
28. Gerhardt, H.; Golding, M.; Fruttiger, M.; Ruhrberg, C.; Lundkvist, A.; Abramsson, A.; Jeltsch, M.; Mitchell, C.; Alitalo, K.; Shima, D.; et al. VEGF guides angiogenic sprouting utilizing endothelial tip cell filopodia. *J. Cell Biol.* **2003**, *161*, 1163–1177. [CrossRef]
29. Ferrara, N.; Henzel, W.J. Pituitary follicular cells secrete a novel heparin-binding growth factor specific for vascular endothelial cells. *Biochem. Biophys. Res. Commun.* **1989**, *161*, 851–858. [CrossRef]
30. Tirpe, A.A.; Gulei, D.; Ciortea, S.M.; Crivii, C.; Berindan-Neagoe, I. Hypoxia: Overview on Hypoxia-Mediated Mechanisms with a Focus on the Role of HIF Genes. *Int. J. Mol. Sci.* **2019**, *20*, 6140. [CrossRef]
31. Shima, D.T.; Adamis, A.P.; Ferrara, N.; Yeo, K.-T.; Yeo, T.-K.; Allende, R.; Folkman, J.; D'Amore, P. Hypoxic Induction of Endothelial Cell Growth Factors in Retinal Cells: Identification and Characterization of Vascular Endothelial Growth Factor (VEGF) as the Mitogen. *Mol. Med.* **1995**, *1*, 182–193. [CrossRef] [PubMed]
32. Carmeliet, P. Mechanisms of angiogenesis and arteriogenesis. *Nat. Med.* **2000**, *6*, 389–395. [CrossRef] [PubMed]
33. Mentzer, S.J.; Konerding, M.A. Intussusceptive angiogenesis: Expansion and remodeling of microvascular networks. *Angiogenesis* **2014**, *17*, 499–509. [CrossRef]
34. Demir, R.; Yaba, A.; Huppertz, B. Vasculogenesis and angiogenesis in the endometrium during menstrual cycle and implantation. *Acta Histochem.* **2010**, *112*, 203–214. [CrossRef] [PubMed]
35. Folkman, J. Angiogenesis in cancer, vascular, rheumatoid and other disease. *Nat. Med.* **1995**, *1*, 27–31. [CrossRef]
36. Priya, S.K.; Nagare, R.; Sneha, V.; Sidhanth, C.; Bindhya, S.; Manasa, P.; Ganesan, T. Tumour angiogenesis—Origin of blood vessels. *Int. J. Cancer* **2016**, *139*, 729–735. [CrossRef]
37. Weckbach, L.T.; Preissner, K.T.; Deindl, E. The Role of Midkine in Arteriogenesis, Involving Mechanosensing, Endothelial Cell Proliferation, and Vasodilation. *Int. J. Mol. Sci.* **2018**, *19*, 2559. [CrossRef]
38. Deindl, E.; Zaruba, M.M.; Brunner, S.; Huber, B.; Mehl, U.; Assmann, G.; Hoefer, I.E.; Mueller-Hoecker, J.; Franz, W.M. G-CSF administration after myocardial infarction in mice attenuates late ischemic cardiomyopathy by enhanced arteriogenesis. *FASEB J.* **2006**, *20*, 956–958. [CrossRef]
39. Deindl, E.; Schaper, W. The Art of Arteriogenesis. *Cell Biophys.* **2005**, *43*, 1–15. [CrossRef]
40. Faber, J.E.; Chilian, W.M.; Deindl, E.; van Royen, N.; Simons, M. A Brief Etymology of the Collateral Circulation. *Arter. Thromb. Vasc. Biol.* **2014**, *34*, 1854–1859. [CrossRef]
41. Rizzi, A.; Benagiano, V.; Ribatti, D. Angiogenesis versus arteriogenesis. *Rom. J. Morphol. Embryol. Rev. Roum. Morphol. Embryol.* **2017**, *58*, 15–19.
42. Heil, M.; Eitenmüller, I.; Schmitz-Rixen, T.; Schaper, W. Arteriogenesis versus angiogenesis: Similarities and differences. *J. Cell. Mol. Med.* **2006**, *10*, 45–55. [CrossRef]
43. Scapini, P.; Morini, M.; Tecchio, C.; Minghelli, S.; Di Carlo, E.; Tanghetti, E.; Albini, A.; Lowell, C.; Berton, G.; Noonan, D.M.; et al. CXCL1/macrophage inflammatory protein-2-induced angiogenesis in vivo is mediated by neutrophil-derived vascular endothelial growth factor-A. *J. Immunol.* **2004**, *172*, 5034–5040. [CrossRef]

44. Gaudry, M.; Brégerie, O.; Andrieu, V.; El Benna, J.; Pocidalo, M.-A.; Hakim, J. Intracellular Pool of Vascular Endothelial Growth Factor in Human Neutrophils. *Blood* **1997**, *90*, 4153–4161. [CrossRef]
45. Gong, Y.; Koh, D.-R. Neutrophils promote inflammatory angiogenesis via release of preformed VEGF in an in vivo corneal model. *Cell Tissue Res.* **2010**, *339*, 437–448. [CrossRef]
46. Ardi, V.C.; Kupriyanova, T.A.; Deryugina, E.I.; Quigley, J.P. Human neutrophils uniquely release TIMP-free MMP-9 to provide a potent catalytic stimulator of angiogenesis. *Proc. Natl. Acad. Sci. USA* **2007**, *104*, 20262–20267. [CrossRef]
47. Du Cheyne, C.; Tay, H.; De Spiegelaere, W. The complex TIE between macrophages and angiogenesis. *Anat. Histol. Embryol.* **2019**. [CrossRef]
48. Aldabbous, L.; Abdul-Salam, V.; McKinnon, T.; Duluc, L.; Pepke-Zaba, J.; Southwood, M.; Ainscough, A.J.; Hadinnapola, C.; Wilkins, M.R.; Toshner, M.; et al. Neutrophil Extracellular Traps Promote Angiogenesis: Evidence from Vascular Pathology in Pulmonary Hypertension. *Arterioscler. Thromb. Vasc. Biol.* **2016**, *36*, 2078–2087. [CrossRef]
49. Takizawa, S.; Murao, A.; Ochani, M.; Aziz, M.; Wang, P. Frontline Science: Extracellular CIRP generates a proinflammatory Ly6G + CD11b hi subset of low-density neutrophils in sepsis. *J. Leukoc. Biol.* **2020**, *109*, 1019–1032. [CrossRef]
50. Murao, A.; Arif, A.; Brenner, M.; Denning, N.-L.; Jin, H.; Takizawa, S.; Nicastro, B.; Wang, P.; Aziz, M. Extracellular CIRP and TREM-1 axis promotes ICAM-1-Rho-mediated NETosis in sepsis. *FASEB J.* **2020**. [CrossRef]
51. Ode, Y.; Aziz, M.; Jin, H.; Arif, A.; Nicastro, J.G.; Wang, P. Cold-inducible RNA-binding Protein Induces Neutrophil Extracellular Traps in the Lungs during Sepsis. *Sci. Rep.* **2019**, *9*, 6252. [CrossRef]
52. Ode, Y.; Aziz, M.; Wang, P. CIRP increases ICAM-1(+) phenotype of neutrophils exhibiting elevated iNOS and NETs in sepsis. *J. Leukoc. Biol.* **2018**, *103*, 693–707. [CrossRef]
53. Rohrbach, A.S.; Slade, D.J.; Thompson, P.R.; Mowen, K.A. Activation of PAD4 in NET formation. *Front. Immunol.* **2012**, *3*, 360. [CrossRef] [PubMed]
54. Idrovo, J.P.; Jacob, A.; Yang, W.L.; Wang, Z.; Yen, H.T.; Nicastro, J.; Coppa, G.F.; Wang, P. A deficiency in cold-inducible RNA-binding protein accelerates the inflammation phase and improves wound healing. *Int. J. Mol. Med.* **2016**, *37*, 423–428. [CrossRef] [PubMed]
55. Welten, S.M.; Bastiaansen, A.J.; de Jong, R.C.; de Vries, M.R.; Peters, E.A.; Boonstra, M.C.; Sheikh, S.P.; La Monica, N.; Kandimalla, E.R.; Quax, P.H.; et al. Inhibition of 14q32 MicroRNAs miR-329, miR-487b, miR-494, and miR-495 Increases Neovascularization and Blood Flow Recovery after Ischemia. *Circ. Res.* **2014**, *115*, 696–708. [CrossRef] [PubMed]
56. Downie Ruiz Velasco, A.; Welten, S.M.J.; Goossens, E.A.C.; Quax, P.H.A.; Rappsilber, J.; Michlewski, G.; Nossent, A.Y. Posttranscriptional Regulation of 14q32 MicroRNAs by the CIRBP and HADHB during Vascular Regeneration after Ischemia. *Mol. Ther. Nucleic Acids* **2019**, *14*, 329–338. [CrossRef]
57. Wang, P.; Luo, Y.; Duan, H.; Xing, S.; Zhang, J.; Lu, D.; Feng, J.; Yang, D.; Song, L.; Yan, X. MicroRNA 329 Suppresses Angiogenesis by Targeting CD146. *Mol. Cell. Biol.* **2013**, *33*, 3689–3699. [CrossRef]
58. Jiang, T.; Zhuang, J.; Duan, H.; Luo, Y.; Zeng, Q.; Fan, K.; Yan, H.; Lu, D.; Ye, Z.; Hao, J.; et al. CD146 is a coreceptor for VEGFR-2 in tumor angiogenesis. *Blood* **2012**, *120*, 2330–2339. [CrossRef]
59. Kübler, M.; Beck, S.; Fischer, S.; Götz, P.; Kumaraswami, K.; Ishikawa-Ankerhold, H.; Lasch, M.; Deindl, E. Absence of Cold-Inducible RNA-Binding Protein (CIRP) Promotes Angiogenesis and Regeneration of Ischemic Tissue by Inducing M2-like Macrophage Polarization. *Biomedicines* **2021**, *9*, 395. [CrossRef] [PubMed]
60. Limbourg, A.; Korff, T.; Napp, L.C.; Schaper, W.; Drexler, H.; Limbourg, F. Evaluation of postnatal arteriogenesis and angiogenesis in a mouse model of hind-limb ischemia. *Nat. Protoc.* **2009**, *4*, 1737–1748. [CrossRef] [PubMed]
61. Baum, O.; Olfert, I.M.; Egginton, S.; Hellsten, Y. Advances and challenges in skeletal muscle angiogenesis. *Am. J. Physiol. Heart Circ. Physiol.* **2016**, *310*, H326–H336. [CrossRef]
62. Chen, K.; Murao, A.; Arif, A.; Takizawa, S.; Jin, H.; Jiang, J.; Aziz, M.; Wang, P. Inhibition of Efferocytosis by Extracellular CIRP–Induced Neutrophil Extracellular Traps. *J. Immunol.* **2020**, *206*, 797–806. [CrossRef] [PubMed]
63. Aziz, M.; Brenner, M.; Wang, P. Extracellular CIRP (eCIRP) and inflammation. *J. Leukoc. Biol.* **2019**, *106*, 133–146. [CrossRef] [PubMed]
64. Zhong, P.; Huang, H. Recent progress in the research of cold-inducible RNA-binding protein. *Future Sci. OA* **2017**, *3*, FSO246. [CrossRef] [PubMed]
65. Seignez, C.; Phillipson, M. The multitasking neutrophils and their involvement in angiogenesis. *Curr. Opin. Hematol.* **2017**, *24*, 3–8. [CrossRef]
66. Wang, J. Neutrophils in tissue injury and repair. *Cell Tissue Res.* **2018**, *371*, 531–539. [CrossRef] [PubMed]
67. Castanheira, F.V.S.; Kubes, P. Neutrophils and NETs in modulating acute and chronic inflammation. *Blood* **2019**, *133*, 2178–2185. [CrossRef]
68. Preissner, K.T.; Fischer, S.; Deindl, E. Extracellular RNA as a Versatile DAMP and Alarm Signal That Influences Leukocyte Recruitment in Inflammation and Infection. *Front. Cell Dev. Biol.* **2020**, *8*. [CrossRef]
69. Wang, J.; Hossain, M.; Thanabalasuriar, A.; Gunzer, M.; Meininger, C.; Kubes, P. Visualizing the function and fate of neutrophils in sterile injury and repair. *Science* **2017**, *358*, 111–116. [CrossRef]
70. Christoffersson, G.; Henriksnäs, J.; Johansson, L.; Rolny, C.; Ahlström, H.; Caballero-Corbalan, J.; Segersvärd, R.; Permert, J.; Korsgren, O.; Carlsson, P.O.; et al. Clinical and experimental pancreatic islet transplantation to striated muscle: Establishment of a vascular system similar to that in native islets. *Diabetes* **2010**, *59*, 2569–2578. [CrossRef]

71. Christoffersson, G.; Vågesjö, E.; Vandooren, J.; Lidén, M.; Massena, S.; Reinert, R.; Brissova, M.; Powers, A.C.; Opdenakker, G.; Phillipson, M. VEGF-A recruits a proangiogenic MMP-9–delivering neutrophil subset that induces angiogenesis in transplanted hypoxic tissue. *Blood* **2012**, *120*, 4653–4662. [CrossRef]
72. Kolaczkowska, E.; Kubes, P. Neutrophil recruitment and function in health and inflammation. *Nat. Rev. Immunol.* **2013**, *13*, 159–175. [CrossRef] [PubMed]
73. Pizza, F.X.; Peterson, J.M.; Baas, J.H.; Koh, T.J. Neutrophils contribute to muscle injury and impair its resolution after lengthening contractions in mice. *J. Physiol.* **2005**, *562 Pt 3*, 899–913. [CrossRef]
74. Toumi, H.; F'Guyer, S.; Best, T.M. The role of neutrophils in injury and repair following muscle stretch. *J. Anat.* **2006**, *208*, 459–470. [CrossRef]
75. Teixeira, C.; Zamuner, S.; Zuliani, J.P.; Fernandes, C.M.; Cruz-Hofling, M.A.; Fernandes, I.; Chaves, F.; Gutiérrez, J.M. Neutrophils do not contribute to local tissue damage, but play a key role in skeletal muscle regeneration, in mice injected withBothrops aspersnake venom. *Muscle Nerve* **2003**, *28*, 449–459. [CrossRef]
76. De Oliveira, S.; Rosowski, E.E.; Huttenlocher, A. Neutrophil migration in infection and wound repair: Going forward in reverse. *Nat. Rev. Immunol.* **2016**, *16*, 378–391. [CrossRef] [PubMed]
77. Jin, H.; Aziz, M.; Ode, Y.; Wang, P. CIRP Induces Neutrophil Reverse Transendothelial Migration in Sepsis. *Shock* **2019**, *51*, 548–556. [CrossRef] [PubMed]
78. Denning, N.-L.; Aziz, M.; Gurien, S.D.; Wang, P. DAMPs and NETs in Sepsis. *Front. Immunol.* **2019**, *10*, 2536. [CrossRef]
79. Lefrancais, E.; Mallavia, B.; Zhuo, H.; Calfee, C.S.; Looney, M.R. Maladaptive role of neutrophil extracellular traps in pathogen-induced lung injury. *JCI Insight* **2018**, *3*. [CrossRef]
80. Wong, S.L.; Demers, M.; Martinod, K.; Gallant, M.; Wang, Y.; Goldfine, A.B.; Kahn, C.R.; Wagner, D.D. Diabetes primes neutrophils to undergo NETosis, which impairs wound healing. *Nat. Med.* **2015**, *21*, 815–819. [CrossRef]
81. Saffarzadeh, M.; Juenemann, C.; Queisser, M.A.; Lochnit, G.; Barreto, G.; Galuska, S.P.; Lohmeyer, J.; Preissner, K.T. Neutrophil Extracellular Traps Directly Induce Epithelial and Endothelial Cell Death: A Predominant Role of Histones. *PLoS ONE* **2012**, *7*, e32366. [CrossRef] [PubMed]
82. Slaba, I.; Wang, J.; Kolaczkowska, E.; McDonald, B.; Lee, W.-Y.; Kubes, P. Imaging the dynamic platelet-neutrophil response in sterile liver injury and repair in mice. *Hepatology* **2015**, *62*, 1593–1605. [CrossRef]
83. Mutua, V.; Gershwin, L.J. A Review of Neutrophil Extracellular Traps (NETs) in Disease: Potential Anti-NETs Therapeutics. *Clin. Rev. Allergy Immunol.* **2020**, *61*, 194–211. [CrossRef] [PubMed]
84. Greenlee-Wacker, M.C. Clearance of apoptotic neutrophils and resolution of inflammation. *Immunol. Rev.* **2016**, *273*, 357–370. [CrossRef] [PubMed]
85. Duffield, J.S.; Forbes, S.; Constandinou, C.M.; Clay, S.; Partolina, M.; Vuthoori, S.; Wu, S.; Lang, R.; Iredale, J.P. Selective depletion of macrophages reveals distinct, opposing roles during liver injury and repair. *J. Clin. Investig.* **2005**, *115*, 56–65. [CrossRef]
86. Lucas, T.; Waisman, A.; Ranjan, R.; Roes, J.; Krieg, T.; Müller, W.; Roers, A.; Eming, S.A. Differential Roles of Macrophages in Diverse Phases of Skin Repair. *J. Immunol.* **2010**, *184*, 3964–3977. [CrossRef]
87. Hong, H.; Tian, X.Y. The Role of Macrophages in Vascular Repair and Regeneration after Ischemic Injury. *Int. J. Mol. Sci.* **2020**, *21*, 6328. [CrossRef]
88. Murray, P.J. Macrophage Polarization. *Annu. Rev. Physiol.* **2017**, *79*, 541–566. [CrossRef]
89. Gordon, S.; Taylor, P. Monocyte and macrophage heterogeneity. *Nat. Rev. Immunol.* **2005**, *5*, 953–964. [CrossRef] [PubMed]
90. Wynn, T.A.; Vannella, K.M. Macrophages in Tissue Repair, Regeneration, and Fibrosis. *Immunity* **2016**, *44*, 450–462. [CrossRef]
91. Gurevich, D.; Severn, C.; Twomey, C.; Greenhough, A.; Cash, J.; Toye, A.M.; Mellor, H.; Martin, P. Live imaging of wound angiogenesis reveals macrophage orchestrated vessel sprouting and regression. *EMBO J.* **2018**, *37*. [CrossRef]
92. Zhang, J.; Muri, J.; Fitzgerald, G.; Gorski, T.; Gianni-Barrera, R.; Masschelein, E.; D'Hulst, G.; Gilardoni, P.; Turiel, G.; Fan, Z.; et al. Endothelial Lactate Controls Muscle Regeneration from Ischemia by Inducing M2-like Macrophage Polarization. *Cell Metab.* **2020**, *31*, 1136–1153.e7. [CrossRef]
93. Willenborg, S.; Lucas, T.; Van Loo, G.; Knipper, J.; Krieg, T.; Haase, I.; Brachvogel, B.; Hammerschmidt, M.; Nagy, A.; Ferrara, N.; et al. CCR2 recruits an inflammatory macrophage subpopulation critical for angiogenesis in tissue repair. *Blood* **2012**, *120*, 613–625. [CrossRef]
94. Dort, J.; Fabre, P.; Molina, T.; Dumont, N.A. Macrophages Are Key Regulators of Stem Cells during Skeletal Muscle Regeneration and Diseases. *Stem Cells Int.* **2019**, *2019*, 4761427. [CrossRef]
95. Zajac, E.; Schweighofer, B.; Kupriyanova, T.A.; Juncker-Jensen, A.; Minder, P.; Quigley, J.P.; Deryugina, E.I. Angiogenic capacity of M1- and M2-polarized macrophages is determined by the levels of TIMP-1 complexed with their secreted proMMP-9. *Blood* **2013**, *122*, 4054–4067. [CrossRef] [PubMed]
96. Gordon, S.; Martinez, F.O. Alternative Activation of Macrophages: Mechanism and Functions. *Immunity* **2010**, *32*, 593–604. [CrossRef] [PubMed]
97. Deshmane, S.L.; Kremlev, S.; Amini, S.; Sawaya, B.E. Monocyte Chemoattractant Protein-1 (MCP-1): An Overview. *J. Interf. Cytokine Res.* **2009**, *29*, 313–326. [CrossRef]
98. Nio, Y.; Yamauchi, T.; Okada-Iwabu, M.; Funata, M.; Yamaguchi, M.; Ueki, K.; Kadowaki, T. Monocyte chemoattractant protein-1 (MCP-1) deficiency enhances alternatively activated M2 macrophages and ameliorates insulin resistance and fatty liver in lipoatrophic diabetic A-ZIP transgenic mice. *Diabetologia* **2012**, *55*, 3350–3358. [CrossRef]

99. Fang, Z.; Wu, D.; Deng, J.; Yang, Q.; Zhang, X.; Chen, J.; Wang, S.; Hu, S.; Hou, W.; Ning, S.; et al. An MD2-perturbing peptide has therapeutic effects in rodent and rhesus monkey models of stroke. *Sci. Transl. Med.* **2021**, *13*, eabb6716. [CrossRef]
100. Troidl, K.; Schubert, C.; Vlacil, A.-K.; Chennupati, R.; Koch, S.; Schütt, J.; Oberoi, R.; Schaper, W.; Schmitz-Rixen, T.; Schieffer, B.; et al. The Lipopeptide MALP-2 Promotes Collateral Growth. *Cells* **2020**, *9*, 997. [CrossRef] [PubMed]

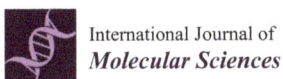

Article

Cold-Inducible RNA-Binding Protein but Not Its Antisense lncRNA Is a Direct Negative Regulator of Angiogenesis In Vitro and In Vivo via Regulation of the 14q32 angiomiRs—microRNA-329-3p and microRNA-495-3p

Eveline A. C. Goossens [1,2,†], Licheng Zhang [2,3,†], Margreet R. de Vries [1,2], J. Wouter Jukema [3,4], Paul H. A. Quax [1,2] and A. Yaël Nossent [1,2,5,6,*]

1. Department of Surgery, Leiden University Medical Center, 2333 ZA Leiden, The Netherlands; eveline@via.demon.nl (E.A.C.G.); M.R.de_Vries@lumc.nl (M.R.d.V.); P.H.A.Quax@lumc.nl (P.H.A.Q.)
2. Einthoven Laboratory for Experimental Vascular Medicine, Leiden University Medical Center, 2333 ZA Leiden, The Netherlands; l.zhang.hlk@lumc.nl
3. Department of Cardiology, Leiden University Medical Center, 2333 ZA Leiden, The Netherlands; J.W.Jukema@lumc.nl
4. Netherlands Heart Institute, 3511 EP Utrecht, The Netherlands
5. Department of Laboratory Medicine, Medical University of Vienna, 1090 Wien, Austria
6. Department of Internal Medicine II, Medical University of Vienna, 1090 Wien, Austria
* Correspondence: a.y.nossent@lumc.nl
† These authors contributed equally.

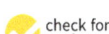

Citation: Goossens, E.A.C.; Zhang, L.; de Vries, M.R.; Jukema, J.W.; Quax, P.H.A.; Nossent, A.Y. Cold-Inducible RNA-Binding Protein but Not Its Antisense lncRNA Is a Direct Negative Regulator of Angiogenesis In Vitro and In Vivo via Regulation of the 14q32 angiomiRs—microRNA-329-3p and microRNA-495-3p. *Int. J. Mol. Sci.* **2021**, *22*, 12678. https://doi.org/10.3390/ijms222312678

Academic Editor: Anne-Catherine Prats

Received: 27 September 2021
Accepted: 20 November 2021
Published: 24 November 2021

Publisher's Note: MDPI stays neutral with regard to jurisdictional claims in published maps and institutional affiliations.

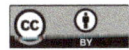

Copyright: © 2021 by the authors. Licensee MDPI, Basel, Switzerland. This article is an open access article distributed under the terms and conditions of the Creative Commons Attribution (CC BY) license (https://creativecommons.org/licenses/by/4.0/).

Abstract: Inhibition of the 14q32 microRNAs, miR-329-3p and miR-495-3p, improves post-ischemic neovascularization. Cold-inducible RNA-binding protein (*CIRBP*) facilitates maturation of these microRNAs. We hypothesized that *CIRBP* deficiency improves post-ischemic angiogenesis via downregulation of 14q32 microRNA expression. We investigated these regulatory mechanisms both in vitro and in vivo. We induced hindlimb ischemia in $Cirp^{-/-}$ and C57Bl/6-J mice, monitored blood flow recovery with laser Doppler perfusion imaging, and assessed neovascularization via immunohistochemistry. Post-ischemic angiogenesis was enhanced in $Cirp^{-/-}$ mice by 34.3% with no effects on arteriogenesis. In vivo at day 7, miR-329-3p and miR-495-3p expression were downregulated in $Cirp^{-/-}$ mice by 40.6% and 36.2%. In HUVECs, *CIRBP* expression was upregulated under hypothermia, while miR-329-3p and miR-495-3p expression remained unaffected. siRNA-mediated *CIRBP* knockdown led to the downregulation of *CIRBP*-splice-variant-1 (*CIRBP-SV1*), *CIRBP* antisense long noncoding RNA (lncRNA-*CIRBP*-AS1), and miR-495-3p with no effects on the expression of *CIRBP-SV2-4* or miR-329-3p. siRNA-mediated *CIRBP* knockdown improved HUVEC migration and tube formation. SiRNA-mediated lncRNA-*CIRBP*-AS1 knockdown had similar long-term effects. After short incubation times, however, only *CIRBP* knockdown affected angiogenesis, indicating that the effects of lncRNA-*CIRBP*-AS1 knockdown were secondary to *CIRBP-SV1* downregulation. *CIRBP* is a negative regulator of angiogenesis in vitro and in vivo and acts, at least in part, through the regulation of miR-329-3p and miR-495-3p.

Keywords: *CIRBP*; 14q32 microRNAs; angiogenesis; peripheral arterial disease; HUVECs

1. Introduction

Peripheral arterial disease (PAD) is caused by occlusions of the arterial vasculature in the lower limbs, mainly the femoral artery, resulting in deprivation of blood flow and, thus, of oxygen and nutrients to the lower extremities [1]. Current treatment options include angioplasty procedures with stent placement and bypass surgery [2]. However, many patients with advanced PAD are not or no longer eligible for these therapies [3,4]. Therefore, novel therapeutic approaches are still required. In patients with PAD, endogenous neovascularization, the collective term for angiogenesis and arteriogenesis, is insufficient to completely recover blood flow to the leg [4]. Hence, enhancing neovascularization is a potential treatment option for patients with PAD. A recent study by Kübler et al. showed that mice deficient in the cold-inducible RNA-binding protein gene (*CIRBP* in humans or *Cirp* in mice) showed increased angiogenesis and decreased hypoxia-induced muscle damage in a hindlimb ischemia model, linked to M2 macrophage polarization [5,6]. *CIRBP* may act on neovascularization via other pathways too, which we investigated more closely in this study.

CIRBP is regulated by differential stress factors, including ischemia [7,8] and, as its name suggests, temperature [7,9–12]. In fact, *CIRBP* was described in 1997 as the first cold shock protein that was induced at mild hypothermia [13], and this effect was conserved both in humans and mice [14]. *CIRBP* is an RNA-binding protein (RBP) that influences post-transcriptional processing of its target RNA [15], and its gene is located at chromosome 19 in humans and at chromosome 10 in mice. *CIRBP* contains an N-terminal RNA-binding domain and a C-terminal domain that has protein binding properties [13,16]. There are various splice variants of *CIRBP* that, in mice, show altered expression patterns in response to hypothermia [17]. The four main splice variants in humans, *CIRBP*-SV1, *CIRBP*-SV2, *CIRBP*-SV3, and *CIRBP*-SV4, have their RNA-binding domain in common but have different C-termini. However, the role of these splice variants, especially the link with microRNAs and neovascularization, needs further investigation. Furthermore, the antisense strand of the human *CIRBP* gene encodes an antisense long non-coding RNA (lncRNA-*CIRBP*-AS1). Antisense long noncoding RNAs (lncRNAs) can have several functions. Antisense lncRNAs have been shown to affect transcription and support function of their respective coding sense-strand [18]. For example, lncRNA MALAT1 has an antisense transcript TALAM1, and together they function as a sense–antisense pair [19,20]. Therefore, it is possible that either sense and antisense strands are co-transcribed and counteract or cooperate in their actions [18] or that one strand affects expression of the other strand. Whether *CIRBP* and lncRNA-*CIRBP*-AS1 have a similar "partnership" remains to be determined.

CIRBP, as an RBP, not only affects processing of messenger RNAs (mRNAs) but also has the ability to act in microRNA processing. Previously, our group showed that a large microRNA cluster, located on chromosome 14 (14q32 locus), plays a regulatory role in different types of vascular remodeling including atherosclerosis and restenosis but also in post-ischemic neovascularization [21–24]. This cluster is also known as the DLK1-DIO3 cluster and is conserved in mice where it is located at the 12F1 locus. *CIRBP* was shown to directly bind two precursors of 14q32 microRNAs, namely, precursor-microRNA (pre-miR)-329 and pre-miR-495 [25], thereby inducing processing into the mature microRNAs miR-329-3p and miR-495-3p. In previous studies, it was found that inhibition of the 14q32 microRNAs, miR-329-3p and miR-495-3p, increased post-ischemic neovascularization [21] and angiogenesis, in particular. At the same time, inhibition of these microRNAs also reduced post-interventional restenosis [22], potentially offering a double advantage for patients with severe PAD. Importantly, inhibition of miR-495-3p affected macrophage influx into the lesions. Therefore, the hypothesis was that inhibition of *CIRBP* leads to a decrease in mature miR-329-3p and miR-495-3p expression and, consequently, promotes post-ischemic neovascularization.

In this study, firstly, the effect of *CIRBP* deficiency on neovascularization in vivo was investigated using a murine hindlimb ischemia model, and the effects on arteriogenesis and angiogenesis were determined, showing that mainly angiogenesis was affected. Next, human umbilical vein endothelial cells (HUVECs) were used to examine the effects of modulating the expression of *CIRBP*, its splice variants, its antisense lncRNA-*CIRBP*-AS1, and its downstream target microRNAs, miR-329-3p and miR-495-3p, and to demonstrate the effects of *CIRBP* and lncRNA-*CIRBP*-AS1 knockdown on in vitro angiogenesis.

2. Results

2.1. Blood Flow Recovery and Neovascularization after Hindlimb Ischemia (HLI) Surgery in Cirp$^{-/-}$ Mice

To investigate the role of *CIRBP* in neovascularization in vivo, an HLI model was induced in *Cirp* knockout (*Cirp$^{-/-}$*) and wild-type (WT) C57BL/6 mice, and blood flow recovery was evaluated over time. No differences were observed in blood flow recovery between WT mice and *Cirp$^{-/-}$* mice over 28 days (Figure 1A,B).

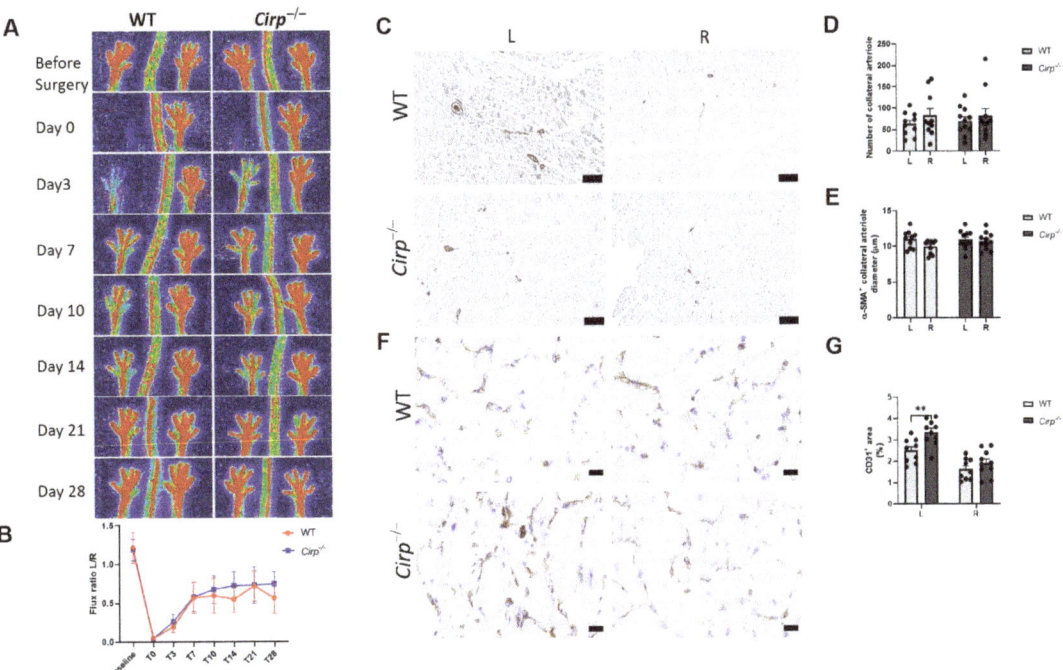

Figure 1. Hindlimb Ischemia (HLI) in mice. (**A**) Representative laser Doppler perfusion imaging (LDPI) of paws of wild-type (WT) mice (*n* = 10) and *Cirp* knockout (*Cirp$^{-/-}$*) mice (*n* = 11) subjected to HLI over time. (**B**) Quantification of LDPI measurements over time, calculated as the ratio of the left (ischemic) over the right (non-ischemic) paw. (**C**) Representative images of α-smooth muscle actin positive (α-SMA$^+$) arterioles in adductor muscle of mice, scale bar = 100 μm. (**D,E**) Quantification of the number and average diameter of α-SMA$^+$ arterioles in adductor muscles. (**F**) Representative images of CD31$^+$ capillaries in the soleus muscle, scale bar = 20 μm. (**G**) Quantification of the CD31$^+$ area in the soleus muscle. Data are presented as the mean ± SEM; ** p < 0.01 by independent sample Student's *t*-tests.

To visualize arteriogenesis, immunohistochemical staining for α-smooth muscle actin (α-SMA) in the adductor muscle was performed (Figure 1C), and the number and diameter of α-SMA positive arterioles were quantified. Collateral density and the size of α-SMA positive arterioles of the ligated paws were similar between WT mice and *Cirp$^{-/-}$* mice (Figure 1D,E), which is in line with the results presented in Figure 1A.

To monitor the effects of *Cirp* deficiency on angiogenesis, capillary formation was evaluated in the soleus muscles at 28 days after induction of ischemia as visualized by CD31 staining (Figure 1F). The CD31$^+$ area represents the density of capillaries in the ischemic muscle. Compared to the unligated (right) paw, there was more capillary formation in the ligated (left) paw as shown in both WT mice (65.2% increase, p = 0.009) and *Cirp$^{-/-}$* mice (100.5% increase, p = 0.003). Moreover, the CD31 positive area in the ligated paw of *Cirp$^{-/-}$*

mice was significantly higher than in WT mice (34.3% increase, p = 0.004), while there was no difference in the unligated paw between the two groups (Figure 1G).

2.2. Ex Vivo Angiogenic Sprouting in Aorta Rings

To study the effects of *Cirp* deficiency on angiogenesis ex vivo, aorta ring assays were performed. Two different vascular endothelial growth factor (VEGF) concentrations (i.e., 10 and 30 ng/mL) were used to induce sprouting in either wild-type or *Cirp* deficient aorta rings. Aorta rings from $Cirp^{-/-}$ mice developed more sprouts compared to the WT control rings, both in rings incubated with 10 (55.4% increase in sprouts) or 30 ng/mL VEGF (79.6% increase in sprouts) (Figure 2). Quantification of the sprouting demonstrated that for both VEGF concentrations, this difference was statistically significant (10 ng/mL VEGF, p = 0.004; 30 ng/mL VEGF, p < 0.001).

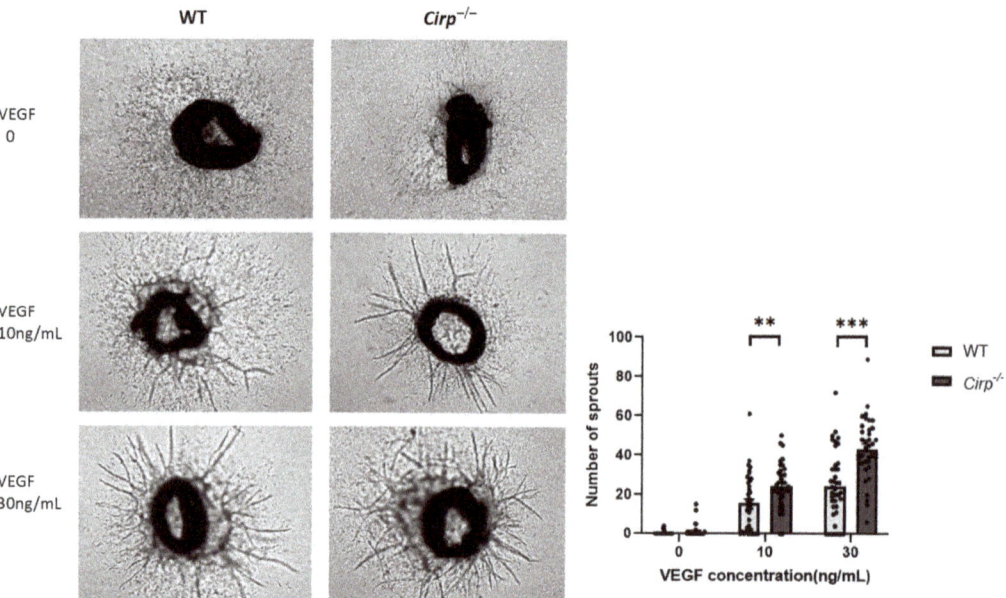

Figure 2. Ex vivo angiogenesis: representative images and quantification of neovessel sprouts from 7 day collagen-embedded aorta rings (40 rings per condition from 3 WT and 3 $Cirp^{-/-}$ mice), treated without or with vascular endothelial growth factor (VEGF) at 10 and 30 ng/mL. Data are presented as the mean ± SEM; ** p < 0.01; *** p < 0.001 by independent sample Student's t-tests.

2.3. MicroRNA Expression in $Cirp^{-/-}$ Mice

MiR-329-3p and miR-495-3p are both highly associated with angiogenesis and regulated by *CIRBP* as has been shown previously [21,25]. To study if and how miR-329-3p and -495-3p expression changes in $Cirp^{-/-}$ mice after induction of hindlimb ischemia, the HLI surgery was repeated, and the mice were sacrificed at 1 day, 3 days, and 7 days after surgery, followed by RNA isolation from the soleus muscle from both the left and right paws. These early timepoints were chosen as ischemia had not resolved yet and angiogenesis was still ongoing. Although the expression of miR-329-3p and miR-495-3p increased in the ischemic soleus muscles of both mouse strains at 7 days, their expression increased significantly less in the $Cirp^{-/-}$ mice (40.6% less, p = 0.028 for miR-329-3p; 36.2% less, p < 0.001 for miR-495-3p; Figure 3A,B). This reduced upregulation became even more clear when looking at the ratio of expression in the ligated over the non-ligated paws, where the ratio only increased in the WT mice and not in the $Cirp^{-/-}$ mice (p = 0.027 for miR-329-3p; $p = 0.0736$ (trend) for miR-495-3p; Figure 3C,D). These differences were most evident at day 7.

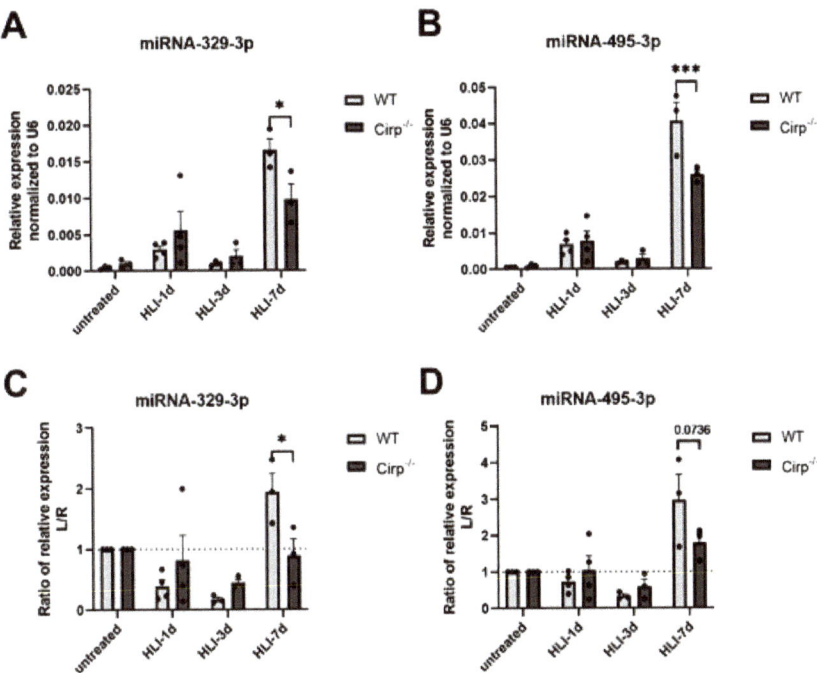

Figure 3. Expression of miRNA-329 and miRNA-495 in soleus muscles. (**A**,**B**) 1, 3, and 7 days after HLI surgery, mature miR-329-3p and -495-3p expression in soleus muscles of the ligated paws from WT mice ($n = 3$ for the untreated group, $n = 4$ for the HLI-1d group, $n = 3$ for the HLI-3d group, and $n = 3$ for the HLI-7d group) and $Cirp^{-/-}$ mice ($n = 3$ for the untreated group, $n = 4$ for the HLI-1d group, $n = 3$ for the HLI-3d group, and $n = 3$ for the HLI-7d group). Expression was normalized to U6. (**C**,**D**) The relative expression of mature miRNA-329 and -495 from mice after HLI surgery at different timepoints, calculated as the ratio of the left (ischemic) over the right (non-ischemic) paw. Data are presented as the mean ± SEM; * $p < 0.05$; *** $p < 0.001$ by two-way ANOVA.

2.4. Total CIRBP, CIRBP Splice Variants, and lncRNA-CIRBP-AS1 Expression in Hypothermia

The gene structure of the human *CIRBP* is shown in Figure 4A. Previous studies showed that *CIRBP* expression increased under cellular stress conditions including mild hypothermia [9]. To demonstrate that hypothermia upregulates *CIRBP*-targeted miRNAs and also the different *CIRBP* splice variants and antisense lncRNAs in HUVECs, HUVECs were subjected to mild hypothermia (32 °C) either for 24 or 48 h. Total *CIRBP* expression increased after both 24 and 48 h compared to the normothermic condition (37 °C) by 205.5% ($p = 0.029$; Figure 4B) and 68.7% ($p = 0.028$; Figure 4F), respectively. *CIRBP-SV1* expression increased by 83.1% at 24 h ($p = 0.12$) and by 67.1% at 48 h ($p = 0.14$) under hypothermia, although this upregulation was not statistically significant. However, the remaining three splice variants were not altered consistently over time under hypothermia, neither were significant changes in microRNA expression observed over time (Figure 4C,D,G,H), indicating that upregulation of *CIRBP* did not lead to additional microRNA processing.

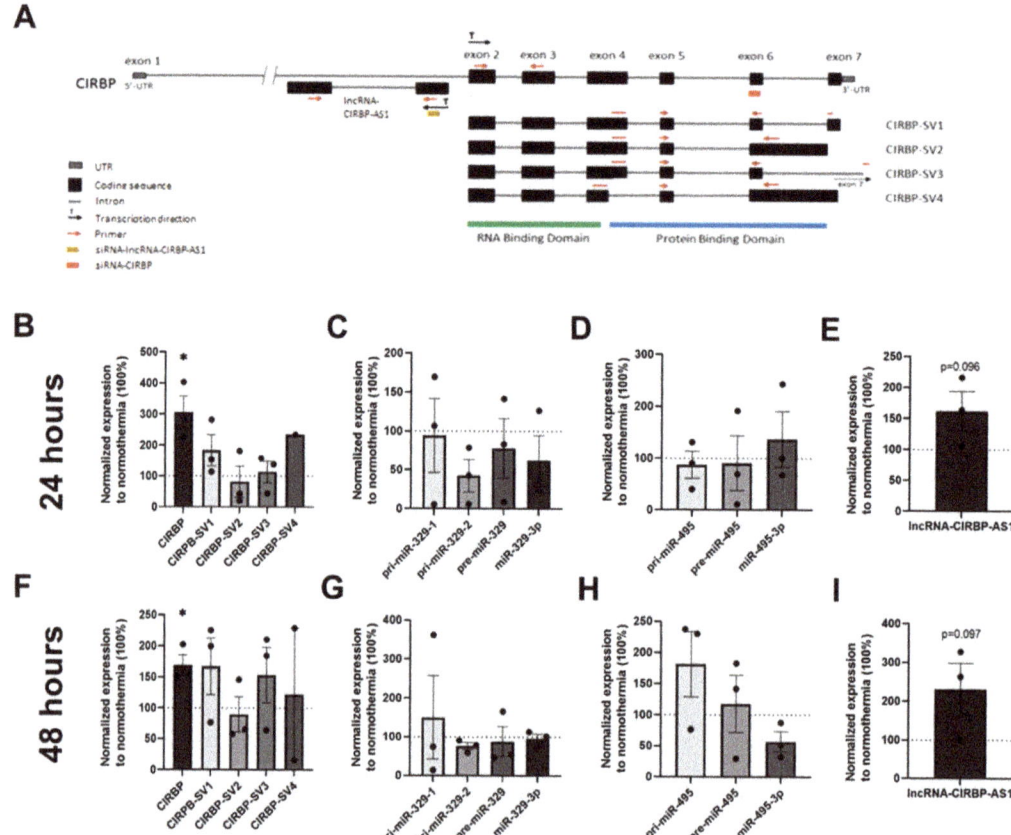

Figure 4. Cold-inducible RNA-binding protein gene (*CIRBP*) expression under hypothermia for 24 and 48 h: (**A**) Schematic representation of the *CIRBP* gene, its splice variants, and lncRNA-*CIRBP*-AS1 with the binding sites of primers and small interfering RNA (siRNA) indicated. Human umbilical vein endothelial cells (HUVECs) were cultured under hypothermic conditions (32 °C) for 24 and 48 h, and (**B,F**) *CIRBP* and *CIRBP* splice variant (*CIRBP-SV*) expression levels were measured and normalized to GAPDH. *CIRBP*-SV4 expression was below the detection limit in several experiments; (**C,D,G,H**) primary microRNA (pri-miR), precursor microRNA (pre-miR), and mature microRNA expression levels of miR-329 and miR-495 were measured and normalized to U6; (**E,I**) *CIRBP* gene antisense long non-coding RNA (lncRNA-*CIRBP*-AS1) expression level was measured and normalized to GAPDH. Data are shown as the relative expression compared to the normothermic group, presented as the mean ± SEM; * $p < 0.05$ by one-sample *t*-tests (one-tail).

lncRNA-*CIRBP*-AS1 did show a trend towards a 61.7% increase in expression under hypothermia after 24 h ($p = 0.096$; Figure 4E) and was even further upregulated by 130.4% after 48 h ($p = 0.097$) compared to normothermia (Figure 4I).

2.5. Angiogenesis Assays and RNA Expression after CIRBP Knockdown

To investigate the role of *CIRBP* in vitro, HUVECs were treated with small interfering RNA (siRNA) targeted to *CIRBP*, and the angiogenic potential was assessed using both scratch-wound healing assays and tube-formation assays. Scratch-wound healing showed an increased (2.8-fold, $p = 0.004$) angiogenic potential after siRNA–*CIRBP* transfection (Figure 5A,B). To exclude any effects of potential *CIRBP* knockdown-induced cell proliferation, the expression of proliferating cell nuclear antigen (*PCNA*) mRNA was assessed and, indeed, no differences were observed compared to the negative control siRNA (Figure 5C). In addition, tube-formation assays also showed improvements in the number of segments

(97.2%, p = 0.046), branches (65.4%, p = 0.016), and total length (27.7%, p = 0.014) after *CIRBP* knockdown (Figure 5H,I).

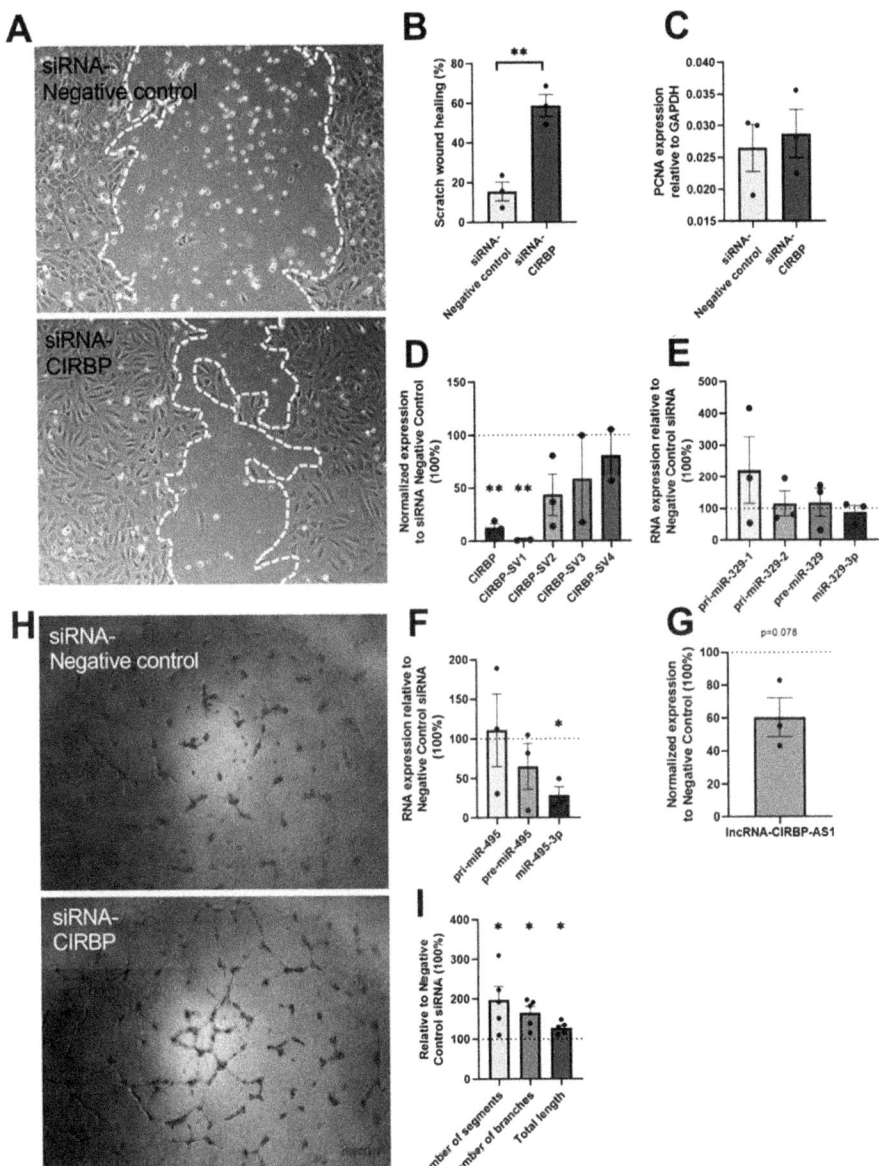

Figure 5. siRNA-*CIRBP* transfection for 24 h in HUVECs: (**A**) Representative images of wound healing (n = 3) and (**B**) quantification of the migration area treated with siRNA targeted to *CIRBP* and negative control for 24 h. White, dotted lines mark the edge of the HUVECs' monolayer. (**C**) Proliferating cell nuclear antigen gene (*PCNA*) expression level in HUVECs as an indicator of cell proliferation. (**D**) Expression of total *CIRBP* and its splice variants after scratch assay, normalized to GAPDH. *CIRBP*-SV3 and *CIRBP*-SV4 expression were below the detection limit in one out of three experiments. (**E**–**G**) pri-miRs, pre-miRs, and mature microRNA expression levels of miR-329 and miR-495 were measured after scratch assay and normalized to U6; lncRNA-*CIRBP*-AS1 expression levels were measured and normalized to GAPDH.

Data show the percentage compared to the siRNA negative control group. (**H**) Representative image of the tube-formation assay ($n = 5$) on HUVECs treated over 24 h with siRNA targeted to *CIRBP* and negative control. (**I**) Quantification of the number of segments, number of branches, and total length of the tubes of the HUVECs after siRNA treatment compared to the negative-control siRNA treatment. Data are presented as the mean ± SEM; * $p < 0.05$; ** $p < 0.01$; independent sample Student's *t*-tests (**B,C**) or one-sample t-tests (two-tail) (**D–G,I**).

After the scratch assays, cells were collected for RNA isolation to assess the expression of total *CIRBP*, *CIRBP-SVs*, and lncRNA-*CIRBP*-AS1 as well as the two microRNAs and their precursors. As shown in Figure 4A, the siRNA-*CIRBP* was designed to target all splice variants. Total *CIRBP* levels were indeed knocked down by 87.3% ($p = 0.002$, Figure 5D). However, when looking at the individual splice variants, only *CIRBP*-SV1 was knocked down (99.0% decrease, $p = 0.002$), whereas the other splice variants remained unaffected (Figure 5D). Furthermore, a trend towards decreased lncRNA-*CIRBP*-AS1 expression (39.5% decrease, $p = 0.078$) was also observed when *CIRBP* was knocked down (Figure 5G). Although upregulation of *CIRBP* expression through hypothermia did not increase microRNA expression, a significant decrease (71.2%; $p = 0.02$; Figure 5F) was observed in the expression of miR-495-3p under *CIRBP* knockdown. Surprisingly, miR-329-3p was not significantly downregulated in response to *CIRBP* knockdown, as it was in Cirp-deficient mice. We did observe a trend towards accumulation of the primary microRNA, pri-miR-329-1, which is in correspondence with *CIRBP*'s effects on microRNA biogenesis [25].

2.6. CIRBP and miRNA Expression in lncRNA-CIRBP-AS1 Knockdown

In order to determine the potential effects of lncRNA-*CIRBP*-AS1 on both angiogenesis and *CIRBP* and microRNA expression, the angiogenesis assays described above were repeated using an siRNA against the lncRNA itself. Knockdown of lncRNA-*CIRBP*-AS1 resulted in a 4.8-fold improvement in HUVEC migration ($p < 0.001$; Figure 6A,B), while no significant difference was observed in the tube formation (Figure 6H,I). The potential effect of cell proliferation on scratch-wound healing was excluded, as there were no differences in the expression of PCNA mRNA between the groups (Figure 6C). Along with the antisense lncRNA (70.0% downregulation; $p = 0.017$; Figure 6G), total *CIRBP* expression was also downregulated by 64.4% ($p = 0.001$; Figure 6D). Both *CIRBP*-SV1 (80.4% downregulation; $p = 0.004$) and *CIRBP*-SV3 (60.0% downregulation; $p = 0.007$) expression decreased, while *CIRBP-SV2* and *-SV4* were unaffected (Figure 6D). Furthermore, knockdown of lncRNA-*CIRBP*-AS1 also resulted in a 53.5% downregulation of mature miR-329-3p ($p = 0.006$; Figure 6E) and an 85.9% decrease in mature miR-495-3p ($p = 0.003$; Figure 6F).

2.7. Scratch-Wound Healing in CIRBP Knockdown or lncRNA-CIRBP-AS1 Knockdown HUVECs after 4 Hours of siRNA Treatment

As knockdown of both *CIRBP* and its antisense had similar effects on microRNA expression and angiogenesis, as well as on each other, it cannot be concluded which of the two was the main effector. Therefore, the scratch-wound healing experiments described above were repeated using a much shorter transfection time of 4 h. We confirmed that a shorter transfection time would allow for direct effects on gene expression but not yet for indirect effects (Supplemental Materials Figure S1).

CIRBP inhibition, again, enhanced HUVEC migration significantly (31.8%, $p = 0.006$ at 4 h; 14.7%, $p = 0.11$ at 8 h; 19.8%, $p = 0.015$ at 12 h; 48.2%, $p = 0.007$ at 20 h, Figure 7A,B).

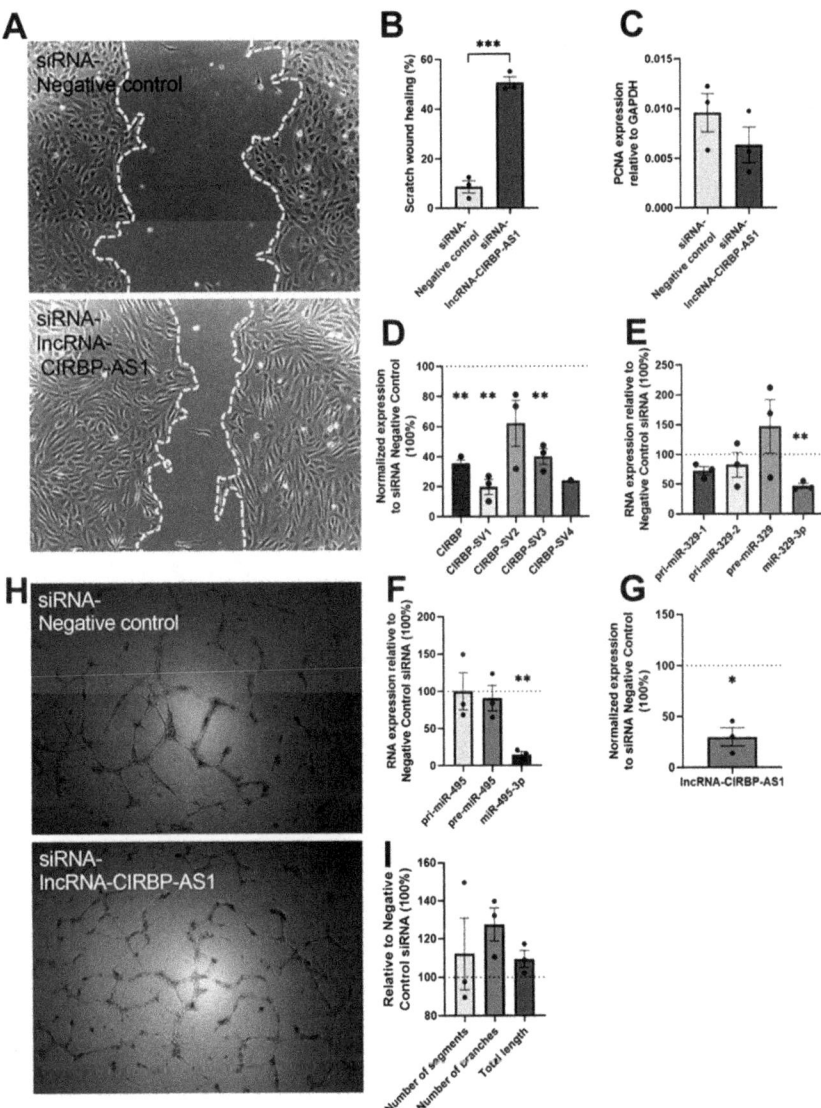

Figure 6. siRNA-lncRNA-*CIRBP*-AS1 transfection over 24 h in HUVECs: (**A**) Representative images of wound healing (*n* = 3) and (**B**) quantification of the migration area, treated with siRNA targeted to lncRNA-*CIRBP*-AS1 and the negative control for 24 h. White, dotted lines mark the edge of the HUVECs' monolayer. (**C**) *PCNA* expression level in HUVECs as an indicator of cell proliferation. (**D**) Total *CIRBP* expression and its splice variant expression after the scratch assay, normalized to GAPDH. *CIRBP*-SV4 expression was below the detection limit in two out of three experiments. (**E–G**) After the scratch assay, pri-miRs, pre-miRs, and mature microRNA expression levels of miR-329 and miR-495 were measured and normalized to U6; lncRNA-*CIRBP*-AS1 expression levels were measured and normalized to GAPDH. Data show the percentage compared to the siRNA negative control group. (**H**) Representative image of the tube formation assay (*n* = 3) on HUVECs treated over 24 h with siRNA targeted to *CIRBP* and the negative control. (**I**) Quantification of the number of segments, number of branches, and total length of the tubes of the HUVECs after siRNA treatment compared to the negative-control siRNA treatment. Data are presented as the mean ± SEM; * $p < 0.05$; ** $p < 0.01$; *** $p < 0.001$; independent sample Student's *t*-tests (**B**,**C**) or one-sample *t*-tests (two-tail) (**D–G**,**I**).

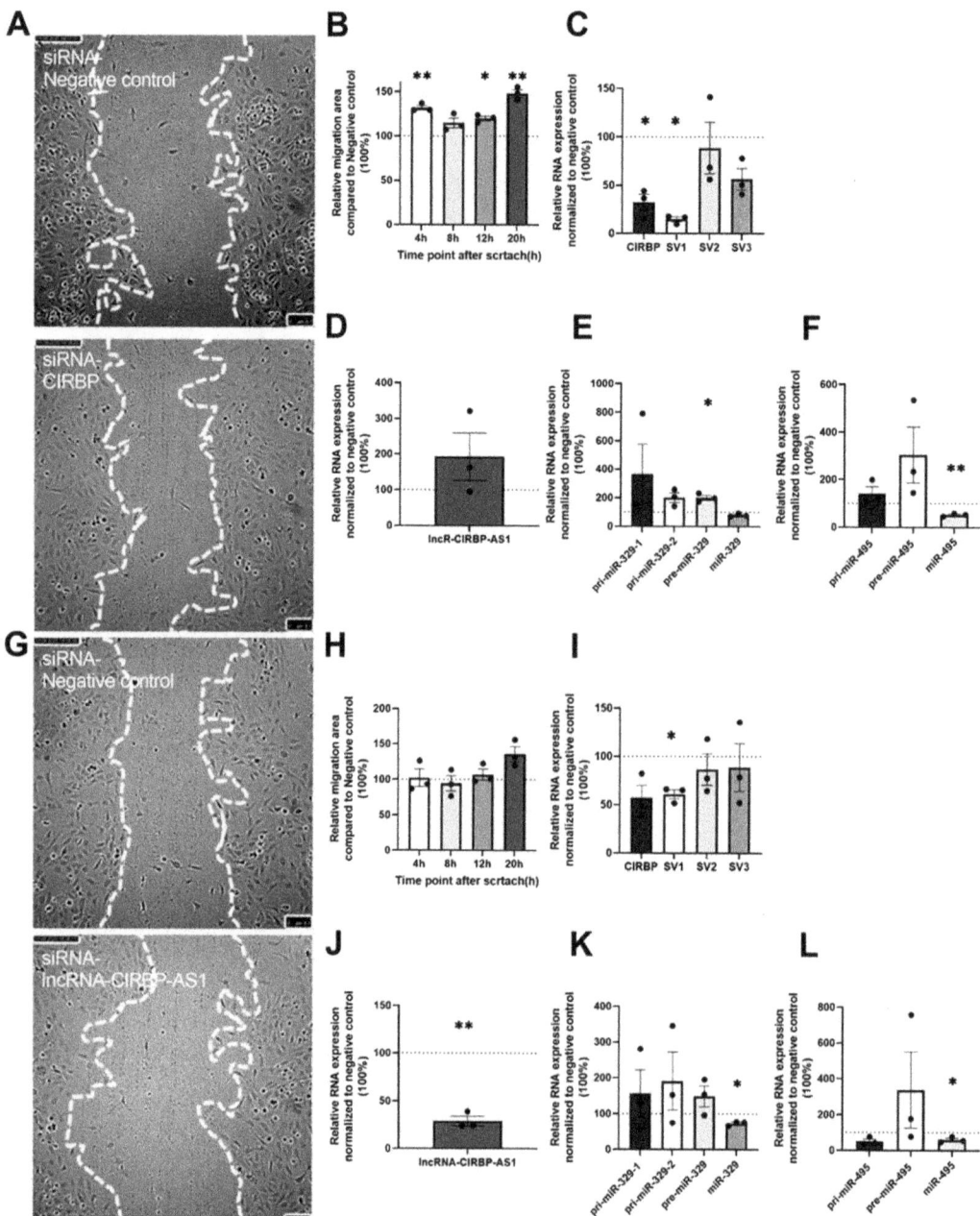

Figure 7. Four-hour transfection of siRNA on HUVECs: (**A**) Representative image of wound healing (n = 3) at 20 h after scratch on HUVECs, and (**B**) quantification of the migration area at different timepoints, treated over 4 h with siRNA targeted to *CIRBP* and the negative control. White, dotted lines mark the edge of the HUVECs' layer. (**C**) Total *CIRBP* expression and its splice variant expressions after the scratch assay, normalized to GAPDH. (**D–F**) After the scratch assay, the pri-miRNA, pre-miRNA, and mature microRNA expression levels of miR-329 and miR-495 were measured and normalized to U6; lncRNA-*CIRBP*-AS1 were measured and normalized to GAPDH. (**G**) Representative image of wound healing (n = 3)

at 20 h after scratch on HUVECs, and (**H**) quantification of the migration area at different timepoints, treated over 4 h with siRNA targeted to *CIRBP* and the negative control. White, dotted lines mark the edge of the HUVECs' layer. (**I**) Total *CIRBP* expression and its splice variant=s after the scratch assay, normalized to GAPDH. (**J–L**) After the scratch assay, the pri-miRNA, pre-miRNA, and mature microRNA expression levels of miR-329 and miR-495 were measured and normalized to U6; lncRNA-*CIRBP*-AS1 were measured and normalized to GAPDH. Data show the percentage compared to siRNA and the negative control group. Data are presented as the mean ± SEM; * $p < 0.05$; ** $p < 0.01$; one-sample *t*-tests (two-tail).

CIRBP and *CIRBP-SV1* expression were downregulated compared to the control siRNA (67.8% decrease, $p = 0.015$; 85.2% decrease, $p < 0.001$, respectively), and *CIRBP-SV3* showed a trend towards decreased expression (43.4%; $p = 0.06$) (Figure 7C). Expression of the lncRNA-*CIRBP*-AS1 was unaffected (Figure 7D); however, both precursors of the microRNAs, pre-miR-329 (101%; $p = 0.03$) and pre-miR-495, appeared upregulated, whereas the mature miR-495-3p was, again, downregulated (46.87%; $p = 0.007$) (Figure 7E,F), indicating reduced processing from precursor to mature microRNA in accordance with our previous study [25]. When HUVECs were transfected with an siRNA against lncRNA-*CIRBP*-AS1 for only 4 h, there was no significant difference in the cell migration area (Figure 7G,H).

Expression of *CIRBP-SV1* and lncRNA-*CIRBP*-AS1 were downregulated by 39.0% ($p = 0.014$) and 71.1% ($p = 0.005$), respectively (Figure 7I,J), and the expression of both miR-329-3p and miR-495-3p also decreased by 26.7% ($p = 0.02$) and 39.9% ($p = 0.045$), respectively (Figure 7K,L).

However, the lack of an effect on cell migration of siRNA-lncRNA-*CIRBP*-AS1 after 4 h of transfection strongly supports the idea that *CIRBP*, and not lncRNA-*CIRBP*-AS1, was the main effector in *CIRBP*-mediated effects on angiogenesis.

3. Discussion

In this study, we confirmed the previous findings that deficiency in *CIRBP* leads to enhanced angiogenesis in a murine hindlimb ischemia model. We demonstrated that during ischemia, *CIRBP* contributed to the regulation of the angiomiRs, miR-329-3p and miR-495-3p, both in vivo and in vitro. Importantly, we demonstrated increased angiogenic activity upon *CIRBP* knockdown in human endothelial cells. Furthermore, we investigated the complex *CIRBP* gene sequence in humans more closely and looked in detail at the regulation of different *CIRBP* splice variants as well as a regulatory antisense lncRNA, lncRNA-*CIRBP*-AS1.

The hindlimb ischemia model is a classical method to investigate post-ischemic neo-vascularization, commonly employed as a model for PAD in humans [26]. Even though $Cirp^{-/-}$ mice display enhanced angiogenesis after induction of ischemia, faster blood flow recovery in $Cirp^{-/-}$ mice compared to wild-type C57/BL6 mice was not observed. Most likely, this can be attributed to the fact that during hindlimb ischemia and PAD, blood flow recovery depends more strongly on arteriogenesis than on angiogenesis [27]. Nonetheless, enhanced angiogenesis can still be highly beneficial for PAD patients, as the available blood is distributed better throughout the affected tissues and as enhanced angiogenesis can prevent non-healing wounds and ulcers, which are a common and serious complication in PAD patients [28]. Indeed, it was shown in $Cirp^{-/-}$ mice that the inflammatory response in tissue wound healing was faster than in wild-type mice. More CD31 expression, as a marker of endothelial cells and, thus, angiogenesis, was observed in the wounds of $Cirp^{-/-}$ mice [29], although the exact mechanism of action for *CIRBP* in wound healing was not elucidated. The pro-inflammatory function of *CIRBP* under stress conditions has already been reported by Qiang et al. [30]. Furthermore, *CIRBP* was reported to influence changes in leukocyte recruitment and macrophage polarization in direction to regenerative M2-like macrophages, thus regulating angiogenesis and tissue regeneration [5]. Moreover, the authors reported that *CIRBP* binds TLR4, MD2, and the TLR4/MD2 complex, which are known to stimulate neovascularization and can be found on both macrophages and neutrophils [31]. However, *CIRBP* acts through other angiogenesis-related pathways as well and, furthermore, the *CIRBP* gene in humans has a more complex structure than in mice, as it has several splice variants that result in different proteins as well as an antisense lncRNA. Their role has not been investigated in angiogenesis yet.

In previous studies, our group showed that *CIRBP* regulates the processing and expression of microRNAs, miR-329-3p and miR-495-3p [25], which both play an important role in angiogenesis [21]. We expected *CIRBP* to affect angiogenesis by regulating the expression of miR-329-3p and miR-495-3p. Importantly, we also reported enhanced macrophage attraction and influx into the vessel wall upon miR-495-3p inhibition [22], which could help explain the effects observed in the studies by Kübler et al. described above. In the current study, we showed that *CIRBP* was regulated under hypothermic conditions as was reported previously [7,9–12]. The novelty of this study, however, is that we showed this in human vascular endothelial cells that were subjected to hypothermic conditions, which frequently occurs in PAD patients [1]. The expression of the 14q32 microRNAs, miR-329-3p and miR-495-3p, did not increase under hypothermia in HUVECs, however, even though the expression of their reported post-transcriptional regulator *CIRBP* increased. In contrast, silencing of *CIRBP*, using an siRNA, did lead to a decrease in miR-495-3p expression. Likely, the processing rate of 14q32 microRNAs was already at an optimum level under normothermic conditions, which can explain that an increase in *CIRBP* did not induce more processing of precursor microRNAs. The dramatic decrease in *CIRBP* expression following siRNA treatment, on the other hand, did result in insufficient processing of miR-495-3p. Surprisingly, expression of miR-329-3p was still unaffected in vitro in human cells, even though we did observe a trend towards accumulation of the primary microRNA, pri-miR-329-1, which would correspond with the inhibition of microRNA biogenesis. In vivo in mice, on the other hand, we could clearly see that ischemia-induced upregulation of both miR-329-3p and miR-495-3p was blocked quite efficiently in $Cirp^{-/-}$ mice.

When we speculate what these findings could mean for human PAD, *CIRBP* expression would likely be increased, as patients suffer from cold extremities [1]. We found that hypothermia caused *CIRBP* expression upregulation. Such an increase in *CIRBP*, likely accompanied by continuously high miR-329-3p and possible miR-495-3p expression, would inhibit efficient angiogenesis and wound healing in PAD patients, with, for example, non-healing ulcers. Meanwhile, others have reported that warm temperatures (42 °C) can decrease *CIRBP* expression in male germ cells [32]. Therefore, one could imagine that hyperthermia leads to decreased *CIRBP* expression in the leg, followed by subsequent increases in angiogenesis. Thus far, heat therapy was shown to be of potential benefit to PAD patients by enhancing leg blood flow and improving muscle function [33,34].

We further assessed the potential pro-angiogenic features of *CIRBP* knockdown in human primary endothelial cells. Indeed, cell-migration assays as well as tube-formation assays in HUVECs showed an increase in angiogenic potential following *CIRBP* downregulation. These findings are in line with those found in vivo. Looking at human cells, however, also allowed us to look into changes in the *CIRBP* splice variants (*CIRBP-SVs*) and its antisense long noncoding RNA (lncRNA-*CIRBP*-AS1). *CIRBP* has four splice variants that alter the coding sequence. Of these four variants, *CIRBP-SV1* specifically showed a trend towards upregulation after 24 and 48 h of hypothermia. When we knocked down *CIRBP* using an siRNA, we again observed specific knockdown of *CIRBP-SV1*. This was unexpected, as the binding site of the siRNA was predicted to target an mRNA sequence that is present in all four splice variants. Although we cannot explain the siRNA's preference for *CIRBP-SV1*, we can conclude that the majority of *CIRBP*'s effects on angiogenesis were elicited through *CIRBP-SV1*.

The antisense strand of the human *CIRBP* gene also encodes a long noncoding RNA, lncRNA-*CIRBP*-AS1, the function of which has not yet been elucidated. We observed a trend towards upregulation of lncRNA-*CIRBP*-AS1 under hypothermic conditions, although the response to hypothermia was slower than that of *CIRBP* itself. After *CIRBP* knockdown, lncRNA-*CIRBP*-AS1 expression decreased, and after lncRNA-*CIRBP*-AS1 knockdown, *CIRBP* expression decreased; inhibition of lncRNA-*CIRBP*-AS1 with an siRNA resulted in simultaneous downregulation of total *CIRBP* and of *CIRBP-SV1*, and *CIRBP-*

SV3 in particular. Furthermore, lncRNA-*CIRBP*-AS1 knockdown resulted in a decreased expression of both mature miR-329-3p and miR-495-3p. More importantly, silencing of lncRNA-*CIRBP*-AS1, like *CIRBP* itself, resulted in increased angiogenesis in HUVECs.

Likely, a positive feedback loop supports the transcription of the *CIRBP* locus, where *CIRBP* and lncRNA-*CIRBP*-AS1 induce each other's expression. In order to elucidate which of the two is the main effector in the enhanced angiogenic potential of HUVECs, we separated their mutual effects by shortening the siRNA transfection duration, and we found that *CIRBP* knockdown still had the same effect on angiogenesis and regulation of microRNA expression, while lncRNA-*CIRBP*-AS1 knockdown could no longer improve angiogenesis, even though miR-329-3p expression was already reduced significantly. Combining these findings, we conclude that the effects of lncRNA-*CIRBP*-AS1 downregulation on angiogenesis were most likely indirect. We can also conclude, however, that lncRNA-*CIRBP*-AS1 can directly impact *CIRBP* expression and, likely, also miR-329-3p expression. The mechanisms behind this regulation remain to be determined.

In conclusion, our findings confirm the previously reported increase in post-ischemic angiogenesis in $Cirp^{-/-}$ mice. We showed that *CIRBP* directly regulated the angiomiRs microRNAs, miR-329-3p and miR-495-3p, in vivo. In addition, we validated these findings in human primary endothelial cells for the first time. Furthermore, we showed that *CIRBP-SV1* was the splice variant that predominantly regulates *CIRBP*'s effects on both microRNA expression and angiogenesis. Finally, the lncRNA-*CIRBP*-AS1 can also impact angiogenesis, but these effects are likely caused by directing changes in *CIRBP-SV1* and, subsequently, miR-329-3p and miR-495-3p.

4. Materials and Methods

4.1. Animal Experiments

All animal experiments were approved by the Committee on Animal Welfare of the Leiden University Medical Center (Leiden, The Netherlands) and were performed in accordance with the Directive 2010/63/EU of the European Parliament and Dutch government guidelines. $Cirp^{-/-}$ embryos on a C57BL6/J background were kindly provided by Jun Fujita's lab (Kyoto University, Kyoto, Japan) [35]. WT C57BL/6 mice (n = 10, male, aged 8–10 weeks) and $Cirp^{-/-}$ mice (n = 11, male, aged 8–10 weeks) were bred in the LUMC's in-house breeding facility and had free access to water and regular chow.

4.2. HLI Model

Before surgery, mice were anesthetized via an intraperitoneal injection of midazolam (5 mg/kg; Roche Diagnostics, Almere, The Netherlands), medetomidine (0.5 mg/kg; Orion, Espoo, Finland), and fentanyl (0.05 mg/kg; Janssen Pharmaceuticals, Beerse, Belgium). Unilateral HLI was induced by double ligation of the left femoral artery, proximal to the superficial epigastric artery and proximal to the bifurcation of the popliteal and saphenous artery. After surgery, mice were given a subcutaneous injection of flumazenil (0.5 mg/kg, Fresenius Kabi, Utrecht, The Netherlands) and atipamezol (2.5 mg/kg, Orion) to antagonize anesthesia. Buprenorphine (0.1 mg/kg, MSD Animal Health, Boxmeer, The Netherlands) was given after surgery for pain relief [36].

4.3. Laser Doppler Perfusion Measurements

Blood flow recovery to the paw was measured over time using laser Doppler perfusion imaging (LDPI) (Moor Instruments, Axminster, United Kingdom) at day 0 (before and after ligation), 3, 7, 10, 14, 21, and 28. Before measurements, mice were anesthetized with an intraperitoneal injection of midazolam (5 mg/kg, Roche Diagnostics) and medetomidine (0.5 mg/kg, Orion). Mice were placed in a double-glassed pot that was perfused with water at 37 °C for 5 min prior to each measurement. LDPI measurements in the ligated paw were normalized to measurements of the unligated paw as an internal control. After LDPI, anesthesia was antagonized by subcutaneous injection of flumazenil (0.5 mg/kg) and atipamezole (2.5 mg/kg).

At day 28, after the last LDPI measurement, mice were injected with fentanyl (0.05 mg/kg) and sacrificed via retro-orbital bleeding. The proximal half of the adductor muscle was harvested and fixed in 4% formaldehyde. The distal half of the adductor muscle and the soleus muscle were harvested and snap-frozen on dry-ice.

4.4. Immunohistochemical Staining

Adductor muscles were embedded in paraffin, and 5 μm thick sections were cut for histological analysis. Smooth muscle cells were stained with primary antibody mouse anti-mouse α-SMA (Dako, 1:1000). Rabbit anti-mouse HRP (Dako, 1:300) was used as the secondary antibody. Slides were scanned with the Pannoramic MIDI digital slide scanner (3DHistech). The number and lumen diameter of α-SMA positive vessels were analyzed by Pannoramic viewer software (3DHistech, version: 2.3) with 20× magnification (3 sections per limb per mouse). The smallest diameter of vessel was measured in the picture as described previously [37].

Six μm-thick frozen soleus sections (3 sections per limb per mouse) were fixed in ice-cold acetone and stained using primary antibody anti-CD31 biotin (Biolegend, 102503, 1:100) and an avidin–biotin complex (ABC) kit (Vector, Burlingame, CA, USA). Slides were scanned with the Pannoramic MIDI digital slide scanner (3DHistech). Random snapshots (3 per section) were taken by the Pannoramic viewer software (3DHistech) with 40× magnification (6–9 images per limb per mouse). The CD31 positive area was quantified by ImageJ as described previously [38].

4.5. Isolation of Venous Endothelial Cells (HUVECs)

Primary human vascular cells were isolated as described earlier by Welten et al. [21]. In brief, for HUVEC isolation, the vein was inserted with a cannula and flushed with sterile PBS. The vessel was infused with 0.075% collagenase type II (Worthington) and incubated at 37 °C for 20 min. The collagenase solution was collected, and the vessel was flushed with PBS in order to collect all detached endothelial cells. The cell suspension was centrifuged at 400× g for 5 min, and the pellet was resuspended in HUVEC culture medium (EBM-2 Basal Medium (CC-3156) and EGMTM-2 SingleQuots™ Supplements (CC-4176), Lonza, Walkersville, MD, USA). HUVECs were cultured in plates coated with 1% fibronectin from bovine plasma (Sigma, Amsterdam, The Netherlands).

4.6. Primary HUVEC Cell Culture

HUVECs were cultured at 37 °C in a humidified 5% CO_2 environment with HUVEC culture medium (EBM-2 Basal Medium (CC-3156) and EGMTM-2 SingleQuots™ Supplements (CC-4176), Lonza). Media were refreshed every 2–3 days. Cells were passed using trypsin (Sigma) at 70–80% confluency. HUVECs were used for the scratch-wound healing assay at passage three. HUVECs were stored up to passage three in 90% heat inactivated New Born Calf Serum (NBSCi) (Sigma) and 10% DMSO (Sigma).

4.7. Hypothermic HUVEC Cell Culture

Primary HUVECs were seeded in 12-well plates coated with 1% fibronectin at 100,000 cells per well in culture medium. After overnight incubation at 37 °C, cells were washed with PBS and new media were applied before putting the plates in the right incubator: the normothermic incubator at 37 °C and the hypothermic incubator at 32 °C, both humidified at 5% CO_2 and 20% O_2. After 24 or 48 h, cells were washed with PBS, and 0.5 mL TRIzol/well was added for RNA isolation. Each single condition was performed in triplicate, and the hypothermia experiment was performed three independent times.

4.8. CIRBP and lncRNA-CIRBP-AS1 Knockdown with siRNA Transfection In Vitro

Primary HUVECs were seeded in 12-well plates coated with 1% fibronectin at 100,000 cells per well in culture medium. After 24 h, cells were washed with PBS, and each well was incubated with 900 μL Opti-MEM medium with 10% NBSCi and 1% penicillin/streptomycin and, after 10 min of incubation, 100 µL of transfection medium (94 µL Opti-MEM with 3 µL of Lipofectamine RNAiMax (Life Technologies, Bleiswijk, The Netherlands) and 3 µL of siRNA) was added. The final siRNA concentration per well was 30 nM. The siRNAs used were siRNA-*CIRBP* (sasi-172352), siRNA-lncRNA-*CIRBP*-AS1 (sasi-208901), and siRNA negative control (Mission Universal Negative Control #1) (all Sigma–Aldrich, Amsterdam, The Netherlands). After addition of transfection agents, cells were put in the incubator at 37 °C for the required time.

4.9. Migration Assay–Scratch Wound Healing

Primary HUVECs were seeded in 12-well plates coated with 1% fibronectin at 150,000 cells per well in HUVEC culture medium. After 24 h, the media were replaced with transfection medium as previously described. Then, transfection was conducted, and a scratch wound was performed across the diameter of each well using a p200 pipette tip. Next, cells were washed with PBS and fresh starving medium, and EBM-2 (Lonza) containing only 0.2% FBS and 1% gentamicin amphotericin of the provided BulletKit was added. In order to monitor scratch-wound closure, live phase-contrast microscopy (Axiovert 40C, Carl Zeiss, Oberkohen, Germany) was used for taking pictures at 0 and 18 h after introducing the scratch wound. In addition, a live cell microscope (Leica AF6000, Leica Microsystems, Tokyo, Japan) was used for taking picture every 4 h after scratch until 20 h in the timeline experiment. Pictures were taken in the same location at two positions in each well. Where necessary, pictures were contrast-enhanced using Microsoft PowerPoint. Scratch size was calculated using the wound healing tool macro for ImageJ. Finally, cells were washed with PBS, and 0.5 mL TRIzol/well was added for RNA isolation. Each single scratch assay condition was performed in triplicate, and the scratch-wound healing assay was performed three independent times.

4.10. Tube-Formation Assay

Tube-formation assay was performed using HUVECs at passage three. At confluence, cells were transfected as described above with Lipofectamine RNAiMax and siRNA-*CIRBP*, lncRNA-*CIRBP*-AS1, or siRNA negative control. After 24 h, cells were counted and seeded on solidified Geltrex™ (ref: A14132-02, Gibco) in a 96-well plate at 15,000 cells per well. Photos were taken using live phase-contrast microscopy at 12 h after seeding and quantified using the ImageJ Angiogenesis Analyzer. Each single tube-formation assay was performed in 6 wells per condition, and the tube-formation assay was performed three independent times.

4.11. Aorta Ring Assay

Thoracic aortas were isolated from $Cirp^{-/-}$ and wild-type mice, aged 4–5 weeks, after exsanguination under anesthesia via an intraperitoneal injection of midazolam (5 mg/kg; Roche Diagnostics), medetomidine (0.5 mg/kg; Orion), and fentanyl (0.05 mg/kg; Janssen Pharmaceuticals). Vessels were washed with Opti-MEM medium containing 1% penicillin/streptomycin and were cut transversely. Consequently, aorta rings were obtained 0.5–1 mm in width and incubated in Opti-MEM medium with 1% penicillin/streptomycin overnight at 37 °C. Collagen (type I, Merck Millipore, Darmstadt, Germany) was diluted to a concentration of 1 mg/mL with DMEM and 1% penicillin/streptomycin, and the pH was adjusted with 5 N NaOH to 7. Aortic rings were placed in 96-well plates coated with 75 µL collagen matrix as described previously [39]. After 1 h, 150 µL Opti-MEM supplemented with 2.5% FBS (PAA Laboratories, Pasching, Austria), penicillin–streptomycin (PAA Laboratories), and with or without vascular endothelial growth factor (in-house production and purification) of 10 or 30 ng/mL were added to the designated wells. Media were refreshed on days 3 and 5. Microvessel outgrowth was quantified after 7 days on photographs taken by live phase-contrast microscopy (Axiovert 40C, Carl Zeiss). The counting of microvessels started from a specific point on the ring, and each microvessel emerging from the ring was counted as a sprout, and individual branches arising from each microvessel counted as a separate sprout, working around the ring clockwise.

4.12. RNA Isolation

RNA isolation of cultured cells or tissue was performed by standard TRIzol–chloroform extraction according to the manufacturer's instructions (Thermo Fisher Scientific, Wilmington, DE, USA). RNA concentrations were measured using the Nanodrop^{TM} 1000 Spectrophotometer (Thermo Fisher Scientific).

4.13. MicroRNA Quantification

For microRNA quantification of miR-329-3p and miR-495-3p, RNA was reversed transcribed using the Taqman^{TM} MicroRNA Reverse-Transcription Kit (Thermo Fisher Scientific) and, subsequently, quantified using microRNA-specific Taqman^{TM} qPCR kits (Thermo Fisher Scientific) on the VIIa7 (Thermo Fisher Scientific). MicroRNA expression was normalized against U6 small nuclear RNA.

4.14. mRNA, pri-microRNA, and pre-microRNA Quantification

For quantification of the expression levels of *CIRBP*, *CIRBP-SVs*, lncRNA-*CIRBP*-AS1, primary microRNAs (pri-miRs), and pre-miRs, RNA was reverse transcribed using a "High-Capacity RNA to cDNA Kit" (Thermo Fisher Scientific) and quantified by qPCR using SybrGreen reagents (Qiagen, Hilden, Germany) on the VIIa7. *CIRBP*, *CIRBP-SVs*, *PCNA*, and lncRNA-*CIRBP*-AS1 expressions were normalized against GAPDH; pri-miRs and pre-miRs expressions were normalized to U6. Primer sequences are provided in Table 1.

Table 1. Sequences of primers used for qPCR and the siRNAs used for knockdown.

Primers	Forward Sequence	Reverse Sequence
HSA-CIRBP	TTGACACCAATGAGCAGTCG	GGCATCCTTAGCGTCGTCAA
HSA-splice variant 1	CGTGGGTTCTCTAGAGGAGGA	CTCGTTGTGTGTAGCGTAACTG
HSA-splice variant 2	CGTGGGTTCTCTAGAGGAGGA	CGCCCTCGGAGTGTGACTTA
HSA-splice variant 3	CGTGGGTTCTCTAGAGGAGGA	TCAACCGTAACTGTCATAACTG
HSA-splice variant 4	GTAGACCAGGCAGGAGGAG	CGCCCTCGGAGTGTGACTTA
HSA-lncRNA-CIRBP-AS1	CAATGGGAAAAGGAGGAAACT	CCTTGTAAAGCTGGTTCTCCA
GAPDH	CACCACCATGGAGAAGGC	AGCAGTTGGTGGTGCAGGA
HSA-pri-miR-329-1	TGGGGAAGAATCAGTGGTGT	GACCAGAAGGCCTCCAAGAT
HSA-pri-miR-329-2	TGTCAAGTTTGGGGAAGGAA	GACCAGAAGGCCTCCAAGAT
HSA-pre-miR-329	TGAAGAGAGGTTTTCTGGGTTT	ACCAGGTGTGTTTCGTCCTC
HSA-pri-miR-495	CTGACCCTCAGTGTCCCTTC	ATGGAGGCACTTCAAGGAGA
HSA-pre-miR-495	GCCCATGTTATTTTCGCTTT	CCGAAAAAGAAGTGCACCAT
U6	AGAAGATTAGCATGGCCCCT	ATTTGCGTGTCATCCTTGCG
siRNA CIRPB	GAGUCAGAGUGGUGGCUAC	
siRNA lncRNA-CIRBP-AS1	CAGGACCCUCACUCACUA	

4.15. Statistical Analyses

Data are presented as the mean ± SEM. Indicated differences had the following levels of significance: * $p < 0.05$; ** $p < 0.01$; *** $p < 0.001$. All tests were performed with a significance level of $\alpha = 0.05$.

One-sample *t*-tests were performed to test differences between treated groups that were expressed relative to the negative control treatment, which was set to 100%. One-sample *t*-tests (two tail) were used in the knockdown experiments, scratch assay, and tube-formation assay. One-sample *t*-tests (one tail) were used in the hypothermia experiment.

Differences in scratch wound healing and PCNA levels between groups were assessed using independent sample Student's *t*-tests.

Two-way ANOVA tests were performed to detect statistically significant differences among multiple groups. These tests were used to compare miRNA-329-3p and -495-3p expression levels of the soleus of mice subjected to HLI surgery at different timepoints.

Supplementary Materials: The following are available online at https://www.mdpi.com/article/10.3390/ijms222312678/s1.

Author Contributions: All authors contributed to the study conception and design. Material preparation, and data collection and analysis were performed by E.A.C.G., L.Z. and M.R.d.V. The first draft of the manuscript was written by E.A.C.G. and L.Z. and revised by M.R.d.V., P.H.A.Q., J.W.J., and A.Y.N. All authors commented on previous versions of the manuscript. All authors have read and approved the final manuscript.

Funding: This research was funded by an LUMC MD/PhD grant (E.A.C. Goossens) and a full research grant by the Austrian Science Fund (FWF) Lise Meitner Fellowship (M-2578-B30, A.Y.N.)

Institutional Review Board Statement: The study was conducted in accordance with the Directive 2010/63/EU of the European Parliament and approved by the Animal Welfare Committee of the Leiden Medical University Center (Project Number: 1160020185764 (Date of approval: 9 April 2020)).

Informed Consent Statement: Not applicable.

Data Availability Statement: All data are included in the manuscript or available upon request.

Acknowledgments: Open Access Funding by the Austrian Science Fund (FWF).

Conflicts of Interest: The authors declare no conflict of interest.

References

1. McDermott, M.M. Lower extremity manifestations of peripheral artery disease: The pathophysiologic and functional implications of leg ischemia. *Circ. Res.* **2015**, *116*, 1540–1550. [CrossRef]
2. Vartanian, S.M.; Conte, M.S. Surgical intervention for peripheral arterial disease. *Circ. Res.* **2015**, *116*, 1614–1628. [CrossRef] [PubMed]
3. Fu, X.; Zhang, Z.; Liang, K.; Shi, S.; Wang, G.; Zhang, K.; Li, K.; Li, W.; Li, T.; Zhai, S. Angioplasty versus bypass surgery in patients with critical limb ischemia-a meta-analysis. *Int. J. Clin. Exp. Med.* **2015**, *8*, 10595–10602. [PubMed]
4. Parvar, S.L.; Ngo, L.; Dawson, J.; Nicholls, S.J.; Fitridge, R.; Psaltis, P.J.; Ranasinghe, I. Long-term outcomes following endovascular and surgical revascularization for peripheral artery disease: A propensity score-matched analysis. *Eur. Heart J.* **2021**, ehab116. [CrossRef] [PubMed]
5. Kubler, M.; Beck, S.; Fischer, S.; Götz, P.; Kumaraswami, K.; Ishikawa-Ankerhold, H.; Lasch, M.; Deindl, E. Absence of Cold-Inducible RNA-Binding Protein (CIRP) Promotes Angiogenesis and Regeneration of Ischemic Tissue by Inducing M2-Like Macrophage Polarization. *Biomedicines* **2021**, *9*, 395. [CrossRef]
6. Kubler, M.; Beck, S.; Peffenköver, L.L.; Götz, P.; Ishikawa-Ankerhold, H.; Preissner, K.T.; Fischer, S.; Lasch, M.; Deindl, E. The Absence of Extracellular Cold-Inducible RNA-Binding Protein (eCIRP) Promotes Pro-Angiogenic Microenvironmental Conditions and Angiogenesis in Muscle Tissue Ischemia. *Int. J. Mol. Sci.* **2021**, *22*, 9484. [CrossRef] [PubMed]
7. Liu, A.; Zhang, Z.; Li, A.; Xue, J. Effects of hypothermia and cerebral ischemia on cold-inducible RNA-binding protein mRNA expression in rat brain. *Brain Res.* **2010**, *134*, 104–110. [CrossRef]
8. Wellmann, S.; Bührer, C.; Moderegger, E.; Zelmer, A.; Kirschner-Schwabe, R.; Koehne, P.; Fujita, J.; Seeger, K. Oxygen-regulated expression of the RNA-binding proteins RBM3 and CIRP by a HIF-1-independent mechanism. *J. Cell Sci.* **2004**, *117*, 1785–1794. [CrossRef]
9. Liao, Y.; Tong, L.; Tang, L.; Wu, S. The role of cold-inducible RNA binding protein in cell stress response. *Int. J. Cancer* **2017**, *141*, 2164–2173. [CrossRef]
10. Al-Fageeh, M.B.; Smales, C.M. Cold-inducible RNA binding protein (CIRP) expression is modulated by alternative mRNAs. *RNA* **2009**, *15*, 1164–1176. [CrossRef]
11. Lleonart, M.E. A new generation of proto-oncogenes: Cold-inducible RNA binding proteins. *Biochim. Biophys. Acta* **2010**, *1805*, 43–52. [CrossRef] [PubMed]
12. Fujita, J. Cold shock response in mammalian cells. *J. Mol. Microbiol. Biotechnol.* **1999**, *1*, 243–255. [PubMed]
13. Nishiyama, H.; Itoh, K.; Kaneko, Y.; Kishishita, M.; Yoshida, O.; Fujita, J. A glycine-rich RNA-binding protein mediating cold-inducible suppression of mammalian cell growth. *J. Cell Biol.* **1997**, *137*, 899–908. [CrossRef]
14. Nishiyama, H.; Higashitsuji, H.; Yokoi, H.; Itoh, K.; Danno, S.; Matsuda, T.; Fujita, J. Cloning and characterization of human CIRP (cold-inducible RNA-binding protein) cDNA and chromosomal assignment of the gene. *Gene* **1997**, *204*, 115–120. [CrossRef]
15. Zhu, X.; Buhrer, C.; Wellmann, S. Cold-inducible proteins CIRP and RBM3, a unique couple with activities far beyond the cold. *Cell. Mol. Life Sci.* **2016**, *73*, 3839–3859. [CrossRef]
16. Zhong, P.; Huang, H. Recent progress in the research of cold-inducible RNA-binding protein. *Future Sci. OA* **2017**, *3*, FSO246. [CrossRef] [PubMed]
17. Horii, Y.; Shiina, T.; Uehara, S.; Nomura, K.; Shimaoka, H.; Horii, K.; Shimizu, Y. Hypothermia induces changes in the alternative splicing pattern of cold-inducible RNA-binding protein transcripts in a non-hibernator, the mouse. *Biomed Res.* **2019**, *40*, 153–161. [CrossRef] [PubMed]
18. Pelechano, V.; Steinmetz, L.M. Gene regulation by antisense transcription. *Nat. Rev. Genet.* **2013**, *14*, 880–893. [CrossRef]

19. Gomes, C.P.; Nóbrega-Pereira, S.; Silva, A.B.D.; Rebelo, K.; Alves-Vale, C.; Marinho, S.P.; Carvalho, T.; Dias, S.; De Jesus, B.B. An antisense transcript mediates MALAT1 response in human breast cancer. *BMC Cancer* **2019**, *19*, 771. [CrossRef]
20. Zong, X.; Nakagawa, S.; Freier, S.M.; Fei, J.; Ha, T.; Prasanth, S.G.; Prasanth, K.V. Natural antisense RNA promotes 3′ end processing and maturation of MALAT1 lncRNA. *Nucleic Acids Res.* **2016**, *44*, 2898–2908. [CrossRef]
21. Welten, S.M.; Bastiaansen, A.J.; de Jong, R.C.; de Vries, M.R.; Peters, E.A.; Boonstra, M.C.; Sheikh, S.P.; La Monica, N.; Kandimalla, E.R.; Quax, P.H.; et al. Inhibition of 14q32 MicroRNAs miR-329, miR-487b, miR-494, and miR-495 increases neovascularization and blood flow recovery after ischemia. *Circ. Res.* **2014**, *115*, 696–708. [CrossRef]
22. Welten, S.M.J.; de Jong, R.C.; Wezel, A.; de Vries, M.R.; Boonstra, M.C.; Parma, L.; Jukema, J.W.; van der Sluis, T.C.; Arens, R.; Bot, I.; et al. Inhibition of 14q32 microRNA miR-495 reduces lesion formation, intimal hyperplasia and plasma cholesterol levels in experimental restenosis. *Atherosclerosis* **2017**, *261*, 26–36. [CrossRef]
23. Wezel, A.; Welten, S.M.J.; Razawy, W.; Lagraauw, H.M.; de Vries, M.R.; Goossens, E.A.C.; Boonstra, M.C.; Hamming, J.F.; Kandimalla, E.R.; Kuiper, J.; et al. Inhibition of MicroRNA-494 Reduces Carotid Artery Atherosclerotic Lesion Development and Increases Plaque Stability. *Ann. Surg.* **2015**, *262*, 841–848. [CrossRef] [PubMed]
24. Welten, S.M.; Goossens, E.; Quax, P.; Nossent, A. The multifactorial nature of microRNAs in vascular remodelling. *Cardiovasc. Res.* **2016**, *110*, 6–22. [CrossRef]
25. Downie Ruiz Velasco, A.; Welten, S.M.; Goossens, E.; Quax, P.; Rappsilber, J.; Michlewski, G.; Nossent, A.Y. Posttranscriptional Regulation of 14q32 MicroRNAs by the CIRBP and HADHB during Vascular Regeneration after Ischemia. *Mol. Ther. Nucleic Acids* **2019**, *14*, 329–338. [CrossRef] [PubMed]
26. Krishna, S.M.; Omer, S.M.; Golledge, J. Evaluation of the clinical relevance and limitations of current pre-clinical models of peripheral artery disease. *Clin. Sci.* **2016**, *130*, 127–150. [CrossRef]
27. Tressel, S.L.; Kim, H.; Ni, C.-W.; Chang, K.; Velasquez-Castano, J.C.; Taylor, W.R.; Yoon, Y.-S.; Jo, H. Angiopoietin-2 stimulates blood flow recovery after femoral artery occlusion by inducing inflammation and arteriogenesis. *Arterioscler. Thromb. Vasc. Biol.* **2008**, *28*, 1989–1995. [CrossRef] [PubMed]
28. Olivieri, B.; Vianna, S.; Adenikinju, O.; Beasley, R.E.; Houseworth, J.; Olivieri, B. On the Cutting Edge: Wound Care for the Endovascular Specialist. *Semin. Intervent. Radiol.* **2018**, *35*, 406–426.
29. Idrovo, J.P.; Jacob, A.; Yang, W.L.; Wang, Z.; Yen, H.T.; Nicastro, J.; Coppa, G.F.; Wang, P. A deficiency in cold-inducible RNA-binding protein accelerates the inflammation phase and improves wound healing. *Int. J. Mol. Med.* **2016**, *37*, 423–428. [CrossRef]
30. Qiang, X.; Yang, W.-L.; Wu, R.; Zhou, M.; Jacob, A.; Dong, W.; Kuncewitch, M.; Ji, Y.; Yang, H.; Wang, H.; et al. Cold-inducible RNA-binding protein (CIRP) triggers inflammatory responses in hemorrhagic shock and sepsis. *Nat. Med.* **2013**, *19*, 1489–1495. [CrossRef]
31. de Groot, D.; Hoefer, I.E.; Grundmann, S.; Schoneveld, A.; Haverslag, R.T.; van Keulen, J.K.; Bot, P.T.; Timmers, L.; Piek, J.J.; Pasterkamp, G.; et al. Arteriogenesis requires toll-like receptor 2 and 4 expression in bone-marrow derived cells. *J. Mol. Cell. Cardiol.* **2011**, *50*, 25–32. [CrossRef]
32. Nishiyama, H.; Danno, S.; Kaneko, Y.; Itoh, K.; Yokoi, H.; Fukumoto, M.; Okuno, H.; Millán, J.L.; Matsuda, T.; Yoshida, O.; et al. Decreased expression of cold-inducible RNA-binding protein (CIRP) in male germ cells at elevated temperature. *Am. J. Pathol.* **1998**, *152*, 289–296. [PubMed]
33. Brunt, V.E.; Weidenfeld-Needham, K.M.; Comrada, L.N.; Francisco, M.A.; Eymann, T.M.; Minson, C.T. Serum from young, sedentary adults who underwent passive heat therapy improves endothelial cell angiogenesis via improved nitric oxide bioavailability. *Temperature* **2019**, *6*, 169–178. [CrossRef] [PubMed]
34. Neff, D.; Kuhlenhoelter, A.M.; Lin, C.; Wong, B.J.; Motaganahalli, R.L.; Roseguini, B.T. Thermotherapy reduces blood pressure and circulating endothelin-1 concentration and enhances leg blood flow in patients with symptomatic peripheral artery disease. *Am. J. Physiol. Regul. Integr. Comp. Physiol.* **2016**, *311*, R392–R400. [CrossRef] [PubMed]
35. Masuda, T.; Itoh, K.; Higashitsuji, H.; Nakazawa, N.; Sakurai, T.; Liu, Y.; Tokuchi, H.; Fujita, T.; Zhao, Y.; Nishiyama, H.; et al. Cold-inducible RNA-binding protein (Cirp) interacts with Dyrk1b/Mirk and promotes proliferation of immature male germ cells in mice. *Proc. Natl. Acad. Sci. USA* **2012**, *109*, 10885–10890. [CrossRef] [PubMed]
36. Aref, Z.; de Vries, M.R.; Quax, P.H.A. Variations in Surgical Procedures for Inducing Hind Limb Ischemia in Mice and the Impact of These Variations on Neovascularization Assessment. *Int. J. Mol. Sci.* **2019**, *20*, 3704. [CrossRef]
37. Bastiaansen, A.J.; Ewing, M.M.; de Boer, H.C.; van der Pouw Kraan, T.C.; de Vries, M.R.; Peters, E.A.; Welten, S.M.; Arens, R.; Moore, S.M.; Faber, J.E.; et al. Lysine acetyltransferase PCAF is a key regulator of arteriogenesis. *Arterioscler. Thromb. Vasc. Biol.* **2013**, *33*, 1902–1910. [CrossRef]
38. Nossent, A.Y.; Bastiaansen, A.J.; Peters, E.A.; de Vries, M.R.; Aref, Z.; Welten, S.M.; de Jager, S.C.A.; van der Pouw Kraan, T.C.T.M.; Quax, P.H.A. CCR7-CCL19/CCL21 Axis is Essential for Effective Arteriogenesis in a Murine Model of Hindlimb Ischemia. *J. Am. Heart Assoc.* **2017**, *6*, e005281. [CrossRef]
39. Parma, L.; Peters, H.A.; Johansson, M.E.; Gutiérrez, S.; Meijerink, H.; De Kimpe, S.; De Vries, M.R.; Quax, P. Bis(maltolato)oxovanadium(IV) Induces Angiogenesis via Phosphorylation of VEGFR2. *Int. J. Mol. Sci.* **2020**, *21*, 4643. [CrossRef]

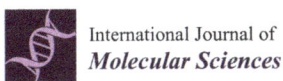

Review

Emerging Role of AP-1 Transcription Factor JunB in Angiogenesis and Vascular Development

Yasuo Yoshitomi *, Takayuki Ikeda, Hidehito Saito-Takatsuji and Hideto Yonekura

Department of Biochemistry, Kanazawa Medical University School of Medicine, 1-1 Daigaku, Uchinada, Kahoku-gun, Ishikawa 920-0293, Japan; tikeda@kanazawa-med.ac.jp (T.I.); saitoh@kanazawa-med.ac.jp (H.S.-T.); yonekura@kanazawa-med.ac.jp (H.Y.)
* Correspondence: yositomi@kanazawa-med.ac.jp; Tel.: +81-76-218-8111

Abstract: Blood vessels are essential for the formation and maintenance of almost all functional tissues. They play fundamental roles in the supply of oxygen and nutrition, as well as development and morphogenesis. Vascular endothelial cells are the main factor in blood vessel formation. Recently, research findings showed heterogeneity in vascular endothelial cells in different tissue/organs. Endothelial cells alter their gene expressions depending on their cell fate or angiogenic states of vascular development in normal and pathological processes. Studies on gene regulation in endothelial cells demonstrated that the activator protein 1 (AP-1) transcription factors are implicated in angiogenesis and vascular development. In particular, it has been revealed that JunB (a member of the AP-1 transcription factor family) is transiently induced in endothelial cells at the angiogenic frontier and controls them on tip cells specification during vascular development. Moreover, JunB plays a role in tissue-specific vascular maturation processes during neurovascular interaction in mouse embryonic skin and retina vasculatures. Thus, JunB appears to be a new angiogenic factor that induces endothelial cell migration and sprouting particularly in neurovascular interaction during vascular development. In this review, we discuss the recently identified role of JunB in endothelial cells and blood vessel formation.

Keywords: AP-1 transcription factors; JunB; angiogenesis; tip cell specification; vascular development; neurovascular interactions

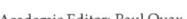

Citation: Yoshitomi, Y.; Ikeda, T.; Saito-Takatsuji, H.; Yonekura, H. Emerging Role of AP-1 Transcription Factor JunB in Angiogenesis and Vascular Development. *Int. J. Mol. Sci.* **2021**, 22, 2804. https://doi.org/10.3390/ijms22062804

Academic Editor: Paul Quax

Received: 19 February 2021
Accepted: 9 March 2021
Published: 10 March 2021

Publisher's Note: MDPI stays neutral with regard to jurisdictional claims in published maps and institutional affiliations.

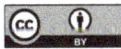

Copyright: © 2021 by the authors. Licensee MDPI, Basel, Switzerland. This article is an open access article distributed under the terms and conditions of the Creative Commons Attribution (CC BY) license (https://creativecommons.org/licenses/by/4.0/).

1. Vascular Endothelial Cells and Activator Protein 1 (AP-1) Transcription Factors

1.1. Endothelial Cell Heterogeneities and Gene Expression

Vascular endothelial cells represent the principal cells of blood vessels in most tissues. They display heterogeneity and different characteristics depending on the state of angiogenesis and tissue type. The differences noted between vascular endothelial cells include the basic properties of arteries, veins, capillaries, tip cells, and stalk cells. In addition, they include a wide variety of tissue-specific endothelial cells, such as the blood-brain barrier structure bearing cerebral blood vessels, and liver sinusoidal vascular endothelial cells that have a loose basement membrane structure. It has been shown that these differences are related to differences in gene expression. For example, blood-brain barrier transporters major facilitator superfamily domain containing 2A (Mfsd2a) and solute carrier family 2 member 1 (Slc2a1) are specifically expressed in endothelial cells of the central nervous system [1]. Moreover, GATA binding protein 4 (GATA4) is involved in the formation of sinusoidal blood vessels in the liver [2]. There is accumulating evidence regarding gene expression in vascular endothelial cells. Recently, a large-scale transcriptome analysis of tissue-type vascular endothelial cells isolated from various tissues identified various tissue-specific vascular endothelial cell gene transcriptomes [3–5]. These data are available in the public vascular endothelial cell transcriptome database EndDB, hosted by VIB-KU Leuven Center for Cancer Biology (Leuven, Belgium; URL: https://vibcancer.be/software-tools/endodb, accessed on 1 February 2021) [6]. The transcription of vascular endothelial cells, similar to that of other cells, is regulated by a number of transcription factors and epigenetic regulation. A recent comprehensive analysis of the chromatin states of human vascular endothelial cells identified 3765 endothelial-specific enhancers [7]. They also identified nine endothelial cell groups divided into two subgroups based on the epigenomic landscape. In addition, numerous homeobox genes and some other transcription factors were differentially activated across the endothelial cell types [7].

The process of vascular development, termed vasculogenesis, is initiated at the early developmental stages by the formation of a primitive vascular plexus, a beehive-like structure of endothelial progenitor cells. In the process of angiogenesis, the primordial vascular plexus invades the vascular-free area in response to angiogenic cues, such as hypoxia and vascular-inducing factors. Budding, branching, and fusion occur repeatedly to create more complex capillary networks. The vascular endothelial growth factor (VEGF) is a primary regulator of angiogenesis and blood vessel formation that controls endothelial cell proliferation, survival, and migration to form blood vessels. VEGFA controls angiogenic sprouting by guiding filopodia extension from tip cells at the vascular-sprouting frontier [8]. At the protrusion tip of the vascular elongation, the first cells which receive VEGF signals, become "tip cells" through VEGF intracellular signaling, thereby forming numerous filopodia and enhancing cell motility. In addition, tip cells express the Notch ligand delta-like canonical Notch ligand 4 (DLL4). Moreover, vascular endothelial cells adjacent to tip cells bind to their membrane receptor Notch1, which transmits signals into the cells and causes them to become stalk cells. Stalk cells lack filopodia, are proliferative, and regulate the number of cells in the subsequent vascular network [8]. Tip and stalk cells maintain plasticity in the formation of the vascular network. Stalk cells may become tip cells or, conversely, tip cells may degenerate into stalk cells by retracting their filopodia. Thus, DLL4-Notch1 signaling regulates the specification of tip cells and stalk cells to maintain proper vessel density [9]. From the primordial vascular plexus, through a process termed remodeling, mature vessels with hierarchical structure are finally constructed in each tissue and organ. These steps include arterial and venous specification, vessel remodeling in the coordination with neurovascular parallel alignment, and formation of functional blood vessels. Numerous previous studies have described the regulation of VEGFA gene expression. Many transcription factors have been identified as VEGF-positive and -negative regulators, including hypoxia-inducible factor 1 subunit alpha (HIF1a) [10,11], Sp transcription factors [12], NF-κB [13], SMAD [14], SRY-box transcription factor 9 (SOX9) [15], forkhead box O3 (FOXO3) [16,17], signal transducer and activator of transcription 3 (STAT3) [18,19], cAMP responsive element binding protein 1 (CREB1) [20], and AP-1 transcription factors [21–28]. In recent years, research has focused on the function of AP-1 factors in endothelial cells. In this review, we focused on the AP-1 transcription factor JunB in endothelial cells in VEGF signaling during angiogenesis.

1.2. AP-1 Transcription Factors in Endothelial Cells

The AP-1transcription factor family consists of Jun (c-Jun, JunB, and JunD), Fos (c-Fos, FosB, Fra-1, and -2), and ATF (ATF-2, -3, -4, and ATFa). These factors form homodimers or heterodimers at the N-terminal leucine zipper common motif, which bind to DNA through the DNA binding motif, thereby regulating the transcription of target genes [29–31]. AP-1 factors control both the basal and inducible transcription of several genes which contain AP-1 sites (consensus sequence 5′-TGAG/CTCA-3′) on their promoter. These consensus sequences are also termed 12-O-tetradecanoylphorbol-13-acetate-responsive elements [29]. In the case of Jun, it is known that the heterodimer Jun/Fos has higher DNA affinity and transcriptional activity than the homodimer Jun/Jun, suggesting that Jun functions as a heterodimer in vivo [30,32]. AP-1 transcription factors are involved in numerous physiological and pathological processes, including the cell cycle, development, and tumor progression. AP-1 transcription factors are also known as immediately early genes, which are transiently and rapidly activated in response to a wide variety of cellular stimuli. These genes are involved in the regulation of gene activity following the primary growth factor response, including VEGFs [33,34]. AP-1 transcription factors are reportedly involved in regulating VEGF expression and endothelial cell gene expression in response to VEGF stimulation [35,36]. In endothelial cells, VEGF stimulation induces its target genes during angiogenesis, and AP-1 transcription factors regulate the expression of these genes by binding to their promoters [26,37–39]. AP-1 transcription factors also reportedly regulate gene expressions implicated in angiogenesis, including VEGFs and matrix metalloproteinases (MMPs) [40–43].

2. AP-1 Transcription Factor JunB in Angiogenesis

2.1. JunB Expression in Endothelial Cells

Previously, it was found that JunB is involved in the differentiation of erythroid cells [44] and T cells [45], as well as tadpole tail regeneration by positively regulating cell proliferation [46]. JunB also positively regulates the proliferation of embryonic fibroblast cells by promoting S to G2/M transition through cyclin A activation [47]. However, the negative regulation of cell proliferation by inhibition of G1-S transition in HeLa cells through inhibition of the cyclin D1 promoter has also been reported [48]. In human umbilical vein endothelial cells (HUVEC), dominant negative c-Fos blocks endothelial cell proliferation by inhibiting cyclin D expression and also inhibits cell migration. In contrast, JunB knockdown in HUVEC attenuated endothelial cell migration but did not affect the proliferation of endothelial cells [33]. These findings indicated that JunB is required primarily for cell migration but may not control the proliferation of endothelial cells.

Expression of JunB in human tissues/organs during different developmental, normal, and pathological conditions has been described. Moreover, human placental JunB expression in JunB/cyclin-D1 imbalance in placental mesenchymal stromal cells derived from pre-eclamptic pregnancies with fetal placental complications has been described [49]. Amplification and overexpression of JunB are associated with primary cutaneous T-cell lymphomas [50]. JunB is an essential transcription factor for the differentiation of inflammatory T-helper 17 (Th17) cells [51–53], which demonstrates that JunB plays roles in T-cell programming. A case study on leukemia demonstrated that JunB expression levels significantly decreased in human chronic myelogenous leukemia (CML) [54]. Abnormally expressed JunB transactivated by IL-6/STAT3 signaling promotes uveal melanoma aggressiveness via epithelial–mesenchymal transition [55]. The role of JunB in psoriasis-like skin disease and arthritis was also reported. The JunB loss in keratinocytes induces chemokine/cytokine expression, attracts neutrophils and macrophages to the epidermis, and contributes to phenotypic changes in psoriasis [56]. A recent study using integrated bulk and single-cell RNA sequencing identified disease-relevant monocytes and a gene network module underlying systemic sclerosis (SSc). Four inflammatory genes from CD16+ monocytes, including JunB, showed the greatest differential expression between SSc and the healthy controls [57]. The defective degradation of JunB in patients with systemic sclerosis contributes to the overproduction of type I collagen and the development of dermatofibrosis [58].

JunB has been implicated in angiogenesis, and its expression is induced by hypoxia and VEGF. In endothelial cells, JunB regulates endothelial cell functions as a downstream factor of VEGF signaling [33]. Moreover, JunB is a hypoxia-inducible factor, its levels are elevated via the translocation and activation of NF-κB under hypoxic conditions [59]. In addition to transcriptional regulation, JunB activities are regulated via its translational regulation and phosphorylation [48,60]. VEGF is an upstream regulator of JunB [33] and also JunB regulates VEGF transcription [26,27,59]. Thus, JunB is implicated in angiogenesis by controlling the transcription upstream and downstream of VEGF-signaling. Mechanistically, the VEGF promoter contains two AP-1 transcription factor-binding sites, and induced JunB binds to the VEGF promoter to positively regulate VEGF expression under hypoxia [59]. In HUVEC, JunB induces VEGF expression, miR-3133 functions as a negative regulator of the JunB/VEGF pathway, thereby affecting angiogenesis [27]. There have also been reports of epigenetic regulation, specifically, JunB exhibits protein–protein interaction with BRG1 in the target gene promoter in HeLa cells [61,62]. Yeast two-hybrid screening has shown that BAF60a of the SWItch Sucrose non-fermentable (SWI/SNF) complex binds to c-Jun, JunB, and c-Fos [63]. In addition, it was reported that breast cancer type 1 susceptibility protein (BRCA1) interacts with JunB and regulates the transcription activity of the activation domain (AD) of BRCA1 in HEK293T cells [64]. In particular, the coiled-coil domain of BRCA1 interacts with the basic leucine zipper (bZIP) domain of JunB, and this interaction enhances BRCA1 AD activity, which affects BRCA1 transcription activity in HEK293T cells [64]. BRCA1 plays important roles in maintaining chromatin stability via its functions in transcriptional regulation and DNA repair [65,66]. BRCA1 is also known to interact with SWI/SNF chromatin remodeling complexes in breast cancer [67]. In retinal vascular development, the genome-wide accessibility of AP-1-binding sites is epigenetically controlled by sphingosine-1-phosphate (S1P) signaling. This process alters the chromatin composition of the AP-1-binding site to become closed and inaccessible, resulting in the inhibition of JunB-related gene expression during vascular maturation in the mouse retina [68].

JunB is expressed in endothelial cells and regulates their morphogenesis by regulating the core-binding factor beta subunit (CBFβ), which controls MMP13 expression, cell migration, and tube formation [42]. In this case, both the JunB–JunB homodimer and JunB–ATF2 heterodimer regulate CBFβ expression in endothelial cells [42].

2.2. JunB Is a Tip Cell Factor in Response to VEGF Signaling

In the sprouting region of the primordial vascular plexus, vascular endothelial cells located at the tip of the growing vessel extend numerous filopodia toward the vessel-free region. The endothelial cells that extend these filopodia are termed tip cells, and the endothelial cells that proliferate behind the tip cells and support vascular growth are called stalk cells [69]. The morphology of tip cells is similar to that of the growth cone in nerve axon elongation. Tip cells migrate by extending their filopodia in response to the concentration gradient of VEGF expressed in vascular-free areas, which determines the direction of vascular growth. However, stalk cells actively proliferate and define the number of cells in the subsequent vascular network. Tip cells and stalk cells maintain plasticity in the construction of the vascular network and can switch morphology. The tip cell and stalk cell specification mechanisms have been clarified [9]. Tip cells express the DLL4, while stalk cells express the Notch receptor Notch1. This DLL4-Notch1 signaling regulates the equilibrium between the tip and stalk cells, as well as the extension of the filopodia of tip cells to maintain a proper vessel density. Therefore, in DLL4-knockout mice, the number of filopodia extending from the tip cells increases along with the ratio of tip cells to stalk cells, resulting in the formation of hyperplasia of the vascular network with compressed vessel spacing. Nevertheless, the growth rate of blood vessels decreases. Eventually, with the emergence of blood flow, the primitive vascular plexus infiltrates the tissue and undergoes a process termed remodeling, resulting in the emergence of a hierarchical mature vascular network.

JunB is reportedly upregulated in tip cells at the angiogenic frontier and contributes to vascular development in mouse embryonic skin [26] and retinal vasculatures [68] (Figure 1). The induction of JunB expression is temporal and spatial in tip cells at the angiogenic frontier or at the branching points during vascular development. In vitro analysis using human primary microvascular endothelial cells (HMVEC) showed that the induced expression of JunB results in marked changes in cell morphology [26]. Specifically, JunB expression has a profound effect on the cell morphology of vascular endothelial cells, causing them to change to a fibroblast-like spindle cell morphology. This morphological change can be positively or negatively regulated by controlling JunB expression alone. In addition, studies using a three-dimensional collagen matrix angiogenesis assay demonstrated that JunB-expressing vascular endothelial cells enhance cell motility and regulate vascular formation. In the development of retinal blood vessels, JunB is strongly induced in the characteristic tip cells located at the angiogenic frontier of the process of radial extension of the primitive vascular plexus into retinal tissue. When JunB expression is abolished by conventional JunB knockout or endothelial cell-specific knockout in mice, the number of tip cells decreased in retinal vasculature, which resulted in a marked suppression of vascular progression and branching [68].

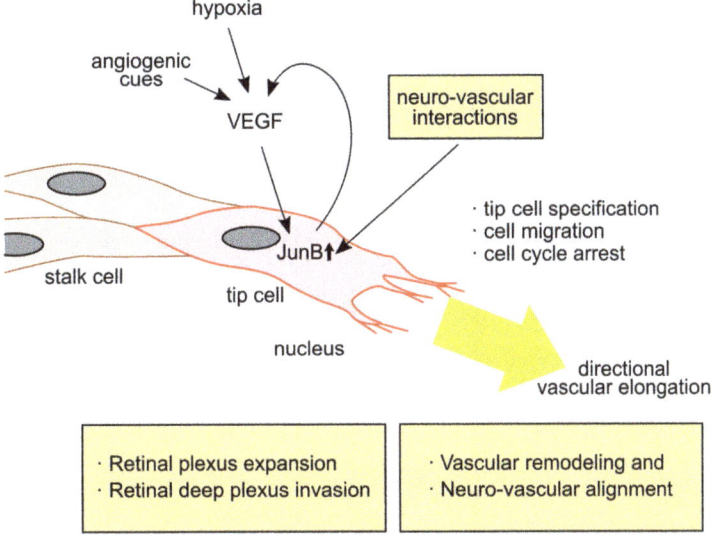

Figure 1. In the event of angiogenesis in embryonic skin and retina, endothelial cells respond to angiogenic cues, such as hypoxia or other signals, to produce new vessel branches at the angiogenic frontier. The vascular endothelial growth factor (VEGF) plays a central role in this process. The VEGF signals that induce JunB expression (small upper arrow) result in the conversion of endothelial cells to tip cells. JunB activation is involved in the vessel parallel alignment with neurons in developing skin, retinal tissue-specific radial vessel expansion, and deep plexus expansion in retinal vessel development. Both vessel-wiring processes in embryonic skin and the retina include neurovascular interactions. The arrows indicate the relationship of signaling directions. Large green arrow indicates direction of vascular elongation.

3. Endothelial JunB Functions in Vascular Development In Vivo

3.1. JunB Is Required for Placentation and Heart Vascular Development in Mice

The in vivo functional study of JunB using conventional JunB knockout mice was the first to describe the loss of JunB resulting in embryonic lethality through placental malformation and failure of cardiac vasculogenesis [70]. More specifically, mouse embryos with conventional JunB knockout die between E8.5 and E10 due to the abnormal formation of the placenta. Knockout of JunB does not affect cell proliferation, however, embryo growth was retarded due to a failed connection of maternal circulation. These results indicated that JunB is a transcription factor required for correct vascular development [42,59,70].

3.2. JunB Is Involved in Retinal Vascular Outgrowth and Retinal Special Vascular Differentiation

Retinal vasculature has been widely used as an analysis system for angiogenic sprouting and vascular development due to its postnatal development and ease of tissue accessibility. VEGF plays a central role in retinal vascular development [8], and it has been shown that VEGF receptor 2 (VEGFR2) and VEGFR receptor 3 (VEGFR3) are required for vessel sprouting [71,72]. VEGFR3 is particularly highly expressed in tip cells and induces angiogenesis and vessel growth in the absence of VEGFR2 in a Notch-independent manner [73]. The VEGFR3 signaling pathway is essential for the development of angiogenesis, with VEGFR3 expression being characteristically induced in developing vascular endothelial cells and is later restricted in lymphatic endothelial cells [74,75]. VEGFR3, which binds to VEGFC and VEGFD, is essential for angiogenesis, particularly in the developmental stages [76] (Figure 2, right). Recently, it was shown that JunB is involved in the pathological process of hypoxia-mediated retinal neovascularization [77]. In retinal endothelial cells, VEGFA signaling phosphorylates intracellular protein kinase C theta (PKCθ), and retinal endothelial cells form tip cells, thereby positively regulating cell migration, sprouting, and tube formation. In hypoxia-induced VEGFA signaling, PKCθ phosphorylation upregulates JunB expression, which induces VEGFR3 expression, thereby inducing tip cell formation, sprouting, and neovascularization of retinal capillaries via STAT3 activation. VEGFR3 is a key regulator of retinal neovascularization, while endothelial-specific knockout of JunB inhibits VEGFR3 expression, inhibiting retinal neovascularization. Mechanistically, it was shown that JunB acts downstream of PKCθ, and JunB directly binds to the promoter of VEGFR3 to regulate VEGFR3 expression (Figure 2).

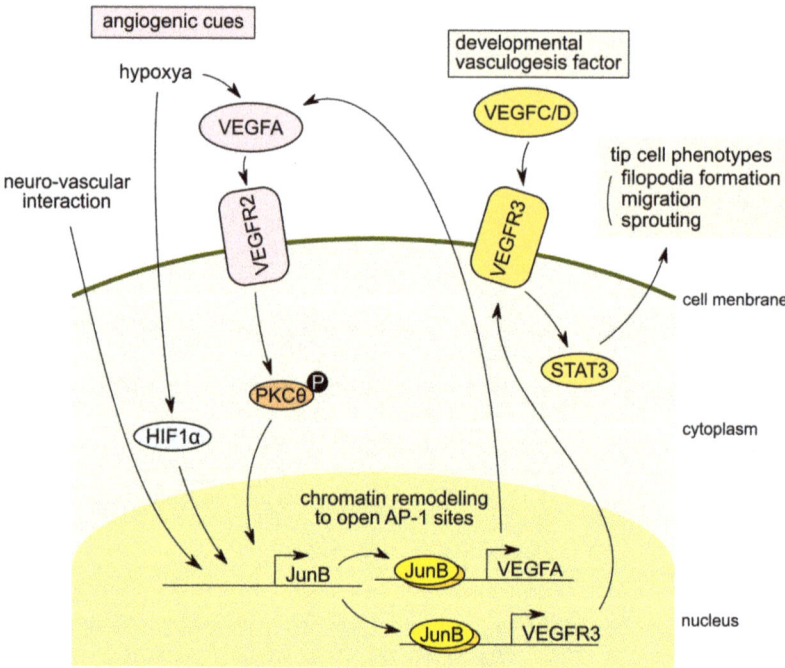

Figure 2. Tip cell phenotype expression in response to angiogenic cues in endothelial cells at the vasculogenesis frontier. In endothelial cells at the angiogenesis frontier during vascular development, JunB expression is induced by angiogenic cues including hypoxia and vascular endothelial growth factor A (VEGFA) through hypoxia-inducible factor 1 subunit alpha (HIF1α) or phosphorylation of protein kinase C theta (PKCθ). "P" indicates phosphorylation of the molecule. (left). In the developing skin vasculatures, the direct interaction of endothelial cells with peripheral neurons can also stimulate JunB expression and coordinate neurovascular parallel alignment (left). In tip cells, JunB is involved in the upregulation of vascular endothelial growth factor receptor 3 (VEGFR3) expression which is a key VEGFR for angiogenesis at specific developmental stages. VEGFR3 binds vascular endothelial growth factor C and D (VEGFC/D), while signaling cascades are required for tip cell migration and sprouting of endothelial cells by signal transducer and activator of transcription 3 (STAT3) activation at the angiogenic frontier (right). The arrows indicate the relationship of signaling directions.

Another study on retinal angiogenesis demonstrated that JunB is involved in the process of retina-specific vascular network development [68]. Retinal blood vessel networks are produced by vascular endothelial cells that invade into the eye retina tissue from the optic nerve papilla. In the early stage of retinal vascular development, radial retinal structures are produced along the superficial nerve fiber layer of the retina to form the superficial plexus. Later, around P8 in mice, retinal blood vessels begin to invade into the retinal nerve tissue vertically toward the retinal deep layer, forming a deep plexus, which is followed by the formation of the middle layer plexus. Yanagida et al. focused on S1P receptor signaling in retinal vascular development and found that it regulates the open-chromatin state of the AP-1 binding motif of retinal endothelial cells genome-wide [68]. Postnatally, following the complete abolishment of S1P receptor signaling by the receptor triple knockout, the AP-1 motif in the open-chromatin region was strongly accumulated. Furthermore, the investigators confirmed that JunB was the AP-1 transcription factor involved in this process. JunB was highly expressed in tip cells at the tip of angiogenesis and promoted angiogenesis until the activation of S1P receptor signaling. Following blood perfusion, the serum-derived S1P induces vascular endothelial-cadherin (VE-cadherin) expression in endothelial cells and results in the suppression of JunB expression in endothelial cells. At the same time, S1P also induces chromatin remodeling to close the AP-1 motif in endothelial cells, which have a lumen structure with blood flow. Reportedly, VE-cadherin is induced by S1P signaling in mature retinal vasculature with lumen structures where blood flow is present, resulting in decreased expression of JunB. In other words, S1P signaling converts the tip cell-like state activated by JunB to a retinal-specific vascular maturation state. Interestingly, in retinal angiogenesis, JunB expression is activated at the sprouting point, i.e., at the branching point where blood vessels extend vertically into the deep retinal layers. Although the initiation of vertical branching is unclear, some stimuli (partial weakening of S1P signaling or interaction of endothelial cells with retinal neurons) causes JunB induction and chromatin remodeling in vascular endothelial cells, thereby exposing the AP-1 site. As a result, JunB target genes (including tip cell genes) can be induced, and the cell converts to a tip cell, extending the retinal plexus invasion into the deeper layers of retinal tissue. During developmental vasculogenesis, JunB expression is specifically observed in endothelial cells. The role of JunB in this directional angiogenesis during retinal vasculature development is consistent with its function in cutaneous vascular development, as described below.

3.3. JunB Regulates Neurovascular Parallel Alignment in Developing Skin Vasculture in Mice

It is established that nerves and blood vessels align parallel to each other. However, until recently, the molecular mechanism involved in this process was unclear. Recent reports described that both neuronal signaling to the blood vessels [78] and vascular signaling to the nerves [79] are involved in the regulation of this juxtaposition process. Moreover, the nerves and blood vessels co-operatively form mature and correct neural and vascular network structures. In zebrafish, it has been reported that inhibition of the function of VEGFR3 results in the loss of nerve-vessel parallelism. Furthermore, the trapping of VEGFC secreted by arterial vascular endothelial cells using VEGFR3-Fc recombinant protein results in abnormal aortic ventral motor nerve function [80]. These findings suggested that VEGFC-VEGFR3 signaling plays an important role in nerve-vessel parallelism. In the development of the subcutaneous vascular network in mouse embryos, peripheral nerve fiber bundles align parallel to arterial blood vessels while retaining a certain distance from nerves, and form a mature vascular network. In 2013, Li et al. reported that VEGF and CXCL12 secreted by nerves act on the primitive vascular plexus, which is the initial structure of blood vessels. This induces vascular remodeling to form neurovascular parallelism, resulting in the formation of a proper mature vascular network [81]. Using a co-culture system of dorsal root ganglion cells and primary HMVEC, it was found that JunB was strongly and specifically induced in endothelial cells during neurovascular interactions [26]. In addition, the knockdown of JunB resulted in disruption of the neurovascular parallelism in vivo. This evidence indicated that induction of JunB in endothelial cells is required for neurovascular parallel alignment during vascular development in mouse embryonic skin [26]. Furthermore, we found that JunB induction is mediated by direct cell-cell contact with nerves-vessels rather than soluble factors secreted by the nerves. Interestingly, vascular endothelial cells with force-induction of JunB expression adopt a spindle-like morphology, show increased motility, and exhibit a unique phenotype which is very similar to that of tip cells found at the angiogenic frontier. In fact, vasculogenesis assays using a three-dimensional collagen matrix and endothelial sphere outgrowth assays revealed that JunB expression is activated in tip cells at the angiogenic frontier [26]. It is clear that JunB is involved in vascular remodeling by conversion of vascular endothelial cells to tip cells, and JunB expression is required for the juxtapositional alignment of the blood vessel to neurons (Figure 2, left). However, the mechanisms through which directional remodeling is induced remains unclear. The candidate molecule(s) of this mechanism may be the upstream molecule(s) of JunB, which are supplied by nerves at the neurovascular interaction.

3.4. JunB also Controls Lymphangiogenesis

During lymphatic vessel development in vertebrates, Prospero homeobox protein 1 (PROX1) expressing endothelial cells in cardinal veins eventually differentiate into lymphatic endothelial cells during lymphangiogenesis, which is considered the master regulator of lymphatic endothelial cell fate specification [82,83]. Forkhead box protein O1 (FOXO1) is required for proper lymphatic vessel development and maturation by upregulating C-X-C chemokine receptor 4 (CXCR4) expression in lymphatic endothelial cells in mouse tail dermis [84]. The functions of JunB in lymphatic vascular development in zebrafish have been described by Kiesow et al. [85]. JunB directly regulates miR-182 expression, which downregulates its downstream FOXO1 expression in lymphatic endothelial cells. The loss of JunB leads to the failure of parachordal lymphangioblast and thoracic duct formation in zebrafish, indicating that JunB plays an important role in lymphatic vascular morphogenesis in zebrafish by negatively regulating JunB/miR-182/Foxo1 axis signaling. The endothelial-specific deletion of Foxo1 in mice results in embryonic lethality at approximately E10.5 due to vascular remodeling defects [86,87]. Its phenotype is similar to that of JunB knockout mice [70]. Nevertheless, currently, the involvement of the JunB–miR-182–FOXO1 axis in blood vessel development remains unknown. In addition, VEGFC–VEGFR3 signaling is implicated in the survival, proliferation, and migration of lymphatic endothelial cells [88,89]. Thus far, the role of JunB in the regulation of VEGFR3 expression in lymphatic endothelial cells is unclear.

4. Conclusions

The main original articles that describe the functions of JunB in angiogenesis and vascular development, discussed in this review, are summarized in Table 1. A variety of angiogenesis-related factors have been identified, including exogenous angiogenesis-inducers (e.g., hypoxia and VEGF), transcription factors in vascular endothelial cells that are induced in response to these inducers, and angiogenesis-related genes transcribed by these transcription factors. Some transcription factors induce the expression of tissue-specific endothelial cell phenotypes in specific endothelial cells. In angiogenesis, tip cells appear at the tip of angiogenesis after receiving angiogenesis-inducing cues (e.g., VEGF) and induce sprouting with migration of vascular endothelial cells to form a proper vascular network. The expression of AP-1 transcription factor JunB is induced in tip cells during vascular development of skin capillaries and retinal vessels, leading to the induction of tip cell-specific characteristics (e.g., cell migration and angiogenic sprouting).

The mechanism of vascular "directional" control appears to be maintained mainly through the signaling balances between attractive and repulsive effectors from various tissues during vascular formation. For example, arterial and venous juxtapositional alignment is controlled by the balance of two types of action: Repulsive effects between arterial EphrinB2 and venous EphB4 [90,91] and attractive action between arterial apelin and the venous apelin receptor (APJ) [92]. The transient induction of tip cells at the frontier of angiogenesis has a dynamic response to various angiogenic attractors (e.g., hypoxia and VEGF), which elongate and remodel the blood vessels according to the location and timing to form a proper vascular network. We and others have shown that JunB induction in tip cells is a novel angiogenic machinery that regulates the motility, filopodia formation, invasion, and remodeling of tip cells in response to angiogenic cues. By controlling the temporal and spatial induction of JunB in tip cells, we may be able to control the elongation of blood vessels. This suggests that the tip cell factor JunB is a determinant of vascular directionality. Nevertheless, the involvement of JunB in tip-stalk cell sorting signaling by Notch-DLL4 intercellular signaling remains unclear.

Table 1. Original articles which describe JunB functions in angiogenesis and vascular development.

JunB Functions in Endothelial Cells	Reference
Angiogenesis	[26,27,42,59,68,70,77]
Neurovascular parallel alignment	[26]
Filopodia formation and tip cell specification	[26,68,77]
Retinal vascular development	[68,77]
Lymphangiogenesis	[85]

In the process of retinal vascular development, JunB is specifically upregulated in tip cells at the angiogenic frontier in the upper layer of retinal nerve tissue and migrates radially on the upper layers of the retina. Expression of JunB is also observed specifically in tip cells vertically protruding into the deep retinal plexus layer, leading to the formation of longitudinally oriented retinal blood vessels [68]. In the remodeling process of mouse embryonic skin vascular development, JunB is induced in endothelial cells in contact with the nerves and enhances the invasiveness of the endothelium to create a vascular network that aligns parallel to the nerves [26]. A common feature of JunB-mediated vascular network formation in both embryonic skin and retina vasculature is that the regulation of the directional vascularization is based on the interaction with nerve cells. Probably, the angiogenic attractors of extracellular matrix produced by neurons or neuronal membrane proteins play a role in determining the direction of blood vessels. In response to this, JunB is induced in vascular endothelial cells to increase migratory activity and determine the direction of extension. However, at present, the factor(s) on the neural side that play a role in this guidance are unknown. Hence, further extensive research is warranted.

Author Contributions: Conceptualization, Y.Y. and H.Y.; writing—original draft preparation, Y.Y.; writing—review and editing, H.S.-T., T.I., and H.Y. All authors have read and agreed to the published version of the manuscript.

Funding: This work was supported in part by JSPS KAKENHI, grant numbers JP18K06924 and JP24790297 to Y.Y.

Institutional Review Board Statement: Not applicable.

Informed Consent Statement: Not applicable.

Data Availability Statement: Not applicable.

Acknowledgments: We thank Kazumi Tanaka (Kanazawa Medical University) for her assistance.

Conflicts of Interest: The authors declare no conflict of interest.

Abbreviations

AP-1	Activator protein 1
HMVEC	Human microvascular endothelial cells
S1P	Sphingosine 1-phosphate
VEGF	Vascular endothelial growth factor
VEGFR	Vascular endothelial growth factor receptor

References

1. Sabbagh, M.F.; Heng, J.S.; Luo, C.; Castanon, R.G.; Nery, J.R.; Rattner, A.; Goff, L.A.; Ecker, J.R.; Nathans, J. Transcriptional and Epigenomic Landscapes of CNS and Non-CNS Vascular Endothelial Cells. *eLife* **2018**, *7*, e36187. [CrossRef] [PubMed]
2. Géraud, C.; Koch, P.-S.; Zierow, J.; Klapproth, K.; Busch, K.; Olsavszky, V.; Leibing, T.; Demory, A.; Ulbrich, F.; Diett, M.; et al. GATA4-Dependent Organ-Specific Endothelial Differentiation Controls Liver Development and Embryonic Hematopoiesis. *J. Clin. Investig.* **2017**, *127*, 1099–1114. [CrossRef]
3. Nolan, D.J.; Ginsberg, M.; Israely, E.; Palikuqi, B.; Poulos, M.G.; James, D.; Ding, B.-S.; Schachterle, W.; Liu, Y.; Rosenwaks, Z.; et al. Molecular Signatures of Tissue-Specific Microvascular Endothelial Cell Heterogeneity in Organ Maintenance and Regeneration. *Dev. Cell* **2013**, *26*, 204–219. [CrossRef]
4. Paik, D.T.; Tian, L.; Williams, I.M.; Rhee, S.; Zhang, H.; Liu, C.; Mishra, R.; Wu, S.M.; Red-Horse, K.; Wu, J.C. Single-Cell RNA Sequencing Unveils Unique Transcriptomic Signatures of Organ-Specific Endothelial Cells. *Circulation* **2020**, *142*, 1848–1862. [CrossRef]
5. Kalucka, J.; de Rooij, L.P.M.H.; Goveia, J.; Rohlenova, K.; Dumas, S.J.; Meta, E.; Conchinha, N.V.; Taverna, F.; Teuwen, L.-A.; Veys, K.; et al. Single-Cell Transcriptome Atlas of Murine Endothelial Cells. *Cell* **2020**, *180*, 764–779.e20. [CrossRef] [PubMed]
6. Khan, S.; Taverna, F.; Rohlenova, K.; Treps, L.; Geldhof, V.; de Rooij, L.; Sokol, L.; Pircher, A.; Conradi, L.-C.; Kalucka, J.; et al. EndoDB: A Database of Endothelial Cell Transcriptomics Data. *Nucleic Acids Res.* **2019**, *47*, D736–D744. [CrossRef] [PubMed]
7. Nakato, R.; Wada, Y.; Nakaki, R.; Nagae, G.; Katou, Y.; Tsutsumi, S.; Nakajima, N.; Fukuhara, H.; Iguchi, A.; Kohro, T.; et al. Comprehensive Epigenome Characterization Reveals Diverse Transcriptional Regulation across Human Vascular Endothelial Cells. *Epigenetics Chromatin* **2019**, *12*, 77. [CrossRef]
8. Gerhardt, H.; Golding, M.; Fruttiger, M.; Ruhrberg, C.; Lundkvist, A.; Abramsson, A.; Jeltsch, M.; Mitchell, C.; Alitalo, K.; Shima, D.; et al. VEGF Guides Angiogenic Sprouting Utilizing Endothelial Tip Cell Filopodia. *J. Cell Biol.* **2003**, *161*, 1163–1177. [CrossRef]
9. Hellström, M.; Phng, L.-K.; Hofmann, J.J.; Wallgard, E.; Coultas, L.; Lindblom, P.; Alva, J.; Nilsson, A.-K.; Karlsson, L.; Gaiano, N.; et al. Dll4 Signalling through Notch1 Regulates Formation of Tip Cells during Angiogenesis. *Nature* **2007**, *445*, 776–780. [CrossRef]
10. Zundel, W.; Schindler, C.; Haas-Kogan, D.; Koong, A.; Kaper, F.; Chen, E.; Gottschalk, A.R.; Ryan, H.E.; Johnson, R.S.; Jefferson, A.B.; et al. Loss of PTEN Facilitates HIF-1-Mediated Gene Expression. *Genes Dev.* **2000**, *14*, 391–396. [CrossRef]
11. Gray, M.J.; Zhang, J.; Ellis, L.M.; Semenza, G.L.; Evans, D.B.; Watowich, S.S.; Gallick, G.E. HIF-1alpha, STAT3, CBP/P300 and Ref-1/APE Are Components of a Transcriptional Complex That Regulates Src-Dependent Hypoxia-Induced Expression of VEGF in Pancreatic and Prostate Carcinomas. *Oncogene* **2005**, *24*, 3110–3120. [CrossRef] [PubMed]
12. Chintharlapalli, S.; Papineni, S.; Ramaiah, S.K.; Safe, S. Betulinic Acid Inhibits Prostate Cancer Growth through Inhibition of Specificity Protein Transcription Factors. *Cancer Res.* **2007**, *67*, 2816–2823. [CrossRef]
13. Xu, C.; Shen, G.; Chen, C.; Gélinas, C.; Kong, A.-N.T. Suppression of NF- κ B and NF- κ B-Regulated Gene Expression by Sulforaphane and PEITC through I κ B α, IKK Pathway in Human Prostate Cancer PC-3 Cells. *Oncogene* **2005**, *24*, 4486–4495. [CrossRef] [PubMed]
14. Kang, H.; Jha, S.; Ivovic, A.; Fratzl-Zelman, N.; Deng, Z.; Mitra, A.; Cabral, W.A.; Hanson, E.P.; Lange, E.; Cowen, E.W.; et al. Somatic SMAD3-Activating Mutations Cause Melorheostosis by up-Regulating the TGF-β/SMAD Pathway. *J. Exp. Med.* **2020**, *217*. [CrossRef]
15. Hattori, T.; Müller, C.; Gebhard, S.; Bauer, E.; Pausch, F.; Schlund, B.; Bösl, M.R.; Hess, A.; Surmann-Schmitt, C.; von der Mark, H.; et al. SOX9 Is a Major Negative Regulator of Cartilage Vascularization, Bone Marrow Formation and Endochondral Ossification. *Dev. Camb. Engl.* **2010**, *137*, 901–911. [CrossRef] [PubMed]
16. Renault, V.M.; Rafalski, V.A.; Morgan, A.A.; Salih, D.A.M.; Brett, J.O.; Webb, A.E.; Villeda, S.A.; Thekkat, P.U.; Guillerey, C.; Denko, N.C.; et al. FoxO3 Regulates Neural Stem Cell Homeostasis. *Cell Stem Cell* **2009**, *5*, 527–539. [CrossRef]
17. Potente, M.; Urbich, C.; Sasaki, K.; Hofmann, W.K.; Heeschen, C.; Aicher, A.; Kollipara, R.; DePinho, R.A.; Zeiher, A.M.; Dimmeler, S. Involvement of Foxo Transcription Factors in Angiogenesis and Postnatal Neovascularization. *J. Clin. Investig.* **2005**, *115*, 2382–2392. [CrossRef]
18. Balic, J.J.; Garama, D.J.; Saad, M.I.; Yu, L.; West, A.C.; West, A.J.; Livis, T.; Bhathal, P.S.; Gough, D.J.; Jenkins, B.J. Serine-Phosphorylated STAT3 Promotes Tumorigenesis via Modulation of RNA Polymerase Transcriptional Activity. *Cancer Res.* **2019**, *79*, 5272–5287. [CrossRef]
19. Kostromina, E.; Gustavsson, N.; Wang, X.; Lim, C.-Y.; Radda, G.K.; Li, C.; Han, W. Glucose Intolerance and Impaired Insulin Secretion in Pancreas-Specific Signal Transducer and Activator of Transcription-3 Knockout Mice Are Associated with Microvascular Alterations in the Pancreas. *Endocrinology* **2010**, *151*, 2050–2059. [CrossRef] [PubMed]
20. Rhee, S.H.; Ma, E.L.; Lee, Y.; Taché, Y.; Pothoulakis, C.; Im, E. Corticotropin Releasing Hormone and Urocortin 3 Stimulate Vascular Endothelial Growth Factor Expression through the CAMP/CREB Pathway. *J. Biol. Chem.* **2015**, *290*, 26194–26203. [CrossRef]
21. Zhao, Y.; Zhou, J.; Liu, D.; Dong, F.; Cheng, H.; Wang, W.; Pang, Y.; Wang, Y.; Mu, X.; Ni, Y.; et al. ATF4 Plays a Pivotal Role in the Development of Functional Hematopoietic Stem Cells in Mouse Fetal Liver. *Blood* **2015**, *126*, 2383–2391. [CrossRef] [PubMed]
22. Park, J.S.; Qiao, L.; Su, Z.Z.; Hinman, D.; Willoughby, K.; McKinstry, R.; Yacoub, A.; Duigou, G.J.; Young, C.S.; Grant, S.; et al. Ionizing Radiation Modulates Vascular Endothelial Growth Factor (VEGF) Expression through Multiple Mitogen Activated Protein Kinase Dependent Pathways. *Oncogene* **2001**, *20*, 3266–3280. [CrossRef]

23. Hu, Y.L.; Tee, M.K.; Goetzl, E.J.; Auersperg, N.; Mills, G.B.; Ferrara, N.; Jaffe, R.B. Lysophosphatidic Acid Induction of Vascular Endothelial Growth Factor Expression in Human Ovarian Cancer Cells. *J. Natl. Cancer Inst.* **2001**, *93*, 762–768. [CrossRef] [PubMed]
24. Ding, J.; Li, J.; Chen, J.; Chen, H.; Ouyang, W.; Zhang, R.; Xue, C.; Zhang, D.; Amin, S.; Desai, D.; et al. Effects of Polycyclic Aromatic Hydrocarbons (PAHs) on Vascular Endothelial Growth Factor Induction through Phosphatidylinositol 3-Kinase/AP-1-Dependent, HIF-1alpha-Independent Pathway. *J. Biol. Chem.* **2006**, *281*, 9093–9100. [CrossRef]
25. Monje, P.; Hernández-Losa, J.; Lyons, R.J.; Castellone, M.D.; Gutkind, J.S. Regulation of the Transcriptional Activity of C-Fos by ERK. A Novel Role for the Prolyl Isomerase PIN1. *J. Biol. Chem.* **2005**, *280*, 35081–35084. [CrossRef]
26. Yoshitomi, Y.; Ikeda, T.; Saito, H.; Yoshitake, Y.; Ishigaki, Y.; Hatta, T.; Kato, N.; Yonekura, H. JunB Regulates Angiogenesis and Neurovascular Parallel Alignment in Mouse Embryonic Skin. *J. Cell Sci.* **2017**, *130*, 916. [CrossRef]
27. Xu, M.; Cao, L.; Zhang, X.; Zhuang, Y.; Zhang, Y.; Wang, Q.; Chen, Y.; Xu, L.; Sun, G. MiR-3133 Inhibits Proliferation and Angiogenesis by Targeting the JUNB/VEGF Pathway in Human Umbilical Vein Endothelial Cells. *Oncol. Rep.* **2020**, *44*, 1699–1708. [CrossRef]
28. Gerald, D.; Berra, E.; Frapart, Y.M.; Chan, D.A.; Giaccia, A.J.; Mansuy, D.; Pouysségur, J.; Yaniv, M.; Mechta-Grigoriou, F. JunD Reduces Tumor Angiogenesis by Protecting Cells from Oxidative Stress. *Cell* **2004**, *118*, 781–794. [CrossRef]
29. Angel, P.; Karin, M. The Role of Jun, Fos and the AP-1 Complex in Cell-Proliferation and Transformation. *Biochim. Biophys. Acta BBA Rev. Cancer* **1991**, *1072*, 129–157. [CrossRef]
30. Eferl, R.; Wagner, E.F. AP-1: A Double-Edged Sword in Tumorigenesis. *Nat. Rev. Cancer* **2003**, *3*, 859–868. [CrossRef]
31. Hess, J.; Angel, P.; Schorpp-Kistner, M. AP-1 Subunits: Quarrel and Harmony among Siblings. *J. Cell Sci.* **2004**, *117*, 5965–5973. [CrossRef]
32. Hai, T.W.; Liu, F.; Coukos, W.J.; Green, M.R. Transcription Factor ATF CDNA Clones: An Extensive Family of Leucine Zipper Proteins Able to Selectively Form DNA-Binding Heterodimers. *Genes Dev.* **1989**, *3*, 2083–2090. [CrossRef] [PubMed]
33. Jia, J.; Ye, T.; Cui, P.; Hua, Q.; Zeng, H.; Zhao, D. AP-1 Transcription Factor Mediates VEGF-Induced Endothelial Cell Migration and Proliferation. *Microvasc. Res.* **2016**, *105*, 103–108. [CrossRef]
34. Chien, M.-H.; Ku, C.-C.; Johansson, G.; Chen, M.-W.; Hsiao, M.; Su, J.-L.; Inoue, H.; Hua, K.-T.; Wei, L.-H.; Kuo, M.-L. Vascular Endothelial Growth Factor-C (VEGF-C) Promotes Angiogenesis by Induction of COX-2 in Leukemic Cells via the VEGF-R3/JNK/AP-1 Pathway. *Carcinogenesis* **2009**, *30*, 2005–2013. [CrossRef]
35. Shih, S.C.; Claffey, K.P. Role of AP-1 and HIF-1 Transcription Factors in TGF-Beta Activation of VEGF Expression. *Growth Factors Chur Switz.* **2001**, *19*, 19–34. [CrossRef]
36. Wang, S.; Lu, J.; You, Q.; Huang, H.; Chen, Y.; Liu, K. The MTOR/AP-1/VEGF Signaling Pathway Regulates Vascular Endothelial Cell Growth. *Oncotarget* **2016**, *7*, 53269–53276. [CrossRef] [PubMed]
37. Kolch, W.; Martiny-Baron, G.; Kieser, A.; Marmé, D. Regulation of the Expression of the VEGF/VPS and Its Receptors: Role in Tumor Angiogenesis. *Breast Cancer Res. Treat.* **1995**, *36*, 139–155. [CrossRef] [PubMed]
38. Singh, N.K.; Quyen, D.V.; Kundumani-Sridharan, V.; Brooks, P.C.; Rao, G.N. AP-1 (Fra-1/c-Jun)-Mediated Induction of Expression of Matrix Metalloproteinase-2 Is Required for 15S-Hydroxyeicosatetraenoic Acid-Induced Angiogenesis. *J. Biol. Chem.* **2010**, *285*, 16830–16843. [CrossRef] [PubMed]
39. Galvagni, F.; Orlandini, M.; Oliviero, S. Role of the AP-1 Transcription Factor FOSL1 in Endothelial Cells Adhesion and Migration. *Cell Adhes. Migr.* **2013**, *7*, 408–411. [CrossRef]
40. Marconcini, L.; Marchio, S.; Morbidelli, L.; Cartocci, E.; Albini, A.; Ziche, M.; Bussolino, F.; Oliviero, S. C-Fos-Induced Growth Factor/Vascular Endothelial Growth Factor D Induces Angiogenesis in Vivo and in Vitro. *Proc. Natl. Acad. Sci. USA* **1999**, *96*, 9671–9676. [CrossRef]
41. Toft, D.J.; Rosenberg, S.B.; Bergers, G.; Volpert, O.; Linzer, D.I. Reactivation of Proliferin Gene Expression is Associated with Increased Angiogenesis in a Cell Culture Model of Fibrosarcoma Tumor Progression. *Proc. Natl. Acad. Sci. USA* **2001**, *98*, 13055–13059. [CrossRef] [PubMed]
42. Licht, A.H.; Pein, O.T.; Florin, L.; Hartenstein, B.; Reuter, H.; Arnold, B.; Lichter, P.; Angel, P.; Schorpp-Kistner, M. JunB Is Required for Endothelial Cell Morphogenesis by Regulating Core-Binding Factor Beta. *J. Cell Biol.* **2006**, *175*, 981–991. [CrossRef]
43. Zhang, G.; Dass, C.R.; Sumithran, E.; Di Girolamo, N.; Sun, L.-Q.; Khachigian, L.M. Effect of Deoxyribozymes Targeting C-Jun on Solid Tumor Growth and Angiogenesis in Rodents. *J. Natl. Cancer Inst.* **2004**, *96*, 683–696. [CrossRef]
44. Jacobs-Helber, S.M.; Abutin, R.M.; Tian, C.; Bondurant, M.; Wickrema, A.; Sawyer, S.T. Role of JunB in Erythroid Differentiation. *J. Biol. Chem.* **2002**, *277*, 4859–4866. [CrossRef]
45. Katagiri, T.; Kameda, H.; Nakano, H.; Yamazaki, S. Regulation of T Cell Differentiation by the AP-1 Transcription Factor JunB. *Immunol. Med.* **2021**, 1–12. [CrossRef]
46. Nakamura, M.; Yoshida, H.; Takahashi, E.; Wlizla, M.; Takebayashi-Suzuki, K.; Horb, M.E.; Suzuki, A. The AP-1 Transcription Factor JunB Functions in Xenopus Tail Regeneration by Positively Regulating Cell Proliferation. *Biochem. Biophys. Res. Commun.* **2020**, *522*, 990–995. [CrossRef]
47. Andrecht, S.; Kolbus, A.; Hartenstein, B.; Angel, P.; Schorpp-Kistner, M. Cell Cycle Promoting Activity of JunB through Cyclin A Activation. *J. Biol. Chem.* **2002**, *277*, 35961–35968. [CrossRef]
48. Bakiri, L.; Lallemand, D.; Bossy-Wetzel, E.; Yaniv, M. Cell Cycle-Dependent Variations in c-Jun and JunB Phosphorylation: A Role in the Control of Cyclin D1 Expression. *EMBO J.* **2000**, *19*, 2056–2068. [CrossRef]

49. Nuzzo, A.M.; Giuffrida, D.; Zenerino, C.; Piazzese, A.; Olearo, E.; Todros, T.; Rolfo, A. JunB/Cyclin-D1 Imbalance in Placental Mesenchymal Stromal Cells Derived from Preeclamptic Pregnancies with Fetal-Placental Compromise. *Placenta* **2014**, *35*, 483–490. [CrossRef] [PubMed]
50. Mao, X.; Orchard, G.; Lillington, D.M.; Russell-Jones, R.; Young, B.D.; Whittaker, S.J. Amplification and Overexpression of JUNB Is Associated with Primary Cutaneous T-Cell Lymphomas. *Blood* **2003**, *101*, 1513–1519. [CrossRef]
51. Carr, T.M.; Wheaton, J.D.; Houtz, G.M.; Ciofani, M. JunB Promotes Th17 Cell Identity and Restrains Alternative CD4 + T-Cell Programs during Inflammation. *Nat. Commun.* **2017**, *8*, 301. [CrossRef]
52. Hasan, Z.; Koizumi, S.; Sasaki, D.; Yamada, H.; Arakaki, N.; Fujihara, Y.; Okitsu, S.; Shirahata, H.; Ishikawa, H. JunB Is Essential for IL-23-Dependent Pathogenicity of Th17 Cells. *Nat. Commun.* **2017**, *8*, 15628. [CrossRef] [PubMed]
53. Yamazaki, S.; Tanaka, Y.; Araki, H.; Kohda, A.; Sanematsu, F.; Arasaki, T.; Duan, X.; Miura, F.; Katagiri, T.; Shindo, R.; et al. The AP-1 Transcription Factor JunB Is Required for Th17 Cell Differentiation. *Sci. Rep.* **2017**, *7*, 17402. [CrossRef]
54. Hoshino, K.; Quintás-Cardama, A.; Radich, J.; Dai, H.; Yang, H.; Garcia-Manero, G. Downregulation of JUNB MRNA Expression in Advanced Phase Chronic Myelogenous Leukemia. *Leuk. Res.* **2009**, *33*, 1361–1366. [CrossRef]
55. Gong, C.; Shen, J.; Fang, Z.; Qiao, L.; Feng, R.; Lin, X.; Li, S. Abnormally Expressed JunB Transactivated by IL-6/STAT3 Signaling Promotes Uveal Melanoma Aggressiveness via Epithelial–Mesenchymal Transition. *Biosci. Rep.* **2018**, *38*. [CrossRef]
56. Zenz, R.; Eferl, R.; Kenner, L.; Florin, L.; Hummerich, L.; Mehic, D.; Scheuch, H.; Angel, P.; Tschachler, E.; Wagner, E.F. Psoriasis-like Skin Disease and Arthritis Caused by Inducible Epidermal Deletion of Jun Proteins. *Nature* **2005**, *437*, 369–375. [CrossRef]
57. Kobayashi, S.; Nagafuchi, Y.; Okubo, M.; Sugimori, Y.; Shirai, H.; Hatano, H.; Junko, M.; Yanaoka, H.; Takeshima, Y.; Ota, M.; et al. Integrated Bulk and Single-Cell RNA-Sequencing Identified Disease-Relevant Monocytes and a Gene Network Module Underlying Systemic Sclerosis. *J. Autoimmun.* **2021**, *116*, 102547. [CrossRef]
58. Ponticos, M.; Papaioannou, I.; Xu, S.; Holmes, A.M.; Khan, K.; Denton, C.P.; Bou-Gharios, G.; Abraham, D.J. Failed Degradation of JunB Contributes to Overproduction of Type I Collagen and Development of Dermal Fibrosis in Patients With Systemic Sclerosis. *Arthritis Rheumatol.* **2015**, *67*, 243–253. [CrossRef]
59. Schmidt, D.; Textor, B.; Pein, O.T.; Licht, A.H.; Andrecht, S.; Sator-Schmitt, M.; Fusenig, N.E.; Angel, P.; Schorpp-Kistner, M. Critical Role for NF-KappaB-Induced JunB in VEGF Regulation and Tumor Angiogenesis. *EMBO J.* **2007**, *26*, 710–719. [CrossRef] [PubMed]
60. Li, B.; Tournier, C.; Davis, R.J.; Flavell, R.A. Regulation of IL-4 Expression by the Transcription Factor JunB during T Helper Cell Differentiation. *EMBO J.* **1999**, *18*, 420–432. [CrossRef]
61. He, H.; Luo, Y. Brg1 Regulates the Transcription of Human Papillomavirus Type 18 E6 and E7 Genes. *Cell Cycle* **2012**, *11*, 617–627. [CrossRef] [PubMed]
62. Henderson, A.; Holloway, A.; Reeves, R.; Tremethick, D.J. Recruitment of SWI/SNF to the Human Immunodeficiency Virus Type 1 Promoter. *Mol. Cell. Biol.* **2004**, *24*, 389–397. [CrossRef]
63. Ito, T.; Yamauchi, M.; Nishina, M.; Yamamichi, N.; Mizutani, T.; Ui, M.; Murakami, M.; Iba, H. Identification of SWI·SNF Complex Subunit BAF60a as a Determinant of the Transactivation Potential of Fos/Jun Dimers. *J. Biol. Chem.* **2001**, *276*, 2852–2857. [CrossRef]
64. Hu, Y.-F.; Li, R. JunB Potentiates Function of BRCA1 Activation Domain 1 (AD1) through a Coiled-Coil-Mediated Interaction. *Genes Dev.* **2002**, *16*, 1509–1517. [CrossRef]
65. Moynahan, M.E.; Chiu, J.W.; Koller, B.H.; Jasin, M. Brca1 Controls Homology-Directed DNA Repair. *Mol. Cell* **1999**, *4*, 511–518. [CrossRef]
66. Scully, R.; Chen, J.; Plug, A.; Xiao, Y.; Weaver, D.; Feunteun, J.; Ashley, T.; Livingston, D.M. Association of BRCA1 with Rad51 in Mitotic and Meiotic Cells. *Cell* **1997**, *88*, 265–275. [CrossRef]
67. Bochar, D.A.; Wang, L.; Beniya, H.; Kinev, A.; Xue, Y.; Lane, W.S.; Wang, W.; Kashanchi, F.; Shiekhattar, R. BRCA1 Is Associated with a Human SWI/SNF-Related Complex: Linking Chromatin Remodeling to Breast Cancer. *Cell* **2000**, *102*, 257–265. [CrossRef]
68. Yanagida, K.; Engelbrecht, E.; Niaudet, C.; Jung, B.; Gaengel, K.; Holton, K.; Swendeman, S.; Liu, C.H.; Levesque, M.V.; Kuo, A.; et al. Sphingosine 1-Phosphate Receptor Signaling Establishes AP-1 Gradients to Allow for Retinal Endothelial Cell Specialization. *Dev. Cell* **2020**, *52*, 779–793.e7. [CrossRef]
69. Carmeliet, P.; Tessier-Lavigne, M. Common Mechanisms of Nerve and Blood Vessel Wiring. *Nature* **2005**, *436*, 193–200. [CrossRef] [PubMed]
70. Schorpp-Kistner, M.; Wang, Z.Q.; Angel, P.; Wagner, E.F. JunB Is Essential for Mammalian Placentation. *EMBO J.* **1999**, *18*, 934–948. [CrossRef] [PubMed]
71. Covassin, L.D.; Villefranc, J.A.; Kacergis, M.C.; Weinstein, B.M.; Lawson, N.D. Distinct Genetic Interactions between Multiple Vegf Receptors Are Required for Development of Different Blood Vessel Types in Zebrafish. *Proc. Natl. Acad. Sci. USA* **2006**, *103*, 6554–6559. [CrossRef]
72. Nilsson, I.; Bahram, F.; Li, X.; Gualandi, L.; Koch, S.; Jarvius, M.; Söderberg, O.; Anisimov, A.; Kholová, I.; Pytowski, B.; et al. VEGF Receptor 2/-3 Heterodimers Detected in Situ by Proximity Ligation on Angiogenic Sprouts. *EMBO J.* **2010**, *29*, 1377–1388. [CrossRef] [PubMed]
73. Benedito, R.; Rocha, S.F.; Woeste, M.; Zamykal, M.; Radtke, F.; Casanovas, O.; Duarte, A.; Pytowski, B.; Adams, R.H. Notch-Dependent VEGFR3 Upregulation Allows Angiogenesis without VEGF-VEGFR2 Signalling. *Nature* **2012**, *484*, 110–114. [CrossRef]

74. Achen, M.G.; Jeltsch, M.; Kukk, E.; Mäkinen, T.; Vitali, A.; Wilks, A.F.; Alitalo, K.; Stacker, S.A. Vascular Endothelial Growth Factor D (VEGF-D) Is a Ligand for the Tyrosine Kinases VEGF Receptor 2 (Flk1) and VEGF Receptor 3 (Flt4). *Proc. Natl. Acad. Sci. USA* **1998**, *95*, 548–553. [CrossRef]
75. Joukov, V.; Pajusola, K.; Kaipainen, A.; Chilov, D.; Lahtinen, I.; Kukk, E.; Saksela, O.; Kalkkinen, N.; Alitalo, K. A Novel Vascular Endothelial Growth Factor, VEGF-C, Is a Ligand for the Flt4 (VEGFR-3) and KDR (VEGFR-2) Receptor Tyrosine Kinases. *EMBO J.* **1996**, *15*, 290–298. [CrossRef]
76. Dumont, D.J.; Jussila, L.; Taipale, J.; Lymboussaki, A.; Mustonen, T.; Pajusola, K.; Breitman, M.; Alitalo, K. Cardiovascular Failure in Mouse Embryos Deficient in VEGF Receptor-3. *Science* **1998**, *282*, 946–949. [CrossRef] [PubMed]
77. Kumar, R.; Mani, A.M.; Singh, N.K.; Rao, G.N. PKCθ-JunB Axis via Upregulation of VEGFR3 Expression Mediates Hypoxia-Induced Pathological Retinal Neovascularization. *Cell Death Dis.* **2020**, *11*, 325. [CrossRef]
78. Mukouyama, Y.; Shin, D.; Britsch, S.; Taniguchi, M.; Anderson, D.J. Sensory Nerves Determine the Pattern of Arterial Differentiation and Blood Vessel Branching in the Skin. *Cell* **2002**, *109*, 693–705. [CrossRef]
79. Saito, D.; Takase, Y.; Murai, H.; Takahashi, Y. The Dorsal Aorta Initiates a Molecular Cascade That Instructs Sympatho-Adrenal Specification. *Science* **2012**, *336*, 1578–1581. [CrossRef]
80. Kwon, H.-B.; Fukuhara, S.; Asakawa, K.; Ando, K.; Kashiwada, T.; Kawakami, K.; Hibi, M.; Kwon, Y.-G.; Kim, K.-W.; Alitalo, K.; et al. The Parallel Growth of Motoneuron Axons with the Dorsal Aorta Depends on Vegfc/Vegfr3 Signaling in Zebrafish. *Development* **2013**, *140*, 4081–4090. [CrossRef] [PubMed]
81. Li, W.; Kohara, H.; Uchida, Y.; James, J.M.; Soneji, K.; Cronshaw, D.G.; Zou, Y.-R.; Nagasawa, T.; Mukouyama, Y. Peripheral Nerve-Derived CXCL12 and VEGF-A Regulate the Patterning of Arterial Vessel Branching in Developing Limb Skin. *Dev. Cell* **2013**, *24*, 359–371. [CrossRef]
82. Wigle, J.T.; Oliver, G. Prox1 Function Is Required for the Development of the Murine Lymphatic System. *Cell* **1999**, *98*, 769–778. [CrossRef]
83. Wigle, J.T.; Harvey, N.; Detmar, M.; Lagutina, I.; Grosveld, G.; Gunn, M.D.; Jackson, D.G.; Oliver, G. An Essential Role for Prox1 in the Induction of the Lymphatic Endothelial Cell Phenotype. *EMBO J.* **2002**, *21*, 1505–1513. [CrossRef]
84. Niimi, K.; Kohara, M.; Sedoh, E.; Fukumoto, M.; Shibata, Y.; Sawano, T.; Tashiro, F.; Miyazaki, S.; Kubota, Y.; Miyazaki, J.-I.; et al. FOXO1 Regulates Developmental Lymphangiogenesis by Upregulating CXCR4 in the Mouse-Tail Dermis. *Dev. Camb. Engl.* **2020**, *147*. [CrossRef]
85. Kiesow, K.; Bennewitz, K.; Miranda, L.G.; Stoll, S.J.; Hartenstein, B.; Angel, P.; Kroll, J.; Schorpp-Kistner, M. Junb Controls Lymphatic Vascular Development in Zebrafish via MiR-182. *Sci. Rep.* **2015**, *5*, 15007. [CrossRef] [PubMed]
86. Furuyama, T.; Kitayama, K.; Shimoda, Y.; Ogawa, M.; Sone, K.; Yoshida-Araki, K.; Hisatsune, H.; Nishikawa, S.; Nakayama, K.; Nakayama, K.; et al. Abnormal Angiogenesis in Foxo1 (Fkhr)-Deficient Mice. *J. Biol. Chem.* **2004**, *279*, 34741–34749. [CrossRef]
87. Sengupta, A.; Chakraborty, S.; Paik, J.; Yutzey, K.E.; Evans-Anderson, H.J. FoxO1 Is Required in Endothelial but Not Myocardial Cell Lineages during Cardiovascular Development. *Dev. Dyn. Off. Publ. Am. Assoc. Anat.* **2012**, *241*, 803–813. [CrossRef] [PubMed]
88. Mäkinen, T.; Veikkola, T.; Mustjoki, S.; Karpanen, T.; Catimel, B.; Nice, E.C.; Wise, L.; Mercer, A.; Kowalski, H.; Kerjaschki, D.; et al. Isolated Lymphatic Endothelial Cells Transduce Growth, Survival and Migratory Signals via the VEGF-C/D Receptor VEGFR-3. *EMBO J.* **2001**, *20*, 4762–4773. [CrossRef]
89. Salameh, A.; Galvagni, F.; Bardelli, M.; Bussolino, F.; Oliviero, S. Direct Recruitment of CRK and GRB2 to VEGFR-3 Induces Proliferation, Migration, and Survival of Endothelial Cells through the Activation of ERK, AKT, and JNK Pathways. *Blood* **2005**, *106*, 3423–3431. [CrossRef]
90. Adams, R.H.; Wilkinson, G.A.; Weiss, C.; Diella, F.; Gale, N.W.; Deutsch, U.; Risau, W.; Klein, R. Roles of EphrinB Ligands and EphB Receptors in Cardiovascular Development: Demarcation of Arterial/Venous Domains, Vascular Morphogenesis, and Sprouting Angiogenesis. *Genes Dev.* **1999**, *13*, 295–306. [CrossRef] [PubMed]
91. Gerety, S.S.; Wang, H.U.; Chen, Z.F.; Anderson, D.J. Symmetrical Mutant Phenotypes of the Receptor EphB4 and Its Specific Transmembrane Ligand Ephrin-B2 in Cardiovascular Development. *Mol. Cell* **1999**, *4*, 403–414. [CrossRef]
92. Kidoya, H.; Naito, H.; Muramatsu, F.; Yamakawa, D.; Jia, W.; Ikawa, M.; Sonobe, T.; Tsuchimochi, H.; Shirai, M.; Adams, R.H.; et al. APJ Regulates Parallel Alignment of Arteries and Veins in the Skin. *Dev. Cell* **2015**, *33*, 247–259. [CrossRef] [PubMed]

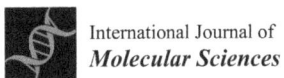

Article

BMP Receptor Inhibition Enhances Tissue Repair in Endoglin Heterozygous Mice

Wineke Bakker [1,†], Calinda K. E. Dingenouts [1,†], Kirsten Lodder [1], Karien C. Wiesmeijer [1], Alwin de Jong [2], Kondababu Kurakula [1], Hans-Jurgen J. Mager [3], Anke M. Smits [1], Margreet R. de Vries [2], Paul H. A. Quax [2] and Marie José T. H. Goumans [1,*]

1. Department of Cell and Chemical Biology, Leiden University Medical Center, 2333 ZC Leiden, The Netherlands; wineke.bakker@gmail.com (W.B.); Calinda.Dingenouts@gmail.com (C.K.E.D.); k.lodder@lumc.nl (K.L.); c.c.wiesmeijer@lumc.nl (K.C.W.); K.B.Kurakula@lumc.nl (K.K.); a.m.smits@lumc.nl (A.M.S.)
2. Department of Surgery, Leiden University Medical Center, 2333 ZC Leiden, The Netherlands; A.de_Jong.HLK@lumc.nl (A.d.J.); m.r.de_vries@lumc.nl (M.R.d.V.); P.H.A.Quax@lumc.nl (P.H.A.Q.)
3. St. Antonius Hospital, 3435 CM Nieuwegein, The Netherlands; jmager@antoniusziekenhuis.nl
* Correspondence: M.J.T.H.Goumans@lumc.nl
† These authors contributed equally to this work.

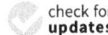

Abstract: Hereditary hemorrhagic telangiectasia type 1 (HHT1) is a severe vascular disorder caused by mutations in the TGFβ/BMP co-receptor *endoglin*. Endoglin haploinsufficiency results in vascular malformations and impaired neoangiogenesis. Furthermore, HHT1 patients display an impaired immune response. To date it is not fully understood how *endoglin* haploinsufficient immune cells contribute to HHT1 pathology. Therefore, we investigated the immune response during tissue repair in *Eng+/−* mice, a model for HHT1. *Eng+/−* mice exhibited prolonged infiltration of macrophages after experimentally induced myocardial infarction. Moreover, there was an increased number of inflammatory M1-like macrophages (Ly6C^{high}/CD206$^-$) at the expense of reparative M2-like macrophages (Ly6C^{low}/CD206$^+$). Interestingly, HHT1 patients also showed an increased number of inflammatory macrophages. In vitro analysis revealed that TGFβ-induced differentiation of *Eng+/−* monocytes into M2-like macrophages was blunted. Inhibiting BMP signaling by treating monocytes with LDN-193189 normalized their differentiation. Finally, LDN treatment improved heart function after MI and enhanced vascularization in both wild type and *Eng+/−* mice. The beneficial effect of LDN was also observed in the hind limb ischemia model. While blood flow recovery was hampered in vehicle-treated animals, LDN treatment improved tissue perfusion recovery in *Eng+/−* mice. In conclusion, BMPR kinase inhibition restored HHT1 macrophage imbalance in vitro and improved tissue repair after ischemic injury in *Eng+/−* mice.

Keywords: transforming growth factor-β; endoglin; neovascularization; tissue repair; myocardial infarction; hind limb ischemia

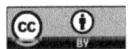

1. Introduction

Endoglin (also known as CD105) is a transmembrane protein that functions as a co-receptor for transforming growth factor-β (TGFβ)1 and TGFβ3. Mutations in *endoglin* resulting in haploinsufficiency are the cause of the autosomal dominant vascular disorder hereditary hemorrhagic telangiectasia type 1 (HHT1). HHT1 is rare life-threatening disorder characterized by local angiodysplasia like arterial venous malformations, telangiectasia, and recurrent epistaxis. Besides vascular dysplasia, an impaired immune response was also observed in HHT1 patients, evident by e.g., increased infection rates in the brain, joints, and liver [1]. To gain more insight into the etiology of HHT1, the murine model for HHT1, the *endoglin* heterozygous (*Eng+/−*) mouse, was extensively studied. Similar to HHT1 patients, *Eng+/−* mice display decreased wound healing [2] and impaired resolution of inflammation [3]. We previously showed that *Eng+/−* mice also have a delay in blood flow recovery and a reduction of collateral artery and capillary formation after hind limb ischemia (HLI) [4]. Furthermore, *Eng+/−* reduced myocardial repair after experimentally induced myocardial infarction (MI) [5], and systemic application of wild type mononuclear cells (MNCs) stimulated revascularization of the injured myocardium and restored cardiac recovery of *Eng+/−* mice, an effect not seen when MNCs of HHT1 patients were used [5]. The exact role of endoglin in inflammation and tissue repair was not yet completely understood, but a rapid increase in expression levels of endoglin during the inflammatory phase of wound healing suggests endoglin was involved in these processes [6–8]. Furthermore, while in healthy individuals the expression of endoglin was upregulated in activated monocytes [9], this response was impaired both in HHT1 patients [10] and *Eng+/−* mice [11], resulting in an increased infection rate and leukopenia [1,3,11,12], for example.

Endoglin exerts its effect by modulating TGFβ and bone morphogenetic protein (BMP) signaling, two pathways proven to be essential during cardiovascular development and disease [13,14], inflammation, and tissue repair [15–20]. TGFβ is the prototypic member of a large family of growth factors to which the activins and BMPs belong [13]. Upon tissue damage, TGFβ is released from the extracellular matrix, or is secreted by activated fibroblasts, endothelial cells, platelets, and macrophages [21–23]. TGFβ signaling is initiated by binding of the ligand to the TGFβ type II (TβRII) transmembrane receptor. In endothelial cells and macrophages, TGFβ can propagate the signal by forming a complex between the TβRII and a type I receptor, also known as activin receptor-like kinase (ALK). Signaling via the type I receptor ALK5 results in phosphorylation of the transcription factors Small mothers against decapentaplegic (SMAD)2 and SMAD3. Complex formation of TβRII with the type I receptor ALK1 is followed by activation of SMAD1 and SMAD5. ALK1 can only signal via TGFβ by forming a heterotetrameric complex consisting of two TβRII receptors, ALK1 and ALK5, in the presence of the co-receptor endoglin damping the TGFβ/ALK5 signaling pathway [13,24,25]. In the absence of endoglin, major vascular defects and impaired angiogenesis are observed, which can only partly be explained by malfunctioning of the endothelial cells by enhanced TGFβ/ALK5 signaling. It is, however, not known what the role of endoglin deficiency in monocytes entails and how this contributes to vascular repair after an ischemic event.

Cardiac wound healing after ischemic injury can be divided in three phases—the ischemic phase, the inflammatory phase, and the repair phase [26]. During the ischemic phase, cells within the obstructed area are devoid of oxygen and nutrients and go into apoptosis or necrosis. In the inflammatory phase, cellular debris within the injured myocardium is resolved by the recruitment of immune cells, inflammatory-like macrophages (M1-like, from here onwards referred to as 'M1'), the secretion of cytokines and degradation of extracellular matrix [26]. Approximately 5 days post-MI, the repair phase starts which is hallmarked by the release of growth factors and cytokines stimulating vascularization, recruitment of endothelial progenitor cells, and differentiation of reparative/regenerative-like macrophages (M2-like, from here onwards referred to as 'M2') [26,27]. The immune cells resolve after 2–3 weeks and a fibrous scar is formed [26]. Although we earlier showed that there is an impaired vascular recovery after ischemic injury in *Eng+/−* mice using two different models [4,5], as well as an imbalance in M1/M2 macrophages [28], the relation between these two observations and *endoglin* heterozygosity is still poorly understood. Therefore, the aim of this study was to elucidate the effect of *endoglin* heterozygosity on M1 and M2 macrophages during the different phases of cardiac wound healing and vascular recovery. We showed that the differentiation of monocytes isolated from the *Eng+/−* mouse into M2 macrophages contributed to the impaired tissue repair. Moreover, the impaired macrophage differentiation was confirmed in monocytes of HHT1 patients, which could be restored in vitro by inhibiting BMP signaling. Finally, BMP receptor kinase inhibition improved tissue repair of both the *Eng+/−* ischemic myocardium as well as the *Eng+/−* ischemic hind limb, by increasing neovascularization.

2. Results

2.1. Endoglin Deficiency Results in Prolonged Inflammation and Reduced M2 Macrophage Presence in the Heart after MI

Recruitment of inflammatory cells and their timely resolution is essential for cardiac tissue repair. An inadequate or excessive inflammatory response is detrimental in injured myocardium and can lead to adverse remodeling. We therefore investigated the effects of *endoglin* heterozygosity on the influx of monocytes during the inflammation phase, after experimentally inducing MI. We first determined if *endoglin* heterozygosity influences MNC composition at baseline. Before induction of MI, we observed no differences in MNC subtypes, like macrophages, lymphocytes, NK-cells, neutrophils, and granulocytes in blood and bone marrow between wild type (WT, *Eng*+/+) and *Eng*+/− mice (data not shown).

Subsequently we induced MI and assessed the number of macrophages present in the heart using immunohistochemical analysis. Four days post-MI, MAC-3 expressing macrophages were present in large numbers in the border zone of the infarcted hearts of both WT and *Eng*+/− mice (Figure 1A,B). Macrophage infiltration in WT hearts was cleared 14 days post MI (Figure 1A,B), confirming previous studies that reported that the inflammatory response is most pronounced at day 3–5 and cleared after approximately two weeks [26]. Interestingly, at 14 days post-MI MAC-3 expressing cells were still easily detectable in the infarct border zone of *Eng*+/− mice (Figure 1B), suggesting a delay in macrophage resolution.

To further characterize the phenotype of these macrophages, we determined the expression of CD11b, a general monocyte/macrophage marker, and CD206, a specific marker for M2 (reparative) macrophages facilitating the healing process. Immunofluorescent analysis of the spleen, used as control tissue, showed the presence of CD11b-positive resident monocytes, while no CD206 staining was observed (Figure 1C). Four days post-MI, hearts of WT mice harbored similar numbers of CD11b and CD206 expressing cells, suggesting that the macrophages present in the heart were M2 macrophages. In contrast, in the hearts of *Eng*+/− mice, CD11b+ cells were easily detectable, while only limited numbers of CD206 expressing cells were present. We quantified these observations using flow cytometry on single cell suspensions of mouse hearts (Figure 1D). At day 4 post-MI, the *Eng*+/− hearts contained significantly less M2 macrophages, while the number of pro-inflammatory M1 macrophages was significantly increased (Figure 1D). This suggests a macrophage polarization in the injured *Eng*+/− heart towards a more inflammatory macrophage phenotype.

2.2. Endoglin Deficiency Reduces In Vitro Differentiation of M2 Macrophages in Both HHT1 Mice and Patients

To gain more insight into how *endoglin* heterozygosity might influence macrophage differentiation, we isolated bone marrow derived CD11b+ monocytes and used immunofluorescence to analyze their differentiation towards macrophages in vitro. Endoglin is expressed on murine macrophages and co-staining of endoglin together with the inflammatory macrophage marker Ly6C, revealed that endoglin is specifically present on murine macrophages with a low expression level of Ly6C (Figure 2A).

Macrophages with high expression levels of Ly6C, known as the inflammatory-like (M1-like) subtype, show low expression levels of endoglin (Figure 2A). More detailed analysis of the different macrophage subtypes in *Eng*+/− mice and HHT1 patients was performed using flow cytometry. Inflammatory (M1) macrophages were identified by the expression of CD11b, high levels of Ly6C and low CD206 expression for mouse macrophages, and the expression of CD14 and absence of CD16 expression for human cells (Figure 2B).

Reparative (M2) macrophages were identified by the expression of CD11b, low levels of Ly6C and high expression of CD206 for mouse, and the expression of both CD14 and CD16 for human cells (Figure 2B). Monocytes isolated from *Eng*+/− mice as well as HHT1 patients showed an increased percentage of inflammatory macrophages and a reduction of reparative macrophages, compared to macrophages from WT mice and healthy volunteers (Figure 2C).

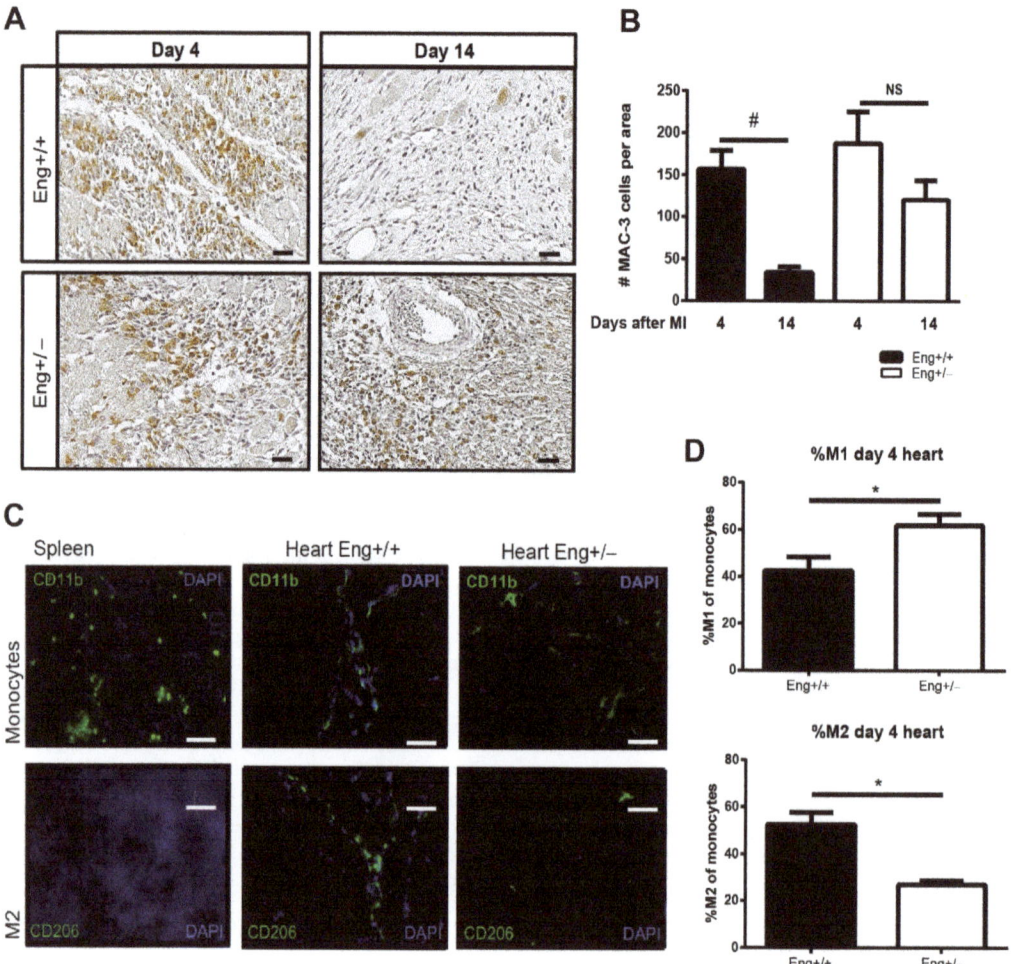

Figure 1. Prolonged macrophage infiltration and decreased number of M2 macrophages after myocardial infarction in *Eng+/−*. (**A**) Cardiac sections of *Eng+/+* and *Eng+/−* mice were stained for MAC-3 expressing macrophage (MAC-3 = brown; nuclei = blue) at day 4 and 14 post MI. Scale bar: 50 µm. (**B**) Quantification of the MAC3 positive cells shown in an N = 5–16 mice per group. (**C**) Splenic and cardiac tissue post-MI were stained for CD11b (general monocyte marker) and CD206 (M2 macrophage marker) 4 days after MI. Scale bar: 50 µm. (**D**) The ratio M1/M2 macrophages was determined by flow cytometry using a single cell suspension of *Eng+/+* and *Eng+/−* mouse hearts 4 days post MI. The inflammatory M1 macrophage was identified by CD11b+/Ly6Chigh/CD206- selection and the regenerative M2 by CD11b+/Ly6Clow/CD206+ selection. N = 5–16 mice per group. *Eng+/+* N = 9, *Eng+/−* N = 5. * $p < 0.05$, # $p < 0.001$, NS: not significant.

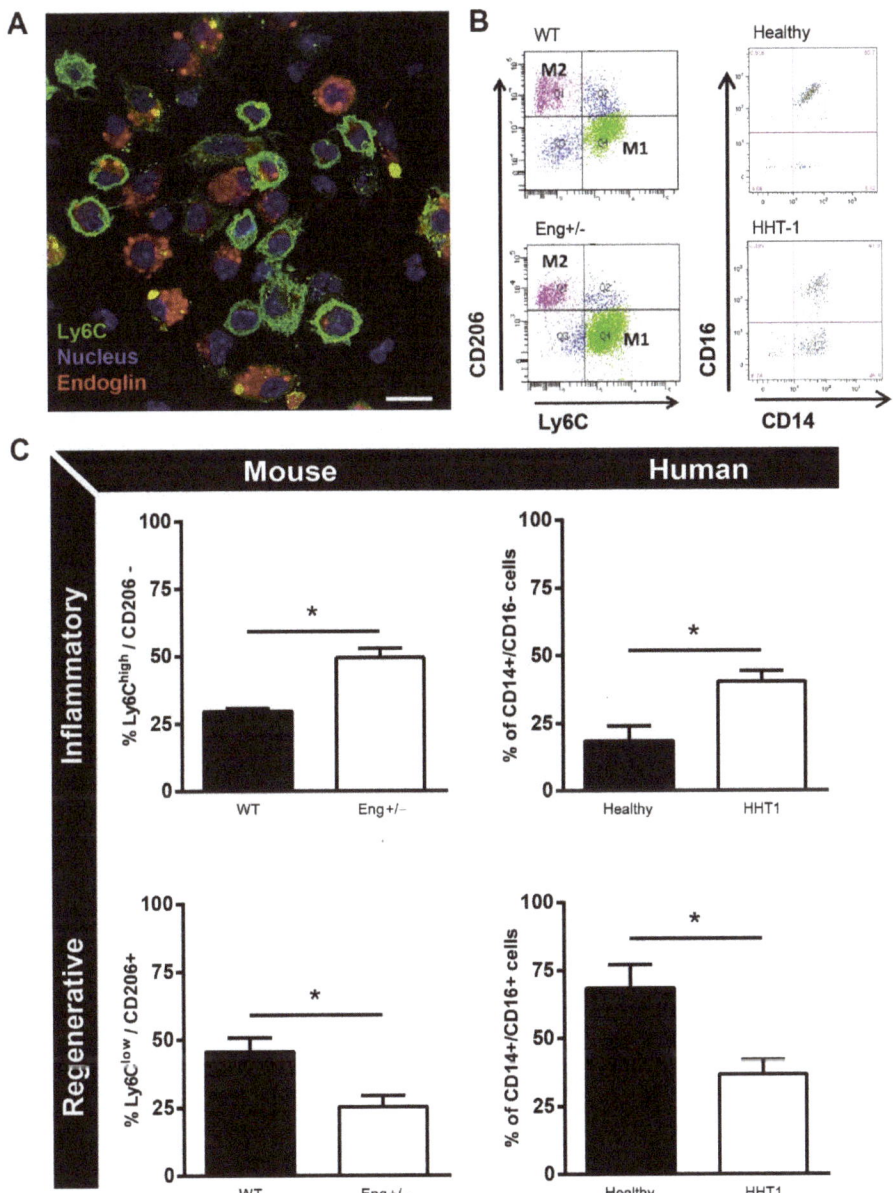

Figure 2. Macrophage phenotype is dependent on endoglin expression. (**A**) Macrophages isolated from *Eng+/+* mice were stained with endoglin (red), Ly6C (green), and dapi (nuclei, blue). Scale bar: 10μm. (**B**) Representative flow charts of mouse and human isolated monocytes of *Eng+/−* mice and HHT1 patients and their healthy controls. Mouse inflammatory monocytes were distinguished by CD11b+/Ly6Chigh/CD206- and regenerative monocytes by CD11b+/Ly6Clow/CD206+ expression. Human inflammatory monocytes were distinguished by CD14+CD16- and regenerative monocytes by CD14+/CD16+ expression. (**C**) Quantification of the flow cytometry data as represented in B, divided in inflammatory and regenerative monocytes for mouse and human. Mouse samples: N = 5–16 mice per group. *Eng+/+* N = 9, *Eng+/−* N = 5. Human samples: 7 HHT1 patients and 5 age- and gender-matched healthy human volunteers. * $p < 0.05$.

Reparative (M2) macrophages were identified by the expression of CD11b, low levels of Ly6C and high expression of CD206 for mice, and the expression of both CD14 and CD16 for human cells (Figure 2B). Monocytes isolated from *endoglin* heterozygous mice as well as HHT1 patients showed an increased percentage of inflammatory macrophages and a reduction of reparative macrophages, compared to macrophages from wildtype mice and healthy volunteers (Figure 2C). Interestingly, monocytes from endoglin heterozygous mice secrete more MCP-1 compared to wild-type cells, confirming their increased inflammatory profile (Supplementary Figure S1).

2.3. In Vitro Switch of Macrophage Differentiation by Adaptation of the TGFβ Signaling Response

As endoglin is a co-receptor for the TGFβ signaling cascade, we next investigated the effect of stimulation and inhibition of the TGFβ-signaling pathway on macrophage differentiation. Monocytes isolated from bone marrow of WT mice were cultured for 3 days in the presence of GM-CSF to stimulate their differentiation into macrophages, after which 1ng/mL of TGFβ ligand was added for either 24 or 96 h. While 24 h of TGFβ stimulation had little effect on the percentage of M1 and M2 macrophages compared to the non-stimulated cells, 96 h of TGFβ stimulation skewed macrophage differentiation towards an M2 phenotype (Figure 3A).

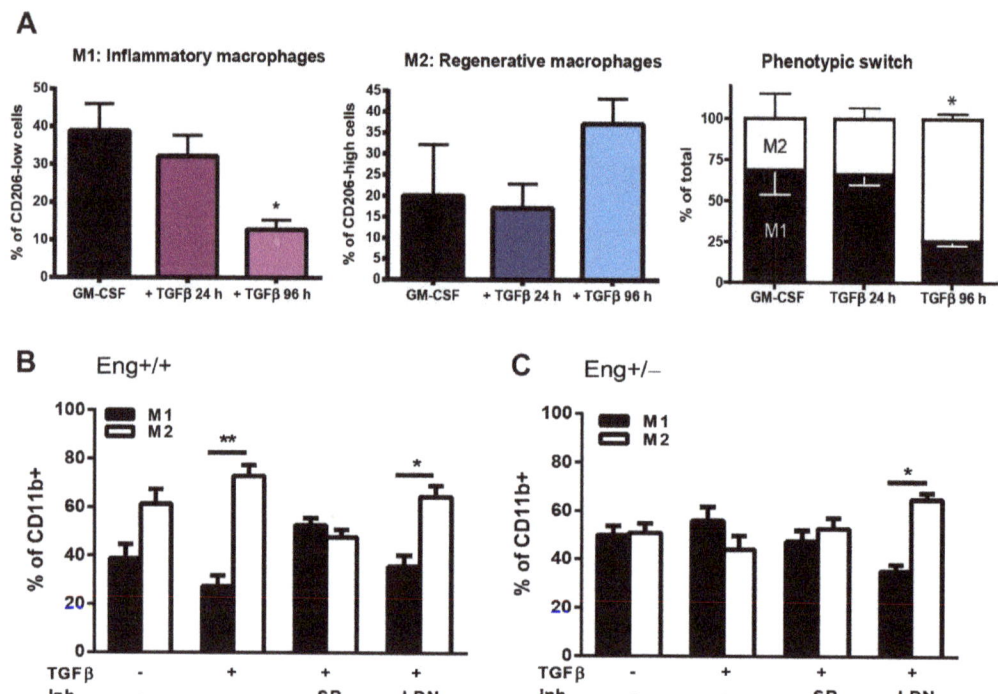

Figure 3. TGFβ signaling influences macrophage subtype differentiation. (**A**) Macrophages from *Eng+/+* mice cultured with either GM-CSF for 7 days or in the presence of TGFβ (2.5 ng/µL) for 24 h and 96 h. The macrophage phenotype was determined based on the expression of Ly6C high (M1) and low (M2) of the CD11b expressing macrophages. * $p = 0.001$ difference in the number of M1 and M2 between GM-CSF vs. TGFβ stimulation for 96 h. (**B,C**) BM isolated monocytes from *Eng+/+* (**B**) and *Eng+/−* (**C**) mice were cultured in the presence of GM-CSF in the presence or absence of TGFβ (2.5 ng/µL), SB (10 µM), or LDN (100 nM). The macrophage subtype was determined based on the expression of Ly6C high (M1) and low (M2) of the CD11b expressing macrophages. * $p = 0.007$; ** $p < 0.0001$.

This TGFβ increase in M2 macrophages was blocked by adding SB-431542 (SB), a potent ALK5 kinase inhibitor, to monocyte cultures from wildtype mice, but was not affected by adding the BMPRI kinase inhibitor LDN-193189 (LDN) (Figure 3B). The M1/M2 macrophage numbers did not change when monocytes isolated from Eng+/− mice were stimulated with TGFβ nor did inhibition of the ALK5 kinase by stimulating the cells with SB. Interestingly, when LDN was added to TGFβ stimulated Eng+/− macrophage cultures, the differentiation towards M1 macrophages was reduced, resulting in a normalization of the ratio of Eng+/− M1–M2 macrophages to WT levels (Figure 3C).

2.4. TGFβ/BMP and Non-Smad Signaling in Eng+/− Macrophages Is Impaired

TGFβ transduces its signal from the membrane to the nucleus by phosphorylation of downstream effectors—canonical Smads and non-canonical signaling proteins Erk and p38. To explore which pathway was used, monocytes from WT and Eng+/− mice were differentiated into macrophages, serum starved, and stimulated for 60 min with TGFβ, in the absence or presence of the indicated inhibitors SB or LDN. TGFβ was not able to detectably phosphorylate SMAD1/5 after serum starvation in either WT or Eng+/− macrophages (data not shown).

Both WT and Eng+/− macrophages showed an induction of SMAD2 phosphorylation upon stimulation with TGFβ, which was blocked when SB was added, but not when treated with LDN (Figure 4A,B). Phosphorylation of SMAD2 was not different between WT and Eng+/− macrophages. Interestingly, while LDN did not influence TGFβ-induced p-SMAD2 in WT macrophages, a significant increase in the phosphorylation of SMAD2 was observed in the Eng+/− macrophages (Figure 4B).

Since TGFβ can also signal via Smad independent pathways [29–31], next, we analyzed the non-canonical pathways known to be involved in stress, inflammation, and differentiation responses—the MAPK and p38 pathways. ERK1/2 phosphorylation was increased in WT macrophages upon stimulation with TGFβ, and was further enhanced when SB or LDN were added to TGFβ-stimulated WT macrophages (Figure 4A,C). Macrophages derived from Eng+/− mice did not show a change in ERK1/2 phosphorylation when stimulated with TGFβ, in the presence or absence of SB or LDN (Figure 4C). Phosphorylation of p38 showed the same trend as ERK; an increase in p-p38 in WT cells upon TGFβ stimulation and further enhancement in the presence of SB or LDN, while there was no response or even a trend towards reduced p-p38 in Eng+/− macrophages (Figure 4A,D). In summary, Eng+/− macrophages showed an increase in SMAD2 phosphorylation when BMP signaling was inhibited, while the non-canonical pathways show a decreased responsiveness.

2.5. LDN Treatment Improves Cardiac Function after Experimentally Induced MI

Since LDN influences the TGFβ response in Eng+/− macrophages in vitro, we next investigated whether LDN might influence the impaired cardiac recovery of Eng+/− mice after MI. LDN was systemically administered 2–14 days after the induction of MI. The efficacy of the LDN treatment was confirmed by a reduction in the number of cells positive for phosphorylated SMAD1 (Figure 5A) and an increased number of cells expressing phosphorylated SMAD2 (Figure 5B), 14 days post-MI.

In both WT and Eng+/− mice, LDN treatment significantly improved cardiac function (Figure 6A) and reduced infarct size (Figure 6B). Investigating the infarct border zone of these animals in more detail revealed that LDN treatment increased capillary density in WT hearts, but had no effect on the number of capillaries in Eng+/− mice. Interestingly, LDN treatment did not change the number of arteries in WT hearts, whereas in Eng+/− animals, the number of arteries increased significantly (Figure 6C–E).

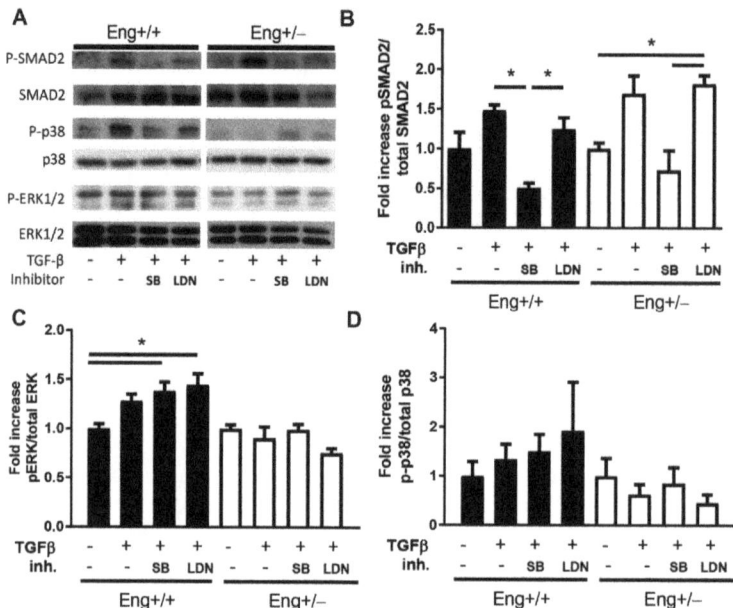

Figure 4. *Eng+/−* macrophages show blunted TGFβ and BMP signaling responses in vitro. (**A**) Western blot analysis of *Eng+/+* and *Eng+/−* cultured murine macrophages with GM-CSF, stimulated 60 min with TGFβ (2.5 ng/uL), SB (10 μM), and LDN (100 nM). Representative blots of N = 3 are shown. (**B**) Densitometric analysis of the blots shown in (A), expressed as percentage of phosphorylated Smad2 relative to total amount of Smad2. N = 3. (**C**) Quantification of the blots as shown in (A), expressed as percentage of phosphorylated ERK relative to total amount of ERK protein. N = 3. (**D**) Quantification of the blots in (A), expressed as the percentage of phosphorylated p38 relative to total amount of p38 protein, N = 3–4. Error bars are SEM. * $p < 0.05$.

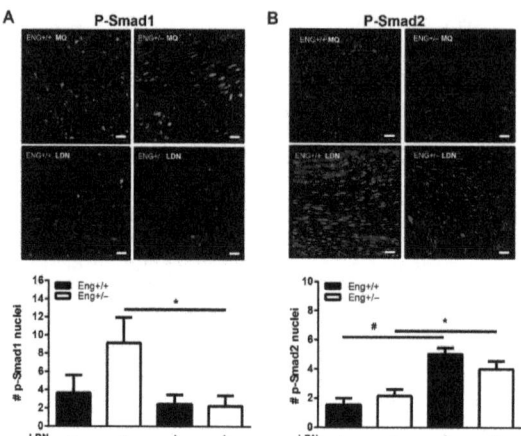

Figure 5. LDN decreases p-Smad1 and induces p-Smad2 in the infarct border zone. Paraffin sections were stained for (**A**) pSmad1 or (**C**) pSmad2 and quantified in (**B**,**D**) for positive stained nuclei in *Eng+/+* and *Eng+/−* mice treated with LDN or placebo. Representative images of heart sections 14 days post-MI are shown. N = 5–16 mice per group. *Eng+/+* control N = 9, *Eng+/−* control N = 5, *Eng+/+* LDN N = 6, *Eng+/−* LDN N = 16. Scale bars: 30 μm. * $p < 0.05$; # $p < 0.001$.

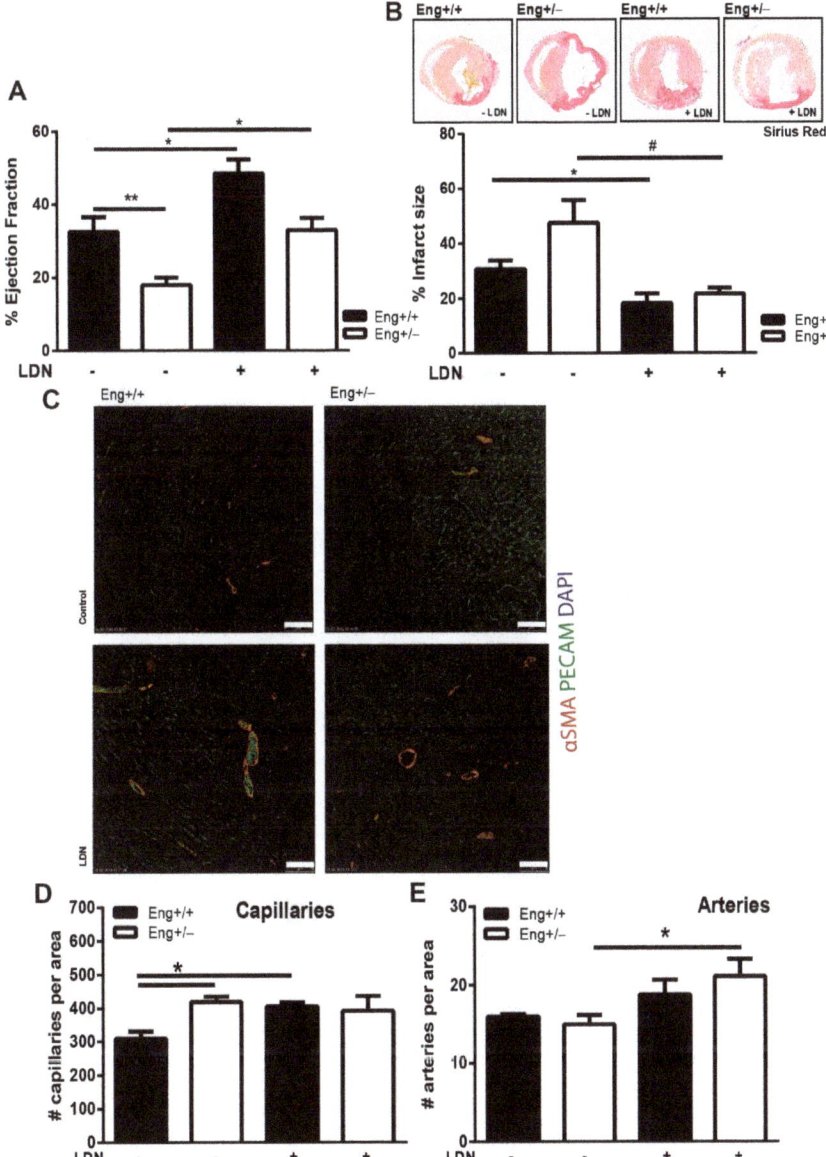

Figure 6. LDN restores cardiac function in *Eng+/−* to normal levels 14 days after MI. (**A**) Cardiac ejection fraction of *Eng+/+* and *Eng+/−* mice 14 days post-MI, treated with LDN or placebo. N = 5–16 mice. (**B**) Infarct size was determined in both *Eng+/+* and *Eng+/−* mice using Picrosirius Red staining. Top row—representative pictures of murine transversal heart sections. 1.0× magnification. Bottom row—quantification of infarcted area as percentage of total LV area. N = 5–16 mice per group. (**C,D**) LDN treatment influences cardiac neo-vascularization post-MI. (**C**) Paraffin sections of mouse hearts were stained for PECAM (green) and αSMA (red). N = 5–16 mice per group. *Eng+/+* control N = 9, *Eng+/−* control N = 5, *Eng+/+* LDN N = 6, *Eng+/−* LDN N = 16. (**D,E**) Quantification of the number of capillaries (**D**) and arteries (**E**) in (**C**). Scale bar: 50 μm. * $p < 0.05$; ** $p < 0.01$; # $p < 0.001$.

2.6. LDN Treatment Improves Perfusion Recovery after Hind Limb Ischemia

$Eng+/-$ mice show a delayed perfusion recovery after induction of ischemia in the mouse hind limb (Figure 7) [4]. Therefore, to determine whether the effect of LDN was specific for the heart or a more general response of endoglin heterozygosity to an ischemic insult, we chose the hind limb ischemia model in addition to the experimentally induced MI. After ligation of the femoral artery, $Eng+/-$ or WT mice were treated with LDN or vehicle, and perfusion recovery was measured by Laser Doppler Perfusion Imaging (LDPI) at day 7 post ligation. Interestingly, while blood flow in the hind limb of WT mice was not different between LDN or vehicle-treated animal, LDN treatment significantly improved the hampered paw perfusion in $Eng+/-$ mice (Figure 7). Overall, we conclude that tissue repair in $Eng+/-$ mice after ischemic damage in both experimentally induced myocardial and hind limb ischemia was improved by LDN treatment.

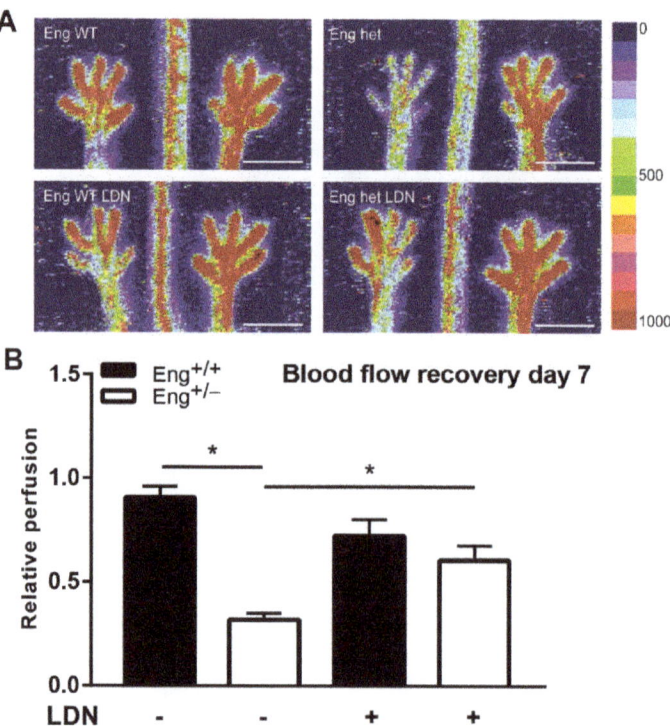

Figure 7. Hind limb blood flow recovery in female mice increases with LDN treatment. (**A**) Representative images of blood flow recovery in the paws as measured by laser Doppler perfusion imaging (LDPI), 7 days after HLI and subsequent treatment with LDN. Colors indicate the level of flow as indicated on the right panel of the figure. The left limb has HLI, the right limb was used as control. Scale bar: 1 cm (**B**) Quantification of LDPI measurements, N = 5–7 female mice per group. Black bars = WT, white bars = $Eng+/-$. * $p < 0.05$.

3. Discussion

The natural response of the body to ischemic injury is to stimulate neovascularization. The influx of circulating monocytes is important for cardiac repair post MI and contributes to the revascularization of ischemic tissue [32,33]. The pro-angiogenic role of endoglin, a TGFβ co-receptor, in vascular development is well established [25,34,35]. We previously reported that the enhanced deterioration of cardiac function after experimentally induced MI in $Eng+/-$ mice, results from impaired capacity of HHT1 MNCs to home to the site of injury and accumulate in the infarct zone to stimulate vessel formation [5,36]. In this study, we showed that monocytes depend on the expression of endoglin to be able to differentiate from an inflammatory M1 macrophage towards a reparative M2 macrophage and that *endoglin* heterozygosity prolongs the inflammatory response after myocardial infarction. This observation might explain why patients [1,37,38] and mice [3,11] haplo-insufficient for *endoglin* show prolonged inflammation and delayed wound healing and tissue repair after injury.

We demonstrated that TGFβ differently influenced the differentiation of wild type versus *Eng*+/− or HHT1 macrophages. Wild type monocytes differentiate to M2 macrophages in an ALK5-dependent manner, while inhibition of the BMP type I receptors did not influence their differentiation. Macrophages heterozygous for *endoglin* did not differentiate towards M2 upon TGFβ stimulation, while inhibition of BMP-signaling resulted in a shift towards M2 macrophages. TGFβ is well-known as an anti-inflammatory/pro-fibrotic cytokine and is mainly secreted by M2 macrophages [39,40]. We previously showed that there was no difference in TGFβ, TβRII, ALK1, and ALK5 expression in WT vs. HHT1 mononuclear cells [5], and endothelial cells deprived of endoglin expression were unable to process and secrete active TGFβ [41]. We hypothesized that the defect in TGFβ/BMP ligand processing due to deficiency in the co-receptor endoglin could play a role in the impaired TGFβ-directed differentiation of *Eng*+/− macrophages and explain why inhibition of BMP signaling could restore defective endoglin/TGFβ signaling. The reduced levels of endoglin might skew the tight balance that often exists between TGFβ and BMP signaling, and inhibition of the BMP type I receptor kinase might push this balance towards enhanced TGFβ signaling, thereby restoring the balance and M2 macrophage differentiation.

The main defect observed in TGFβ signaling in *Eng*+/− monocytes was related to the non-Smad signaling pathway. *Eng*+/− macrophages were still able to signal via the canonical TGFβ/SMAD pathway and phosphorylation of Smad2 was significantly increased when TGFβ was present in combination with LDN. Endoglin has two splice isoforms, a long form (L-Endoglin) and a short form (s-endoglin), containing a 33 amino acid shorter cytoplasmic tail [42]. Both isoforms are able to bind TGFβ but differ in phosphorylation status and their ability to interact with ALK1 and ALK5 [43,44]. A recent study showed that hypoxia-induced expression of S-endoglin stimulates signaling via TGFβ/ALK5/Smad2, causing impaired angiogenesis in the pulmonary vasculature of the developing lung [45]. Although we analyzed the impact of *endoglin* heterozygosity, determining which isoform of endoglin is involved in the pathology of HHT is an interesting topic for future research.

We observed reduced activation of the non-canonical MAPK/ERK pathway. An overall imbalance in the ERK and p38 signaling has a pronounced effect on the inflammation status and in reaction to stress [46]. Previous studies reported the involvement of endoglin in the MAPK/ERK pathway. In dermal fibroblasts, *endoglin* haploinsufficiency did not affect the basal or TGFβ induced pERK1/2, while the basal levels of Akt show a higher degree of phosphorylation [47]. In endothelial cells, the activation levels of Akt was not different between WT and *Eng*+/− cells, while ERK and p38 signaling was more active in *Eng*+/− endothelial cells [48]. We showed that in macrophages heterozygous for *endoglin*, ERK1/2 phosphorylation was impaired and neither stimulation nor inhibition of TGFβ signaling resulted in the phosphorylation of ERK1/2. ERK signaling is involved in cell growth and differentiation [49], and might affect apoptosis [50]. Defects in these aforementioned processes could explain the prolonged inflammatory status we observed in *Eng*+/− mice. In addition to impaired ERK activation, *Eng*+/− macrophages showed decreased phosphorylation of p38 in response to TGFβ stimulation and BMP inhibition. P38 is involved in TGFβ-directed monocyte migration and inhibits monocyte proliferation [51], has anti-angiogenic properties, and is reported to be involved in maintaining a proper balance in the angiogenic response [52]. Phosphorylated p38 was reported to inhibit VEGF signaling [53], and *Eng*+/− cells exhibit increased VEGF expression [48]. Therefore, the reduced levels of p-p38 could explain the endothelial hyperplasia and impaired angiogenesis found in HHT1 patients [54,55].

In the present study we showed that the inability of MNCs from HHT1 patients to induce neoangiogenesis post MI was not solely due to an impaired recruitment of the MNCs to the site of injury [36], but was also a result of impaired macrophage differentiation, mainly towards an inflammatory phenotype, which would intervene with myocardial repair [56]. High levels of inflammatory macrophages correlate with ventricular dysfunction after MI, in both mice and patients [57,58]. Selective depletion of M2 macrophages resulted in a nine-fold increase in cardiac rupture [59], and interfered with differentiation into M2 macrophages by knocking out tribbles pseudokinase 1 impaired ventricular function, 7 days post MI [60]. These studies, support our observation that M2 macrophages show a beneficial role in tissue remodeling. The impaired differentiation towards the reparative macrophage subtype due to *endoglin* heterozygosity could be restored by inhibiting the BMP type I receptor kinase with the small molecule inhibitor LDN, confirming both a BMP-dependent and non-canonical modulation of macrophage function in HHT1. Furthermore, cardiac ejection fraction after MI and reperfusion recovery after HLI were improved when *endoglin* heterozygous mice were treated with LDN. An important limitation of our study is that we used a non-reperfused myocardial infarction model, causing the infarct zone to be cut off from the circulation. The main effect of our LDN inhibitor is therefore likely of greatest impact at the infarct border zone, where blood vessels are still intact and tissue is perfused. Future research should include ischemia-reperfusion models to assess the effect of LDN on cardiac repair. Cumulatively, our results imply that treating HHT1 patients with a BMP type I receptor kinase inhibitor would improve tissue repair, and could be considered as a novel therapeutic target in patients with ischemic tissue damage.

4. Materials and Methods

4.1. Clinical Studies

The procedures performed were approved by the Medical Ethics Committee of the St. Antonius Hospital Nieuwegein, The Netherlands. The study conformed to the principles outlined in the 1964 Declaration of Helsinki and its later amendments. All persons gave their informed consent prior to their inclusion in this study. Venous blood samples from 7 HHT1 patients and 5 age- and gender-matched healthy human volunteers were collected. Peripheral blood MNCs were isolated by density gradient centrifugation using Ficoll Paque Plus (GE Life sciences, Zwijndrecht, The Netherlands, #17-1440-02), according to the manufacturer's protocol.

4.2. Animals

All mouse experiments were approved by the regulatory authorities of Leiden University, The Netherlands (ADEC nr 14-141) and were in compliance with the guidelines from Directive 2010/63/EU of the European Parliament, on the protection of animals used for scientific purposes, approved date 16 September 2014. Experiments were conducted in 10–12 weeks old *Eng+/+* and *Eng+/−* male or female C57BL/6Jico mice (Charles River, Leiden, The Netherlands).

4.3. Myocardial Infarction and BMPRI-Inhibitor Treatment

Myocardial infarction (MI) was induced in male mice, as described before [36]. Briefly, mice were anesthetized with isoflurane (1.5–2.5%), intubated and ventilated, after which the left anterior descending coronary artery was permanently ligated. The mice were given the analgesic drug Temgesic, both pre-operative and 24 h post-operative to relieve pain. Mice were randomly allocated to the treatment or placebo control groups. Placebo or BMPRI-inhibitor [61] LDN-193189 was reported to inhibit the kinase activity of the BMP type I receptors ALK1/2 (IC50 = 5 nM) [62], leaving the TGFβ/ALK5 pathway unaffected. LDN-193189 (2.0 mg/kg, Axon Medchem, Groningen, The Netherlands, #Axon1509) was administered twice daily via intraperitoneal injection from 2 days after MI till day 14. Heart function was measured by echocardiography 14 days post-MI, after which the hearts were isolated and fixated in 4% paraformaldehyde (in PBS) and embedded in paraffin.

Mice were monitored daily by the researchers or animal care staff to check their health and behavior for human endpoints. All were trained in animal care and handling and determining the following criteria and symptoms—impaired reaction to external stimuli, reduced mobility, or decreased grooming. Furthermore, for 3 days post-MI and onwards—bleeding, swelling, redness, or discharge of the incision area. Mice were weighed at day of surgery and prior to echocardiography and euthanized by carbon dioxide, when losing more than 15% weight. Animals dropped out prior just after MI or within 10 days post-MI-due to cardiac rupture.

4.4. Cardiac Function Measurements

Echocardiography was performed after mice were anesthetized with 1.5–2.5% isoflurane using the Vevo 770 (VisualSonics, Inc., Toronto, ON, Canada) system, with a 30 MHz transducer (RMV707B). We imaged the longitudinal axis of the left ventricle using the Electrocardiography-based Kilohertz Visualization (EKV) imaging mode. The ejection fraction was determined by tracing the left ventricular volume during the systolic and diastolic phase, using the Vevo770 V3.0 imaging software (VisualSonics, Inc., Toronto, ON, Canada).

4.5. Hind Limb Ischemia and Perfusion Imaging

Hind limb ischemia (HLI) was induced as described before [63]. In brief, male and female mice were anesthetized by intraperitoneal injection of midazolam (8.0 mg/kg, Roche Diagnostics, Almere, The Netherlands), medetomidine (0.4 mg/kg, Orion, Espoo, Finland), and fentanyl (0.08 mg/kg, Janssen Pharmaceuticals, Beerse, Belgium). Ischemia of the left hind limb was induced by electrocoagulation of the left femoral artery, the right hind limb served as control. After surgery, anesthesia was antagonized with flumazenil (0.7 mg/kg, Fresenius Kabi), atipamezole (3.3 mg/kg, Orion), and buprenorphine (0.2 mg/kg, MSD Animal Health, Boxmeer, The Netherlands).

Blood flow recovery to the hind limb was measured using laser Doppler perfusion imaging (LDPI, Moore Instruments, Axminster, UK), at 7 days post injury. During LDPI measurements, mice were anesthetized by intraperitoneal injection of midazolam (8.0 mg/kg, Roche Diagnostics) and medetomidine (0.4 mg/kg, Orion). After LDPI, anesthesia was antagonized by subcutaneous injection of flumazenil (0.7 mg/kg, Fresenius Kabi, Bad Homburg vor der Höhe, Germany) and atipamezole (3.3 mg/kg, Orion). Humane endpoints after induction of HLI were considered when mice were less mobile, showed impaired reaction to external stimuli, or decreased grooming. Furthermore, when the incision wound area was bleeding, swollen, or discharged, animals would be euthanized by carbon dioxide.

4.6. Immunohistochemistry

After euthanasia by carbon dioxide, mouse hearts were dissected, fixated overnight in 4% paraformaldehyde (in PBS) at 4 °C, dehydrated, and embedded in paraffin wax. Six μm sections were baked onto coated glass slides (VWR, Amsterdam, The Netherlands, SuperFrost Plus), and stained for the presence of macrophages in the infarct border zone, using rat anti-mouse MAC3 (CD107b, dilution 1:200, BD Biosciences, San Jose, CA, USA, #550292) and goat anti-rat biotinylated secondary antibody (1:300, Vector Laboratories, Burlingame, CA, USA, #BA-9400). An avidin/biotin based DAB peroxidase staining was used (Vectastain ABC system, Vector Laboratories, #PK-4000) to detect antibody binding, next to a hematoxylin counterstain for cell nuclei.

Infarct size was determined by Picrosirius Red (PSR) collagen staining; slides were deparaffinized and hydrated, followed by 1 h incubation with PSR solution; 0.1gram Sirius Red F3B (Merck, Zwijndrecht, The Netherlands) dissolved in 100 mL saturated picric acid solution (pH = 2.0) (Sigma, Zwijndrecht, The Netherlands, #P6744). Slides were washed in acidified water, dehydrated in ethanol and mounted with Entellan (Merck) mountant.

Immunofluorescent stainings were performed using standard protocol as previously described [64] for visualization of capillaries by PECAM (CD31, dilution 1:800, Santa Cruz, #sc-1506), arteries by both PECAM (CD31, dilution 1:800, Santa Cruz Biotechnology Inc. Heidelberg, Germany) and αSMA (alpha smooth muscle actin, dilution 1:500, Abcam). Macrophages were stained with CD11b (MAC-1, dilution 1:200, Biolegend, London, UK #1012505, clone M1/70), MAC-3 (CD107b, dilution 1:200, BD Biosciences, #550292), and CD206 (dilution 1:300, Abcam, #ab64693). Simultaneously, detection of p-Smad1/5/8 (dilution 1:100, Cell signaling, Bioke, Leiden The Netherlands, #9511) was performed by 30 min antigen retrieval and subsequently p-Smad2 (dilution 1:200, Cell signaling, #3101) was amplified using a TSATM-Biotin System (Tyramide Signal Amplification) Kit (Perkin Elmer Life Science, Waltham Massachusetss, USA, #NEL700A). Fluorescent-labelled secondary antibodies (ThermoFisher Scientific, Bleiswijk, The Netherlands) were incubated for 1.5 h, at 1:250 dilutions. Sections were mounted with Prolong® Gold Antifade mountant with DAPI (ThermoFisher Scientific, # P36931).

4.7. Isolation of Immune Cells from Murine Hearts

Hearts were harvested from the mice 4 days post- MI and put in PBS buffer on ice. After excision of the left ventricle, the tissue was put into 1-mL digestion buffer (450U Collagenase A, Sigma Aldrich, Zwijndrecht, The Netherlands, # 10103578001, 60U hyaluronidase, Sigma Aldrich, #H3506, 60U DNAse-1, Roche, #10104159001) at 37 °C for 1 h. The tissue homogenate was filtered through an 80-μm cell strainer (Falcon # 352350) and MNCs were isolated using Ficoll density gradient, specific for small mammalians (Histopaque-1083, Sigma Aldrich # 10831). Flow cytometry and staining was performed as described below.

4.8. Flow Cytometry

Mouse monocytes from either 50 μL of whole blood, bone marrow mononuclear cells, or from heart lysates were stained for CD11b (with anti-mouse CD11b, BD Biosciences, #561114), Ly6C (Bio-rad Laboratories, Veenendaal, The Netherlands # MCA2389A647T or BD Biosciences, #561085), and CD206 (Bio-rad Laboratories, #MCA2235A488T), to identify M1 and M2 macrophages, respectively.

Human monocytes were isolated from peripheral blood, through Ficoll gradient separation. Total MNCs (3×10^5 cells per sample) were stained with anti-CD14-ECD (Beckman Coulter, Woerden, The Netherlands IM2707U) and anti-CD16-APC (Beckman Coulter, # A66330). Fluorescence was measured with LSRII flow cytometer (BD Biosciences) and analyzed by FACS Diva (BD Biosciences) and the FlowJo software (FlowJo LLC V9.4).

4.9. Cultured Macrophages from Mouse Bone Marrow

Monocytes were isolated from the bone marrow using CD11b+ magnetic beads (Miltenyi Biotec MACS #130-049-601) and subsequently cultured in the RPMI medium (Gibco RPMI 1640 Medium, #11875-093), supplemented with 10% FBS (Fetal Bovine Serum, Gibco, ThermoFisher Scientific, #10270), and 1 ng/mL GM-CSF (Peprotech, #315-03), to induce differentiation into macrophages. After 3 days, the attached cells were stimulated with TGFβ3 (1 ng/mL, kind gift of Dr. K. Iwata), ALK5 kinase was inhibited using SB-431542 (10 μM, Tocris, Abingdon, UK #1614), and BMPR type I (ALK1/2/3) were inhibited using LDN-193189 (100 nM, Axon Medchem, #Axon1509) addition for 4 days.

4.10. Western Blot Analysis

For intracellular protein analysis, at day 6 of culture, the macrophages were serum starved overnight, after which they were either stimulated or not for 1 h with TGFβ or inhibitors at the indicated concentrations, after which cells were lysed with RIPA lysis buffer (5 M NaCl, 0.5 M EDTA, pH 8.0, 1 M Tris, pH 8.0, NP-40 (IGEPAL CA-630), 10% sodium deoxycholate, 10% SDS, in dH2O) supplemented with phosphatase inhibitors (1M NaF Sigma Aldrich # S7920, 10% NaPi Avantor #3850-01, 0.1M NaVan Sigma Aldrich #

S6508) and protease inhibitors (complete protease inhibitor cocktail tablets, Roche Diagnostics, #11697498001). Protein concentration was measured using Pierce BCA protein assay (ThermoFisher Scientific, #23225). Equal amounts of protein were loaded onto 10% SDS-polyacrylamide gel and transferred to an Immobilon-P transfer membrane (PVDF membrane, Millipore, # IPVH00010). The blots were blocked for 1 h using 5% milk in TBST (Tris-buffered saline, 0.1% Tween20) solution and incubated O/N with rabbit anti-mouse phosphorylated Smad2 (Cell signaling, #3101), total Smad2/3 (BD Biosciences, BD610842), mouse anti-mouse phosphorylated ERK1/2 (Sigma-Aldrich, #M8159), rabbit anti-mouse total ERK1/2 (p44/42 MAPK, Cell Signaling, #4695, clone 137F5), rabbit anti-mouse phosphorylated p38 (Cell Signaling Technology, #9211), and mouse anti-rabbit total p38 (Santa Cruz Biotechnology Inc. #535). Blots were incubated for 60 min with horse radish peroxidase anti-rabbit (ECL rabbit IgG, HRP-linked whole Ab, GE Healthcare, #NA934V) or anti-mouse (ECL mouse IgG, HRP-linked whole Ab, GE Healthcare, #NA931V) antibodies. Blots were developed in an X-omat 1000 processor (Kodak) with SuperSignal West Dura Extended Duration Substrate (ThermoFisher Scientific, #37071) or SuperSignal West Pico Chemiluminescent Substrate (ThermoFisher Scientific, # 34080AB), and exposed to SuperRX medical X-ray film (Fujifilm Corporation). Analysis was performed using ImageJ (Version 1.51, https://imagej.nih.gov/ij/index.html (accessed on 17 February 2021), National Institutes of Health, Bethesda, MD, USA).

4.11. Morphometry

Tissues were sectioned using a cryotome (hind limb muscle) or microtome (cardiac tissue) at approximately 300 μm intervals along the ischemic area. Cardiac infarct size was determined using Picrosirius Red staining and calculating the percentage of the infarct area to the total area of the left ventricle. Cell infiltration was determined by manual quantification of 2 to 4 digital images per heart at the border zone facing the infarcted area or hind limb, taken at 40× magnification (CaseViewer 3D Histech). The quantification of the number of capillaries and arteries present was done manually in the border zone surrounding the ischemic area, where (cardio)myocytes were still viable. Data were blinded to the investigator and quantified by using ImageJ v1.46r (https://imagej.nih.gov/ij/index.html (accessed on 17 February 2021), National Institutes of Health, Bethesda, MD, USA).

4.12. Statistical Analysis

Statistical significance was evaluated by the D'Agostino-Pearson normality test, followed by Mann-Whitney (non-parametric) or unpaired Student's t-test (parametric) between 2 groups. To perform testing between multiple groups, ANOVA (parametric) with Bonferroni correction or Kruskal-Wallis (non-parametric) test was used. Analysis was performed with GraphPad Prism 6 software. Values are represented as mean ± SD or SEM when otherwise indicated. Values of $p < 0.05$ are denoted as statistically significant.

4.13. Data Availability

No datasets were generated or analyzed during the current study. The results generated during or analyzed during the current study are available from the corresponding author on reasonable request.

Supplementary Materials: The following are available online at https://www.mdpi.com/1422-0067/22/4/2010/s1, Figure S1: *Endoglin* heterozygous macrophages secrete more MCP-1 compared to wild type cells. MNC cells were cultured for 24 h after which the amount of MCP-1 present in the medium was determined using an ELISA assay.

Author Contributions: Conceptualization, W.B., A.M.S., P.H.A.Q., and M.J.T.H.G.; formal analysis, W.B., C.K.E.D., M.R.d.V., P.H.A.Q., and M.J.T.H.G.; investigation, W.B., C.K.E.D., K.L., K.C.W., K.K., and A.d.J.; H.-J.J.M., providing HHT patient samples; resources, M.J.T.H.G., and P.H.A.Q.; writing—original draft preparation, W.B. and C.K.E.D.; writing—review and editing, W.B., C.K.E.D., A.M.S., H.-J.J.M., M.R.d.V., P.H.A.Q., and M.J.T.H.G.; supervision, M.J.T.H.G. and P.H.A.Q. All authors have read and agreed to the published version of the manuscript.

Funding: This work was financially supported by The Netherlands Institute for Regenerative Medicine (NIRM, FES0908), the Dutch Heart Foundation (NHS2009B063), and by the Dutch Cardiovascular Alliance (CVON-PHAEDRA-Impact consortium (http://www.phaedraresearch.nl (accessed on 17 February 2021))).

Institutional Review Board Statement: Ethical review and approval were waived for this study in 2011, since blood drawn was part of the routine medical check-up and only 1 additional tube was collected for this study.

Informed Consent Statement: Informed consent was obtained from all subjects involved in the study.

Data Availability Statement: The data presented in this study are available on request from the corresponding author.

Conflicts of Interest: The authors declare no conflict of interest.

References

1. Guilhem, A.; Malcus, C.; Clarivet, B.; Plauchu, H. Immunological abnormalities associated with hereditary haemorrhagic telangiec-tasia. *J. Intern. Med.* **2013**, 351–362. [CrossRef] [PubMed]
2. Pérez-Gómez, E.; Jerkic, M.; Prieto, M.; Del Castillo, G.; Martín-Villar, E.; Letarte, M.; Bernabeu, C.; Pérez-Barriocanal, F.; Quintanilla, M.; López-Novoa, J.M. Impaired wound repair in adult endoglin heterozygous mice associated with lower NO bioavailability. *J. Investig. Dermatol.* **2014**, *134*, 247–255. [CrossRef] [PubMed]
3. Peter, M.R.; Jerkic, M.; Sotov, V.; Douda, D.N.; Ardelean, D.S.; Ghamami, N.; Lakschevitz, F.; Khan, M.A.; Robertson, S.J.; Glogauer, M.; et al. Impaired resolution of inflammation in the endoglin heterozygous mouse model of chronic colitis. *Mediat. Inflamm.* **2014**, *2014*, 1–13. [CrossRef]
4. Seghers, L.; De Vries, M.R.; Pardali, E.; Hoefer, I.E.; Hierck, B.P.; Dijke, P.T.T.; Goumans, M.J.; Quax, P.H.A. Shear induced collateral artery growth modulated by endoglin but not by ALK1. *J. Cell. Mol. Med.* **2012**, *16*, 2440–2450. [CrossRef] [PubMed]
5. van Laake, L.W.; van den Driesche, S.; Post, S.; Feijen, A.; Jansen, M.A.; Driessens, M.H.; Mager, J.J.; Snijder, R.J.; Westermann, C.J.J.; Doevendans, P.A.; et al. Endoglin has a crucial role in blood cell-mediated vascular repair. *Circulation* **2006**, *114*, 2288–2297. [CrossRef]
6. Torsney, E.; Charlton, R.; Parums, D.; Collis, M.; Arthur, H. Inducible expression of human endoglin during inflammation and wound healing in vivo. *Inflamm. Res. Off. J. Eur. Histamine Res. Soc.* **2002**, *51*, 464–470. [CrossRef] [PubMed]
7. Rossi, E.; Sanz-Rodriguez, F.; Eleno, N.; Düwell, A.; Blanco, F.J.; Langa, C.; Botella, L.M.; Cabañas, C.; Lopez-Novoa, J.M.; Bernabéu, C. Endothelial endoglin is involved in inflammation: Role in leukocyte adhesion and transmigration. *Blood* **2013**, *121*, 403–415. [CrossRef]
8. Rossi, E.; Lopez-Novoa, J.M.; Bernabéu, C. Endoglin involvement in integrin-mediated cell adhesion as a putative pathogenic mechanism in hereditary hemorrhagic telangiectasia type 1 (HHT1). *Front. Genet.* **2015**, *5*, 457. [CrossRef]
9. Aristorena, M.; Blanco, F.J.; Casas-Engel, M.D.L.; Ojeda-Fernandez, L.; Gallardo-Vara, E.; Corbi, A.; Botella, L.M.; Bernabéu, C. Expression of endoglin isoforms in the myeloid lineage and their role during aging and macrophage polarization. *J. Cell Sci.* **2014**, *127*, 2723–2735. [CrossRef]
10. Sanz-Rodríguez, F.; Fernández, L.A.; Zarrabeitia, R.; Perez-Molino, A.; Ramírez, J.R.; Coto, E.; Bernabéu, C.; Botella, L.M. Mutation analysis in spanish patients with hereditary hemorrhagic telangiectasia: Deficient endoglin up-regulation in activated monocytes. *Clin. Chem.* **2004**, *50*, 2003–2011. [CrossRef]
11. Ojeda-Fernández, L.; Recio-Poveda, L.; Aristorena, M.; Lastres, P.; Blanco, F.J.; Sanz-Rodríguez, F.; Gallardo-Vara, E.; de las Casas-Engel, M.; Corbí, Á.; Arthur, H.M.; et al. Mice lacking endoglin in macrophages show an impaired immune response. *PLoS Genet.* **2016**, *12*, e1005935. [CrossRef]
12. Zhang, R.; Han, Z.; Degos, V.; Shen, F.; Choi, E.-J.; Sun, Z.; Kang, S.; Wong, M.; Zhu, W.; Zhan, L.; et al. Persistent infiltration and pro-inflammatory differentiation of monocytes cause unresolved inflammation in brain arteriovenous malformation. *Angiogenesis* **2016**, *19*, 451–461. [CrossRef]
13. Goumans, M.J.; ten Dijke, P. TGF-β signaling in control of cardiovascular function. *Cold Spring Harb. Perspect. Biol.* **2018**, *10*, a022210. [CrossRef]
14. Goumans, M.-J.; Zwijsen, A.; ten Dijke, P.; Bailly, S. Bone morphogenetic proteins in vascular homeostasis and disease. *Cold Spring Harb. Perspect. Biol.* **2018**, *10*, a031989. [CrossRef] [PubMed]
15. Doetschman, T.; Barnett, J.V.; Runyan, R.B.; Camenisch, T.D.; Heimark, R.L.; Granzier, H.L.; Conway, S.J.; Azhar, M. Transforming growth factor beta signaling in adult cardiovascular diseases and repair. *Cell Tissue Res.* **2011**, *347*, 203–223. [CrossRef] [PubMed]
16. Ishida, Y.; Kondo, T.; Takayasu, T.; Iwakura, Y.; Mukaida, N. The essential involvement of cross-talk between IFN-γ and TGF-beta in the skin wound-healing process. *J. Immunol.* **2004**, *172*, 1848–1855. [CrossRef]
17. Kulkarni, A.B.; Huh, C.G.; Becker, D.; Geiser, A.; Lyght, M.; Flanders, K.C.; Roberts, A.B.; Sporn, M.B.; Ward, J.M.; Karlsson, S. Transforming growth factor β 1 null mutation in mice causes excessive inflammatory response and early death. *Proc. Natl. Acad. Sci. USA* **1993**, *90*, 770–774. [CrossRef] [PubMed]

18. Larsson, J.; Goumans, M.; Sjöstrand, L.J.; Van Rooijen, M.A.; Ward, D.; Levéen, P.; Xu, X.; ten Dijke, P.; Mummery, C.L.; Karlsson, S. Abnormal angiogenesis but intact hematopoietic potential in TGF-beta type I receptor-deficient mice. *EMBO J.* 2001, *20*, 1663–1673. [CrossRef]
19. Russell, N.S.; Floot, B.; Van Werkhoven, E.; Schriemer, M.; De Jong-Korlaar, R.; Woerdeman, L.A.; Stewart, F.A.; Scharpfenecker, M. Blood and lymphatic microvessel damage in irradiated human skin: The role of TGF-β, endoglin and macrophages. *Radiother. Oncol.* 2015, *116*, 455–461. [CrossRef] [PubMed]
20. Shull, M.M.; Ormsby, I.; Kier, A.B.; Pawlowski, S.; Diebold, R.J.; Yin, M.; Allen, R.; Sidman, C.; Proetzel, G.; Calvint, D.; et al. Targeted disruption of the mouse transforming growth factor-β1 gene results in multifocal inflammatory disease. *Nat. Cell Biol.* 1992, *359*, 693–699. [CrossRef]
21. Grainger, D.J.; Mosedale, D.E.; Metcalfe, J.C. TGF-β in blood: A complex problem. *Cytokine Growth Factor Rev.* 2000, *11*, 133–145. [CrossRef]
22. Wan, M.; Li, C.; Zhen, G.; Jiao, K.; He, W.; Jia, X.; Wang, W.; Shi, C.; Xing, Q.; Chen, Y.-F.; et al. Injury-Activated Transforming Growth Factor β Controls Mobilization of Mesenchymal Stem Cells for Tissue Remodeling. *Stem Cells* 2012, *30*, 2498–2511. [CrossRef]
23. de Sousa Lopes, S.M.C.; Feijen, A.; Korving, J.; Korchynskyi, O.; Larsson, J.; Karlsson, S.; ten Dijke, P.; Lyons, K.M.; Goldschmeding, R.; Doevendans, P.; et al. Connective tissue growth factor expression and Smad signaling during mouse heart development and myocardial infarction. *Dev. Dyn.* 2004, *231*, 542–550. [CrossRef] [PubMed]
24. Goumans, M.-J.; Van Zonneveld, A.J.; Dijke, P.T. Transforming growth factor β-induced endothelial-to-mesenchymal transition: A switch to cardiac fibrosis? *Trends Cardiovasc. Med.* 2008, *18*, 293–298. [CrossRef]
25. Lebrin, F.; Goumans, M.-J.; Jonker, L.; Carvalho, R.L.C.; Valdimarsdottir, G.; Thorikay, M.; Mummery, C.; Arthur, H.M.; ten Dijke, P. Endoglin promotes endothelial cell proliferation and TGF-β/ALK1 signal transduction. *EMBO J.* 2004, *23*, 4018–4028. [CrossRef] [PubMed]
26. Nahrendorf, M.; Swirski, F.K.; Aikawa, E.; Stangenberg, L.; Wurdinger, T.; Figueiredo, J.-L.; Libby, P.; Weissleder, R.; Pittet, M.J. The healing myocardium sequentially mobilizes two monocyte subsets with divergent and complementary functions. *J. Exp. Med.* 2007, *204*, 3037–3047. [CrossRef] [PubMed]
27. Mills, C.D.; Harris, R.A.; Ley, K. Macrophage polarization: Decisions that affect health. *J. Clin. Cell. Immunol.* 2015, *6*. [CrossRef]
28. Dingenouts, C.K.E.; Bakker, W.; Lodder, K.; Wiesmeijer, K.C.; Moerkamp, A.T.; Maring, J.A.; Arthur, H.; Smits, A.M.; Goumans, M.-J. Inhibiting DPP4 in a mouse model of HHT1 results in a shift towards regenerative macrophages and reduces fibrosis after myocardial infarction. *PLoS ONE* 2017, *12*, e0189805. [CrossRef]
29. Massagué, J. How cells read TGF-β signals. *Nat. Rev. Mol. Cell Biol.* 2000, *1*, 169–178. [CrossRef] [PubMed]
30. Nakagawa, T.; Lan, H.Y.; Glushakova, O.; Zhu, H.J.; Kang, D.; Schreiner, G.F.; Böttinger, E.P.; Johnson, R.J.; Sautin, Y.Y. Role of ERK1/2 and p38 mitogen-activated protein kinases in the regulation of thrombospondin-1 by TGF-β1 in rat proximal tubular cells and mouse fibroblasts. *J. Am. Soc. Nephrol. JASN* 2005, *16*, 899–904. [CrossRef]
31. Zhang, Y.E. Non-Smad Signaling Pathways of the TGF-β Family. *Cold Spring Harb. Perspect. Biol.* 2017, *9*. [CrossRef] [PubMed]
32. Frangogiannis, N.G. The inflammatory response in myocardial injury, repair, and remodelling. *Nat. Rev. Cardiol.* 2014, *11*, 255–265. [CrossRef]
33. Gombozhapova, A.; Rogovskaya, Y.; Shurupov, V.; Rebenkova, M.; Kzhyshkowska, J.; Popov, S.V.; Karpov, R.S.; Ryabov, V. Macrophage activation and polarization in post-infarction cardiac remodeling. *J. Biomed. Sci.* 2017, *24*, 1–11. [CrossRef] [PubMed]
34. ten Dijke, P.; Goumans, M.-J.; Pardali, E. Endoglin in angiogenesis and vascular diseases. *Angiogenesis* 2008, *11*, 79–89. [CrossRef] [PubMed]
35. Tual-Chalot, S.; Mahmoud, M.; Allinson, K.R.; Redgrave, R.E.; Zhai, Z.; Oh, S.P.; Fruttiger, M.; Arthur, H.M. Endothelial depletion of Acvrl1 in mice leads to arteriovenous malformations associated with reduced endoglin expression. *PLoS ONE* 2014, *9*, e98646. [CrossRef] [PubMed]
36. Post, S.; Smits, A.M.; Broek, A.J.V.D.; Sluijter, J.P.; Hoefer, I.E.; Janssen, B.J.; Snijder, R.J.; Mager, J.J.; Pasterkamp, G.; Mummery, C.; et al. Impaired recruitment of HHT-1 mononuclear cells to the ischaemic heart is due to an altered CXCR4/CD26 balance. *Cardiovasc. Res.* 2009, *85*, 494–502. [CrossRef] [PubMed]
37. Dupuis-Girod, S.; Giraud, S.; Decullier, E.; Lesca, G.; Cottin, V.; Faure, F.; Merrot, O.; Saurin, J.; Cordier, J.; Plauchu, H. Hemorrhagic hereditary telangiectasia (Rendu-Osler disease) and infectious diseases: An underestimated association. *Clin. Infect. Dis.* 2007, *44*, 841–845. [CrossRef] [PubMed]
38. Mathis, S.; Dupuis-Girod, S.; Plauchu, H.; Giroud, M.; Barroso, B.; Ly, K.H.; Ingrand, P.; Gilbert, B.; Godeneche, G.; Neau, J.-P. Cerebral abscesses in hereditary haemorrhagic telangiectasia: A clinical and microbiological evaluation. *Clin. Neurol. Neurosurg.* 2012, *114*, 235–240. [CrossRef] [PubMed]
39. Braga, T.T.; Agudelo, J.S.H.; Camara, N.O.S. Macrophages during the fibrotic process: M2 as friend and foe. *Front. Immunol.* 2015, *6*, 602. [CrossRef] [PubMed]
40. Vernon, M.A.; Mylonas, K.J.; Hughes, J. Macrophages and renal fibrosis. *Semin. Nephrol.* 2010, *30*, 302–317. [CrossRef]
41. Carvalho, R.L.; Jonker, L.; Goumans, M.; Larsson, J.; Bouwman, P.; Karlsson, S.; ten Dijke, P.; Arthur, H.M.; Mummery, C.L. Defective paracrine signalling by TGFβ in yolk sac vasculature of endoglin mutant mice: A paradigm for hereditary haemorrhagic telangiectasia. *Development* 2004, *131*, 6237–6247. [CrossRef] [PubMed]

42. Pérez-Gómez, E.; Eleno, N.; López-Novoa, J.M.; Ramirez, J.R.; Velasco, B.; Letarte, M.; Bernabéu, C.; Quintanilla, M. Characterization of murine S-endoglin isoform and its effects on tumor development. *Oncogene* **2005**, *24*, 4450–4461. [CrossRef]
43. Velasco, S.; Alvarez-Muñoz, P.; Pericacho, M.; Dijke, P.T.; Bernabéu, C.; López-Novoa, J.M.; Rodríguez-Barbero, A. L- and S-endoglin differentially modulate TGFβ1 signaling mediated by ALK1 and ALK5 in L6E9 myoblasts. *J. Cell Sci.* **2008**, *121*, 913–919. [CrossRef] [PubMed]
44. Blanco, F.J.; Grande, M.T.; Langa, C.; Oujo, B.; Velasco, S.; Rodriguez-Barbero, A.; Pérez-Gómez, E.; Quintanilla, M.; López-Novoa, J.M.; Bernabéu, C. S-Endoglin expression is induced in senescent endothelial cells and contributes to vascular pathology. *Circ. Res.* **2008**, *103*, 1383–1392. [CrossRef] [PubMed]
45. Lee, Y.; Lee, J.; Nam, S.K.; Hoon Jun, Y. S-endoglin expression is induced in hyperoxia and contributes to altered pulmonary angi-ogenesis in bronchopulmonary dysplasia development. *Sci. Rep.* **2020**, *10*, 3043. [CrossRef]
46. Kebir, D.E.; Filep, J.G. Modulation of neutrophil apoptosis and the resolution of inflammation through β2 integrins. *Front. Immunol.* **2013**, *4*, 1–15. [CrossRef]
47. Pericacho, M.; Velasco, S.; Prieto, M.; Llano, E.; López-Novoa, J.M.; Rodríguez-Barbero, A. Endoglin haploinsufficiency promotes fibroblast accumulation during wound healing through Akt activation. *PLoS ONE* **2013**, *8*, e54687. [CrossRef]
48. Park, S.; DiMaio, T.A.; Liu, W.; Wang, S.; Sorenson, C.M.; Sheibani, N. Endoglin regulates the activation and quiescence of endothelium by participating in canonical and non-canonical TGF-β signaling pathways. *J. Cell Sci.* **2013**, *126*, 1392–1405. [CrossRef] [PubMed]
49. Monick, M.M.; Powers, L.S.; Barrett, C.W.; Hinde, S.; Ashare, A.; Groskreutz, D.J.; Nyunoya, T.; Coleman, M.; Spitz, D.R.; Hunninghake, G.W. Constitutive ERK MAPK activity regulates macrophage ATP production and mitochondrial integrity. *J. Immunol.* **2008**, *180*, 7485–7496. [CrossRef] [PubMed]
50. Sawatzky, D.A.; Willoughby, D.A.; Colville-Nash, P.R.; Rossi, A.G. The Involvement of the Apoptosis-Modulating Proteins ERK 1/2, Bcl-xL and Bax in the Resolution of Acute Inflammation in Vivo. *Am. J. Pathol.* **2006**, *168*, 33–41. [CrossRef]
51. Olieslagers, S.; Pardali, E.; Tchaikovski, V.; ten Dijke, P.; Waltenberger, J. TGF-β1/ALK5-induced monocyte migration involves PI3K and p38 pathways and is not negatively affected by diabetes mellitus. *Cardiovasc. Res.* **2011**, *91*, 510–518. [CrossRef]
52. Aguirre-Ghiso, J.A. Models, mechanisms and clinical evidence for cancer dormancy. *Nat. Rev. Cancer* **2007**, *7*, 834–846. [CrossRef] [PubMed]
53. Gomes, E.; Rockwell, P. p38 MAPK as a negative regulator of VEGF/VEGFR2 signaling pathway in serum deprived human SK-N-SH neuroblastoma cells. *Neurosci. Lett.* **2008**, *431*, 95–100. [CrossRef]
54. Abdalla, S.A. Hereditary haemorrhagic telangiectasia: Current views on genetics and mechanisms of disease. *J. Med. Genet.* **2005**, *43*, 97–110. [CrossRef] [PubMed]
55. Thalgott, J.; Dos-Santos-Luis, D.; Lebrin, F. Pericytes as targets in hereditary hemorrhagic telangiectasia. *Front. Genet.* **2015**, *6*, 1–16. [CrossRef]
56. Peet, C.; Ivetic, A.I.; Bromage, D.; Shah, A.M. Cardiac monocytes and macrophages after myocardial infarction. *Cardiovasc. Res.* **2020**, *116*, 1101–1112. [CrossRef] [PubMed]
57. Panizzi, P.; Swirski, F.K.; Figueiredo, J.-L.; Waterman, P.; Sosnovik, D.E.; Aikawa, E.; Libby, P.; Pittet, M.; Weissleder, R.; Nahrendorf, M. Impaired Infarct Healing in Atherosclerotic Mice With Ly-6ChiMonocytosis. *J. Am. Coll. Cardiol.* **2010**, *55*, 1629–1638. [CrossRef] [PubMed]
58. Maekawa, Y.; Anzai, T.; Yoshikawa, T.; Asakura, Y.; Takahashi, T.; Ishikawa, S.; Mitamura, H.; Ogawa, S. Prognostic significance of peripheral monocytosis after reperfused acute myocardial infarction:a possible role for left ventricular remodeling. *J. Am. Coll. Cardiol.* **2002**, *39*, 241–246. [CrossRef]
59. Shintani, Y.; Shintani, Y.; Shintani, Y.; Ishida, H.; Saba, R.; Yamaguchi, A.; Adachi, H.; Yashiro, K.; Suzuki, K. Alternatively activated macrophages determine repair of the infarcted adult murine heart. *J. Clin. Investig.* **2016**, *126*, 2151–2166.
60. Ma, Y.; Halade, G.V.; Zhang, J.; Ramirez, T.A.; Levin, D.; Voorhees, A.; Jin, Y.-F.; Han, H.-C.; Manicone, A.M.; Lindsey, M.L. Matrix Metalloproteinase-28 Deletion Exacerbates Cardiac Dysfunction and Rupture After Myocardial Infarction in Mice by Inhibiting M2 Macrophage Activation. *Circ. Res.* **2013**, *112*, 675–688. [CrossRef]
61. De Vinuesa, A.G.; Bocci, M.; Pietras, K.; ten Dijke, P. Targeting tumour vasculature by inhibiting activin receptor-like kinase (ALK)1 function. *Biochem. Soc. Trans.* **2016**, *44*, 1142–1149. [CrossRef] [PubMed]
62. Yu, P.B.; Deng, D.Y.; Lai, C.S.; Hong, C.C.; Cuny, G.D.; Bouxsein, M.L.; Hong, D.W.; McManus, P.M.; Katagiri, T.; Sachidanandan, C.; et al. BMP type I receptor inhibition reduces heterotopic ossification. *Nat. Med.* **2008**, *14*, 1363–1369. [CrossRef] [PubMed]
63. Welten, S.M.; Bastiaansen, A.J.; De Jong, R.C.; De Vries, M.R.; Peters, E.A.; Boonstra, M.C.; Sheikh, S.P.; La Monica, N.; Kandimalla, E.R.; Quax, P.H.; et al. Inhibition of 14q32 MicroRNAs miR-329, miR-487b, miR-494, and miR-495 Increases Neovascularization and Blood Flow Recovery After Ischemia. *Circ. Res.* **2014**, *115*, 696–708. [CrossRef] [PubMed]
64. Duim, S.N.; Kurakula, K.; Goumans, M.-J.; Kruithof, B.P. Cardiac endothelial cells express Wilms' tumor-1. Wt1 expression in the developing, adult and infarcted heart. *J. Mol. Cell. Cardiol.* **2015**, *81*, 127–135. [CrossRef]

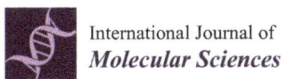

Article

Proangiogenic Effect of 2A-Peptide Based Multicistronic Recombinant Constructs Encoding VEGF and FGF2 Growth Factors

Dilara Z. Gatina [1], Ekaterina E. Garanina [1], Margarita N. Zhuravleva [1], Gulnaz E. Synbulatova [1], Adelya F. Mullakhmetova [1], Valeriya V. Solovyeva [1], Andrey P. Kiyasov [1], Catrin S. Rutland [2], Albert A. Rizvanov [1,*] and Ilnur I. Salafutdinov [1,*]

[1] Institute of Fundamental Medicine and Biology, Kazan Federal University, 420008 Kazan, Russia; gatina_dilara@mail.ru (D.Z.G.); kathryn.cherenkova@gmail.com (E.E.G.); k.i.t.t.1807@gmail.com (M.N.Z.); gulnazgg12@gmail.com (G.E.S.); mullahmetovaadela@gmail.com (A.F.M.); solovyovavv@gmail.com (V.V.S.); kiassov@mail.ru (A.P.K.)

[2] School of Veterinary Medicine and Science, University of Nottingham, Nottingham LE12 5RD, UK; Catrin.Rutland@nottingham.ac.uk

* Correspondence: rizvanov@gmail.com (A.A.R.); sal.ilnur@gmail.com (I.I.S.)

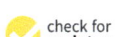

Citation: Gatina, D.Z.; Garanina, E.E.; Zhuravleva, M.N.; Synbulatova, G.E.; Mullakhmetova, A.F.; Solovyeva, V.V.; Kiyasov, A.P.; Rutland, C.S.; Rizvanov, A.A.; Salafutdinov, I.I. Proangiogenic Effect of 2A-Peptide Based Multicistronic Recombinant Constructs Encoding VEGF and FGF2 Growth Factors. *Int. J. Mol. Sci.* **2021**, *22*, 5922. https://doi.org/10.3390/ijms22115922

Academic Editors: Paul Quax and Elisabeth Deindl

Received: 29 April 2021
Accepted: 27 May 2021
Published: 31 May 2021

Publisher's Note: MDPI stays neutral with regard to jurisdictional claims in published maps and institutional affiliations.

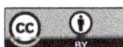

Copyright: © 2021 by the authors. Licensee MDPI, Basel, Switzerland. This article is an open access article distributed under the terms and conditions of the Creative Commons Attribution (CC BY) license (https:// creativecommons.org/licenses/by/ 4.0/).

Abstract: Coronary artery disease remains one of the primary healthcare problems due to the high cost of treatment, increased number of patients, poor clinical outcomes, and lack of effective therapy. Though pharmacological and surgical treatments positively affect symptoms and arrest the disease progression, they generally exhibit a limited effect on the disease outcome. The development of alternative therapeutic approaches towards ischemic disease treatment, especially of decompensated forms, is therefore relevant. Therapeutic angiogenesis, stimulated by various cytokines, chemokines, and growth factors, provides the possibility of restoring functional blood flow in ischemic tissues, thereby ensuring the regeneration of the damaged area. In the current study, based on the clinically approved plasmid vector pVax1, multigenic constructs were developed encoding vascular endothelial growth factor (VEGF), fibroblast growth factors (FGF2), and the DsRed fluorescent protein, integrated via picornaviruses' furin-2A peptide sequences. In vitro experiments demonstrated that genetically modified cells with engineered plasmid constructs expressed the target proteins. Overexpression of VEGF and FGF2 resulted in increased levels of the recombinant proteins. Concomitantly, these did not lead to a significant shift in the general secretory profile of modified HEK293T cells. Simultaneously, the secretome of genetically modified cells showed significant stimulating effects on the formation of capillary-like structures by HUVEC (endothelial cells) in vitro. Our results revealed that when the multicistronic multigene vectors encoding 2A peptide sequences are created, transient transgene co-expression is ensured. The results obtained indicated the mutual synergistic effects of the growth factors VEGF and FGF2 on the proliferation of endothelial cells in vitro. Thus, recombinant multicistronic multigenic constructs might serve as a promising approach for establishing safe and effective systems to treat ischemic diseases.

Keywords: angiogenesis; gene expression; non-viral vectors; 2A-peptides; growth factors; tube formation; VEGF; FGF2; cytokines

1. Introduction

Currently, ischemic diseases remain one of the leading causes of death in the world's developed countries [1]. This disease group is characterized by a lack of oxygen and nutrient supply due to impaired micro- and macro-blood supply to a tissue, organ, or limb [2]. Simultaneously, the lack of an adequate blood supply stimulates the activation of angiogenesis processes due to the release of proangiogenic factors [3]. In this regard, a strategy of supportive angiogenic therapy was proposed, which underlies the introduction of exogenous growth factors that promote vasculogenesis and blood circulation restoration [4].

Angiogenesis depends on complex interactions including spatial-temporal interaction of cells and various proangiogenic factors, particularly vascular endothelial growth factor (VEGF) and fibroblast growth factor (FGF2). As the most critical angiogenic factor, vascular endothelial growth factor (VEGF) remains one of the promising candidates for proangiogenic therapy [5–7]. The results of numerous in vitro and in vivo experiments have demonstrated that VEGF promotes de novo new blood vessel formation, improves blood flow, and supports myogenesis [8,9]. In addition, binding to the VEGFR1 and VEGFR2 receptors increases vascular permeability and induces proliferation and migration of endothelial cells [10]. It is known that VEGF contributes to the survivability of endothelial cells preventing apoptosis via the PI3K/AKT-signaling pathway and induces expression of the antiapoptotic proteins A1 and Bcl-2 [11–13]. The crucial role of VEGF in angiogenic processes has been confirmed in numerous investigations. The knockout of even one allele of the VEGF gene led to embryonic lethality and disorders in the cardiovascular system [14]. VEGF-A inhibitors are widely used in the therapy of solid tumors, thus indicating the significant role of VEGF in both normal and pathological angiogenesis [15]. Over the last decade, several randomized controlled trials have also utilized plasmid and viral vectors with the VEGF gene to treat severe coronary heart disease (Euroinject One, KAT, REVASC, NOTHERN, NOVA, VEGF-A Neupogen, and GENASIS) [6,16]. In 2011, the drug Neovasculgen was approved in Russia (ClinicalTrials.gov identifier: NCT03068585) to treat lower limb ischemia of atherosclerotic genesis, including chronic critical lower limb ischemia. This drug represents a highly purified, supercoiled form of the plasmid pCMV-VEGF165-encoding isoform 165 (a) of vascular endothelial growth factor [17,18].

The basic fibroblast growth factor (FGF2) is the second of the most characterized mitogens utilized in gene therapy protocols to induce therapeutic angiogenesis [19]. FGF2 interacts with the FGFR1 and FGFR2 receptors and with heparan sulfate proteoglycans, which results in proliferation and migration of endothelial cells, protease production, and angiogenesis. Proangiogenic effects of FGF2 have been confirmed in numerous experimental in vivo models of angiogenesis, including the chick embryo chorioallantoic membrane model, the cornea of the eye, and matrigel implants [20]. Moreover, positive effects of FGF2 have been reported in cases of pressure sores, diabetic foot ulcers, and burns. In 2001, Trafermin, a medicine based on human FGF2 for treating pressure ulcers and skin ulcers, was approved in Japan [21]. Likewise, the application of FGF2 has been successful in the treatment of second-degree burns. In the randomized study, patients with deep burns received local injections of either a placebo or bovine FGF2. All patients treated with FGF2 demonstrated faster granulation tissue formation and epidermal regeneration than patients in the placebo group [22]. Similar to VEGF, FGF2 has an affinity for heparin, increases neuronal survival, and reduces apoptotic cell death [23,24]. Unlike VEGF, FGF2 is capable of stimulating the proliferation of not only endothelial cells but also smooth muscle cells and fibroblasts. FGF2 also regulates the recruitment of immune cells such as monocytes, macrophages, and neutrophils, affecting the production of various chemokines [25,26].

The synergetic effects of VEGF and FGF2 were demonstrated in a broad range of studies dedicated to induction of angiogenesis and blood flow restoration [27,28]. For example, it has been described that FGF2 can induce endogenic VEGF expression and its receptors in endothelial cells where VEGFR2 inhibitors had arrested FGF2-induced angiogenesis [29]. Numerous studies have also shown that coordinated activity of VEGF and FGF2 is crucial in all stages of angiogenesis, especially during early embryogenesis, to increase vascular permeability and recruitment of endothelial cells. Stimulation of endothelial cells initiates protease production and plasminogen secretion, destroying basement membrane and activating the invasion of cells in the surrounding matrix [30,31]. Though the exact synergetic mechanism remains unclear, there are several potential signaling pathways involved in both VEGF and FGF2 interactions and interactions with their receptors. Interaction between VEGF–VEGFR is known to activate the Ras-MEK-MAPK and AKT, P38, and PKC signaling pathways, which in turn modulate FGF2 expression and proangiogenic cellular responses [32]. The interaction between FGF2–FGFR also activates Ras-MEK-MAPK signaling pathways and induces VEGF expression [33]. SRC cascade, AKT/P13K, and PKC pathways are known to participate in FGF2-dependent angiogenesis [34]. Thus, interaction between VEGF and FGF2 activate numerous signaling cascades and ultimately stimulate the angiogenic processes in endothelial cells.

Augmented concentrations of proangiogenic factors are known to cause aberrant vessel formation and hemangiomas as well [35]. These results were obtained when viral constructions were used providing longitudinal transgene expression [36]. It is common knowledge that viral vectors represent an efficient vehicle for target gen delivery due to their natural infection capacity of various cell types [37,38]. However, uncontrolled gene expression, immune responses to the constituent components of viral particles, and some viral genomes' relatively small packaging capacities restrict the feasibility of constructs based on recombinant viruses [39,40]. Compared to viruses, the application of non-viral gene therapy approaches using plasmid vectors do not provoke systemic reactions in the organism, and plasmids could be easily manufactured in preparative amounts [41]. Additionally, the development of new delivery systems has made it possible to achieve high efficiency of transfection both in vitro and in vivo. Continuous improvement of non-viral gene therapy techniques therefore contributes to their widespread use in clinical practice [9].

Currently, several strategies have been proposed to ensure simultaneous gene expression [42,43]: independent internal promoters [44], internal ribosomal entry sites (IRES) [45], mRNA splicing [46], bi-directional promoters, and 2A-peptides [47,48]. However, utilizing several promoters might significantly decrease transcriptional activity and reduce the vector's packaging capacity. In turn, IRESs provide effective co-expression of a few genes, but their large molecular weight (up to 1 kb) presents a limiting factor [49]. Moreover, the level of transgene expression depends on the location and spatial organization of the transgene. Downstream genes are transcribed less effectively in multicistronic constructions than cistrons located upstream of IRES [50–54].

Picornoviral 2A-sequences represent short peptides, composed of 14-21 amino acid residues, and contain a functional consensus motif Asp-Val/Ile-Glu-Asn-X-Pro-Gly -Pro [55]. This motif interrupts translation, "skipping" the formation of the last glycine-proline bond and releasing an upstream polypeptide that is attached to the C-terminal sequence of 2A. When translating the next polypeptide, proline is used as the first amino acid [56,57]. After 2A-mediated cleavage, the newly synthesized proteins contain a small N-terminal proline and a C-terminal residue of the 2A peptide; however, the proteins usually remain functionally active [57]. Currently, four types of 2A-peptide sequences are utilized in biomedical applications: foot-and-mouth disease virus FMDV 2A (F2A); equine rhinitis virus A (ERAV) 2A (E2A); porcine tospovirus 1 2A (P2A); and asigna virus 2A (T2A) [51]. Mostly, 2A peptide dedicated studies focus on the efficiency of cleavage of various proteins in multicistronic vectors. For example, it has been demonstrated that T2A usually has the most efficient cleavage compared to other types of 2A-peptides. In contrast, other results have also revealed higher efficiencies of P2A-mediated cleavage in comparison to T2A [51,58]. It is quite important to consider post-translational conformation of target proteins to achieve the most effective transgene expression. For example, the secretion of TGF-β was arrested due to the coding sequence's upstream position to 2A peptide [59]. Incorporation of the furin cleavage site (Fu) upstream to the 2 sequence enables polyprotein convertase specifically to hydrolyze C-terminal peptide bonds of arginine and cleavage the proteins downstream of R-X-K/R-R motif. This sequence has been discovered in various human proteins, plays a crucial role in protein formation, and enables active secretion and membrane-associated proteins [60,61].

In the present study, using a clinically approved plasmid vector, we designed recombinant constructions containing picornavirus peptide sequences, codon-optimized sequences of VEGF and FGF2, and a reporter DsRed fluorescent protein under the control of a cytomegalovirus promoter. Expression of recombinant proteins, the secretome of modified cells, and the synergetic effects of the target proteins on the formation of capillary-like structures by HUVECs were investigated.

2. Materials and Methods

2.1. Recombinant Constructs, Isolation, and Restriction Analysis of Plasmid DNA

Based on a clinically approved plasmid vector pVax1 (Thermo Fisher Scientific) [62], multicistronic constructions encoding various gene combinations (pVax1-VEGF-FGF2-DsRed, pVax1-VEGF-DsRed, pVax1-FGF2-DsRed, pVax1-DsRed) were designed and developed (Figure 1). Nucleotide sequences of the VEGF (GeneBank AF486837.1) and FGF2 (GeneBank #DD406196.1) genes were obtained from the NCBI database and cloned under a single CMV promoter. The Fu-cleavage site (AGAAACAGAAGA) and p2A skipping motif (CCACGAAGCAAGCAGGAGATGTTGAAGAAAACCCCGGGCCT) were incorporated between the target genes [63]. To enhance gene expression and reduce restriction sites, an Optimum Gene™ (GenScript, Piscataway, NJ, USA) algorithm was applied. Synthesis of plasmid constructions de novo were carried out using GenScript (https://www.genscript.com/).

2.2. Genetic Modification of the Cells with Recombinant Plasmids

Human embryonic kidney cells HEK293T (ATCC CRL-11268) were cultivated on Dulbecco's modified media supplemented with 10% fetal bovine serum (FBS), 100 U/mL penicillin/streptomycin, and 4 mM L-glutamine. A total of 2.5×10^5 cells were seeded per well in a 24-well plate in two ml medium. Transfections were carried once 70% confluence had been achieved using Turbofect transfection reagent (Thermo Fisher Scientific, Waltham, MA, USA). Transfection efficiency was analyzed after 48 h using DsRed expression by the modified cells as an indicator using a fluorescent inverted micro-scope AxioObserver Z1 Carl Zeiss AG, Oberkochen, Germany).

2.3. Quantitative Analysis of mRNA Expression

Total RNA from genetically modified cells was isolated using TRIZOL (Thermo Fisher Scientific, Waltham, MA, USA) according to manufacturer's instructions. Concentrations of isolated RNA were evaluated using a spectrophotometer NanoDrop 2000 (Thermo Fisher Scientific, Waltham, MA, USA). Complementary DNA (cDNA) was synthesized using a RevertAid kit (Thermo Fisher Scientific, Waltham, MA, USA), also in accordance with the recommended protocol. Expression of target genes was assessed by Real-time PCR and TaqMan technology on a CFX96 Touch Real-Time PCR Detection System (Bio-Rad, Hercules, CA, USA). Non-transfected 293 cells (NTC—non-transfected cells) served as negative controls for quantitative analysis of transgene expression. The relative amount of mRNA for the target genes was normalized to 18S rRNA and calculated using the $2^{-\Delta\Delta CT}$. Nucleotide sequences of primers specific to codon-optimized sequences of target genes are presented in Table 1.

2.4. Immunofluorescent Assays for Transfected HEK293T Cells

Transfected HEK293T cells were primarily fixed with chilled methanol for 20 min at 20°. Cell membranes were permeabilized by adding 0.1% Triton-100 (Helicon, Russia) and then incubated with primary antibodies at a dilution of 1:100, VEGF (Santa Cruze Biotechnology, CA, USA) and FGF2 (Santa Cruze Biotechnology, Santa Cruz, CA, USA), in Tris-buffer saline (TBS) for one hour. Following the primary antibody incubation period, the cells were washed with TBS and coated with the species-specific secondary. Nuclei were stained using a DAPI solution (4′,6-diamidino-2-phenylindole;62248, Thermo Fisher Scientific, Waltham, MA, USA) and photomicrographs for analysis were captured on a fluorescent microscope AxioObserver Z1 (Carl Zeiss AG, Oberkochen, Germany).

Table 1. Nucleotide sequences of primers and probes used for qPCR.

Primer Name	Nucleotide Sequence
rmh-18s-TMF	GCCGCTAGAGGTGAAATTCTTG
rmh-18s-TMR	CATTCTTGGCAAATGGTTTCG
rmh-18s-prode	(HEK)-ACCGGCGCAAGACGGACCA-(BHQ)
co-VEGF165-F	CAGATCATGGGGATCAAGCC
co-VEGF165-R	CATGGATTCTCCTGCCTTGC
co-VEGF165-Probe	(6-FAM)-CCAGGGCCAGCACATCGGCG -(BHQ1)
co-FGF2-F	GAGGCTGTACTGCAAGAACG
co-FGF2-R	TGATAGACACCAACGCCTCTC
co-FGF2-R	(6-FAM)-CCTCGGCCTGCAGCTGCTGCAGC -(BHQ1)

2.5. Enzyme-Linked Immunosorbent Assay (ELISA) of Target Genes

The concentrations of VEGF and FGF2 in cell lysates and supernatants of transfected and native cells were evaluated using Human VEGF (DY293B) and Human FGF2 (DY233) kits (R&D Systems, DuoSet, Minneapolis, MN, USA) in accordance with the manufacturers' recommended protocol. The calibration curve was created based on seven different concentrations in the range of 31.1–2000 pg/mL. Optical densities were measured using BioRadxMark at OD 450. The resulting standard curve was utilized for quantitative analysis of the recombinant proteins.

2.6. Multiplex Analysis

Quantitative assessment of secreted soluble factors in conditioned media and cell lysates was measured using a Bio-Plex200 System. based on xMAP Luminex technology, with Bio-Plex Pro Human Cytokine 27-plex Assay (M500KCAF0Y) including the following analytes: IL-1, IL-1ra, IL-2, IL-4, IL-5, IL-6, IL-7, IL-8, IL-9, IL-10, IL-12, IL-13, IL-15, IL-17, FGF2, Eotaxin, G-CSF, GM-CSF, IFN-γ, IP-10, MP-1, MIP-1, MIP-1, PDGF-BB, RANTES, TNF-α, and VEGF. Data collection and analysis was performed using Bio-Plex Manager 4.1 software.

2.7. Tube Formation Assay Using Matrigel Matrix

Human Umbilical Vein Endothelial Cells (HUVEC) were isolated and cultivated according to the previously described protocol [43]. Wells in a chilled 96-well plate were coated with 50 µL of Matrigel matrix (with a reduced concentration of growth factors (Becton Dickinson, Franklin Lakes, NJ, USA)) and incubated at 37 °C for an hour. After the matrix had solidified, 1×10^4 endothelial cells were seeded in 100 µL onto the Matrigel surface by adding conditioned medium from the HEK293T cells previously transfected with various plasmid constructs. Non-transfected HEK293T medium and poor medium containing 10% FBS were used as a negative control. Complete medium containing 10% FBS and Endothelial Cell Growth Supplement (ECGS) 30 µg/mL (Sigma-Aldrich, St. Louis, MO, USA) was used as a positive control. The formation of capillary-like structures was assessed after 6 h using phase-contrast microscopy. The total tube length and the number of formed branch nodes were calculated using the WimTube software package in the Wimamsis system (Available online: https://www.wimasis.com/en/WimTube, accessed on 19 March 2019)

2.8. Statistical Analysis

Each experiment was performed three times in replicates. All data are presented as mean with standard error of the mean ($\pm$s.e.). Multiple comparisons were tested by one-way analysis of variance (ANOVA) followed by a post-hoc Tukey test using the

GraphPad Prism 7 software (GraphPad Software, California, USA). The *p*-value $p < 0.05$ was considered statistically significant. Significant probability values were denoted as follows: * $p < 0.05$, ** $p < 0.01$, *** $p < 0.001$, **** $p < 0.0001$, ns—no statistically significant difference.

3. Results

3.1. Characterization of Multigenic Constructs Containing Picornavirus 2A-Peptide Sequences

In the current study, recombinant plasmid vectors were designed, encoding codon-optimized sequences of VEGF and FGF2 genes and DsRed under the single control CMV promoter. In bi-cistronic (pVax1-VEGF-DsRed, pVax1-FGF2-DsRed) and tri-cistronic vectors (pVax1-VEGF-FGF2-DsRed) the Fu-2A-peptide sequence was incorporated between the target genes. All vectors were constructed based on widely used and clinically approved plasmid pVax1. The primary structure of DNA was verified via routine sequencing (data not shown). The quality of both the purified plasmids, and the presence of target inserts, were confirmed by restriction analysis. The resulting fragments corresponded to the expected molecular size (Figure 1).

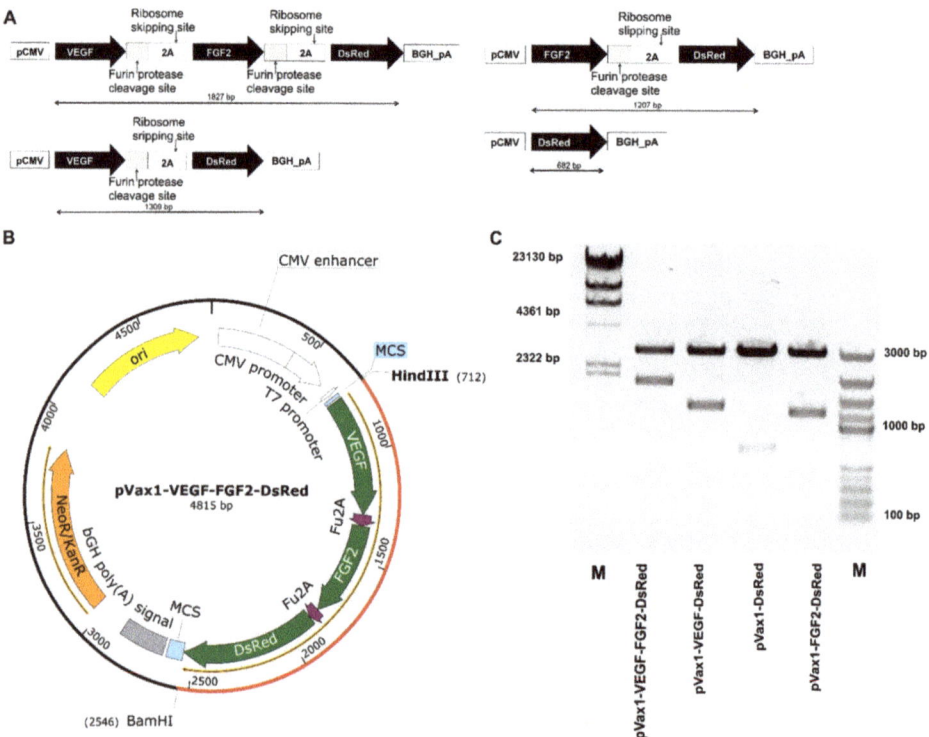

Figure 1. Design and characterization of plasmid vectors. (**A**) Schematic of the genetic cassettes, containing therapeutic genes (Vascular Endothelial Growth Factor (VEGF165), Basic Fibroblast Growth Factor (FGF2)) and reporter fluorescent protein (Red fluorescent protein (DsRed)). (**B**) Schematic diagrams of the expression vectors. (**C**) Analysis of enzymatic digestion. Agarose gel electrophoresis. M—marker/HindIII (SM0103) and GeneRuler DNA LadderMix (SM0331).

3.2. VEGF, FGF2 and DsRed Expression in Genetically Modified Cells In Vitro

To confirm the expression of target genes, HEK293T cells were transfected with recombinant plasmid constructs. We found that the expression plasmids increase the expression of mRNA VEGF- and FGF2-modified cells compared with the empty vector (pVax1-Dsred) and non-transfected cells. Fluorescent microscopy analysis revealed DsRed expression in all experimental groups. The immunofluorescent assay demonstrated a positive reaction for antibodies to VEGF and FGF2 in transfected cells (Figure 2A).

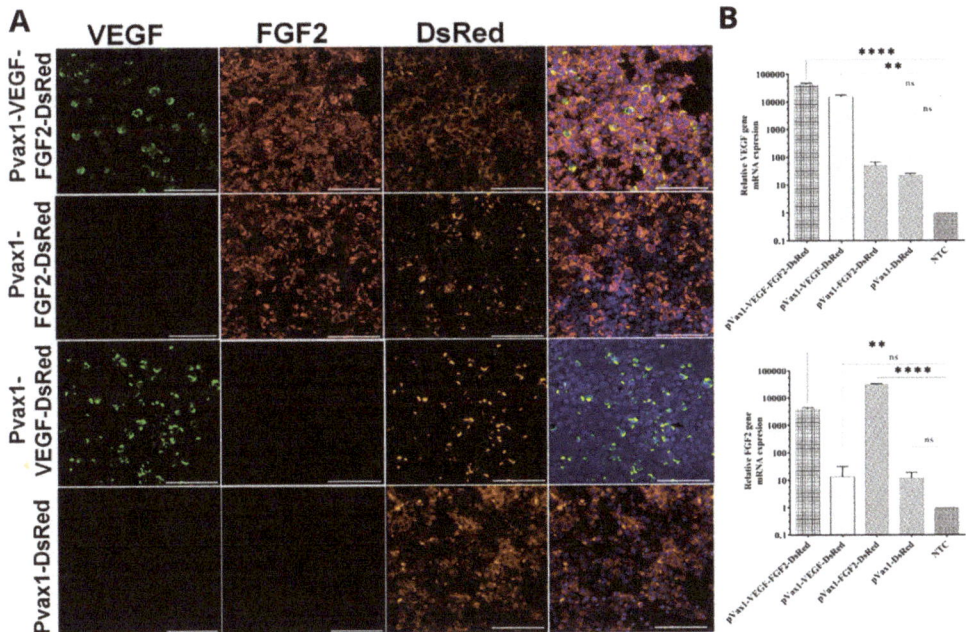

Figure 2. Expression of recombinant angiogenic factors in transfected HEK293T cells. (**A**) Immunofluorescent analysis of genetically modified HEK293T cells. Staining for VEGF (green) and FGF2 (red). Nuclei were counterstained using a DAPI solution (4′,6-diamidino-2-phenylindole) (blue). Scale bar 100 μm. (**B**) mRNA expression of target genes (VEGF, FGF2) in HEK293T cells transfected with plasmids pVax1-VEGF-FGF2-Dsred, pVax1-VEGF-Dsred, pVax1-FGF2-Dsred, pVax1-Dsred. mRNA from cells was assayed by RT–PCR and quantified relative to 18S rRNA mRNA levels. mRNA expression in non-transfected cells (NTC) was considered as control. Data presented as average ± s.e.; $p < 0.05$ * regarded as statistical significant differences ($n = 3$; ** $p < 0.01$; **** $p < 0.0001$ compared with control; ns—non-significant).

3.3. Production of VEGF and FGF2 by Genetically Modified Cells

The efficiency of VEGF and FGF2 secretion ex vivo was confirmed using indirect ELISA of cell lysates and supernatants collected from genetically modified cells. The ELISA results revealed statistically significant upregulation of VEGF secretion in both the supernatants and lysates of the cells modified with pVax1-VEGF-FGF2-DsRed (3629.68 ± 125.05 pg/mL). Increased VEGF production was also registered in supernatants of the cells transfected with pVax1-VEGF-DsRed (3530.00 ± 291.15 pg/mL) compared to non-transfected control (61.77 ± 3.03 pg/mL) (Figure 3A). Cells transfected with pVax1-VEGF-FGF2-DsRed (1396.00 ± 29.06 pg/mL) and pVax1-FGF2-DsRed (1728.00 ± 85.18 pg/mL) produced increased amounts of FGF2 compared to the cells modified with pVax1-VEGF-DsRed (16.73 ± 6.09 pg/mL) and in comparison to pVax1-DsRed and naïve cells as well (Figure 3B).

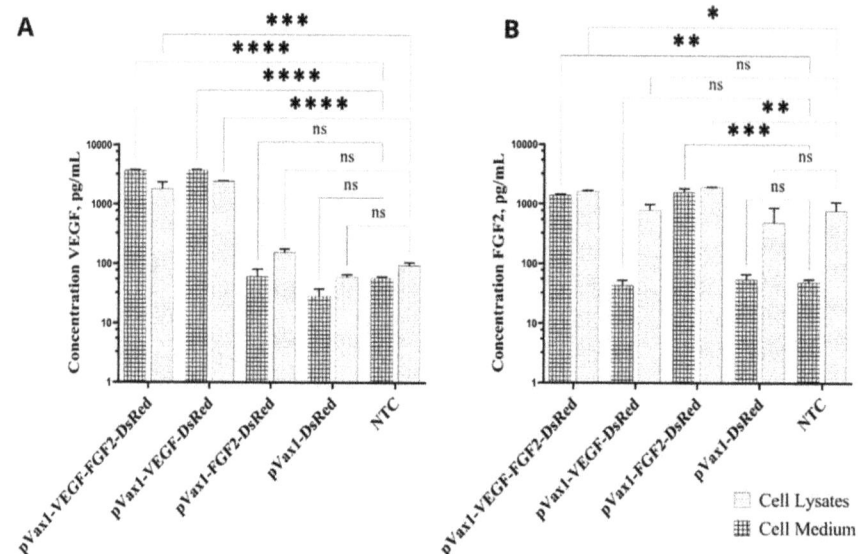

Figure 3. Analysis of VEGF and FGF2 concentrations in HEK293T cells transfected with obtained plasmid constructions. A total of 2.5×10^5 were seeded per well in a 12-well plate, and transfections were conducted after letting the cells adhere overnight. (**A**) VEGF concentration in supernatants and cell lysates of modified cells (pVax1-VEGF-FGF2-DsRed, pVax1-VEGF-DsRed, pVax1-FGF2-DsRed, pVax1-DsRed) and non-transfected controls (NTC); (**B**) FGF2 concentration in supernatants and cell lysates of modified cells (pVax1-VEGF-FGF2-DsRed, pVax1-VEGF-DsRed, pVax1-FGF2-DsRed, pVax1-DsRed) and non-transfected controls (NTC). Data presented as average ± s.e. of three independent repeats in independent samples, statistically significant differences * $p < 0.05$; ** $p < 0.01$; *** $p < 0.0001$, **** $p < 0.0001$; ns—non-significant.

3.4. Cytokine Profile Study of Genetically Modified Cells

The effect of the upregulated expression on cytokine pattern was investigated by multiplex analysis of cell lysates and supernatants collected from genetically modified cells. A total of 27 proteins were analyzed and the expression of 15 proteins was detected. Non-transfected cells were shown to express soluble receptor (IL-1ra), pro-inflammatory (IFN-γ, IL-6, IL-7, IL-12(p70),), anti-inflammatory cytokines (IL-8, IL-10), chemokines (IP-10, MCP-1, RANTES), and growth factors (G-CSF, FGF2, GM-CSF, PDGF-bb, VEGF). Secretion levels of several cytokines were insignificantly higher in modified cells. Notably, in cell lysates and supernatants from pVax1-VEGF-FGF2-DsRed group, upregulated IL-1ra, IL-7, IL-8, IL-12(p70), IL-6, IL-10, IFN-γ, IP-10, RANTES, MCP-1, and growth factors G-CSF, GM-CSF, PDGF-bb were observed at levels 3–7 times higher compared to NTC. However, it was statistically not significant ($p > 0.05$). Increased production of the aforementioned factors was also observed in cells transfected with pVax1-VEGF-DsRed. Slight augmentation of IL-6, IL-8, MCP-1, IFN-γ, and PDGF-bb were registered in cell lysates in the pVax1-FGF2-DsRed group ($p > 0.05$). An expected augmentation of VEGF and FGF2 ($p < 0.01$) was scored in pVax1-VEGF-DsRed, pVax1-FGF2-DsRed, and pVax1-VEGF-FGF2-DsRed transfected cells (Figure 4) that coincided with the above-mentioned ELISA data (Figure 3).

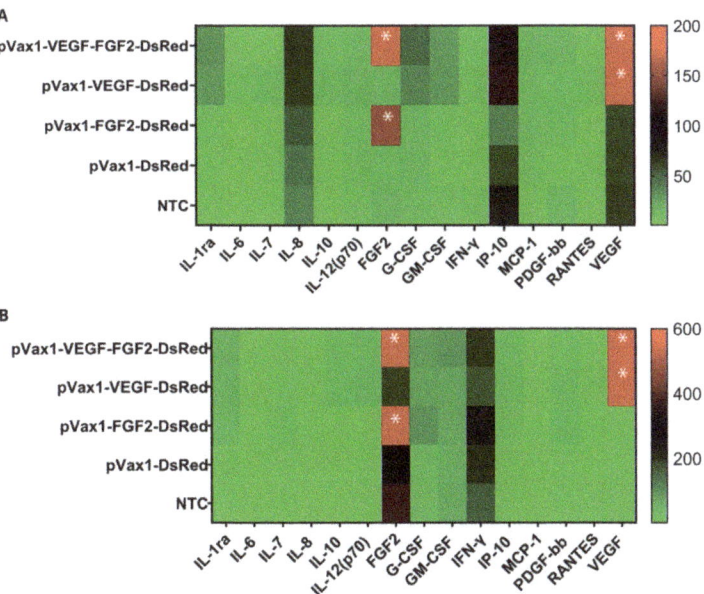

Figure 4. Protein array analysis of cytokine, chemokine, and growth factor in genetically modified HEK293T cells (pg/mL). (**A**) Concentration of soluble molecules, secreted by transfected HEK293T cells. (**B**) Concentrations produced from factors in lysates from transfected HEK293T cells. Analytes was measured 48 h after cell transfection. Data presented as average (n = 4), asterisks (*) indicate statistical significance compared with the control, as determined by one-way analysis of variance (ANOVA) followed by a post-hoc Tukey test (** $p < 0.01$).

3.5. Effect of Increased VEGF and FGF2 Expression on Capillary-Like Structures Formation by HUVEC In Vitro

To evaluate the proangiogenic potency of plasmid constructs and the synergetic effect of secreted VEGF and FGF2, HUVEC cells were cultured on a three-dimensional Matrigel matrix supplemented with conditioned media from transfected cells (Figure 5). Conditioned media collected from cells transfected with pVax1-VEGF-FGF2-DsRed provoked the most significant stimulation on tube formation by HUVEC compared with cells supplemented with media obtained from pVax1-VEGF-DsRed, pVax1-FGF2-DsRed, pVax1-DsRed, and control HEK293T cells. Meanwhile, in the control groups (pVax1-DsRed and NTC), a few cellular structures that were not connected were observed. In contrast, other groups demonstrated a higher level of organization of capillary-like structures (tubule area and total length) and a higher level of tubular organization (number of loops and bifurcations). In the pVax1-VEGF-DsRed group the total length of formed tubes was less (166640.30 ± 1297.53px) compared to pVax1-VEGF-FGF2-DsRed (21409.00 ± 2183.81px). However, in the pVax1-FGF2-DsRed group (20150.30 ± 1289.05px), the total length of the formed tubes was not significantly different from the pVax1-VEGF-FGF2-DsRed group21409.00 ± 2183.81px) (Figure 5B). Similar results were obtained concerning the number of branch points discovered; in the pVax1-VEGF-FGF2-DsRed (190 ± 28.86), pVax1-VEGF-DsRed (139.00 ± 15.30), and pVax1-FGF2-DsRed (187.66 ± 16.259), the numbers were higher in comparison to the control groups pVax1-DsRed (86.66 ±15.45) and NTC (70.00 ± 3.7) (Figure 5C). Thus, augmented expression of VEGF and FGF2 contributed to the formation of a denser network of capillary structures compared to other groups, resulting in increased amount of loops forms, with pVax1-VEGF-FGF2-DsRed (71.5 ± 11.61), pVax1-VEGF-DsRed (44.25 ± 6.00), and pVax1-FGF2-DsRed (69.66 ± 11002) showing higher numbers than control groups pVax1-DsRed (20.33 ± 7.12) and NTC (11.33 ± 2.18)

(Figure 5D). In the pVax1-VEGF-FGF2-DsRed and pVax1-FGF2-DsRed groups, the percentage of cell coverage increased by 10% compared to control groups pVax1-DsRed and NTC. This up-regulation was statistically significant and correlated with other indexes, including the differential number of loops, branch points, and total tube length (Figure 5E).

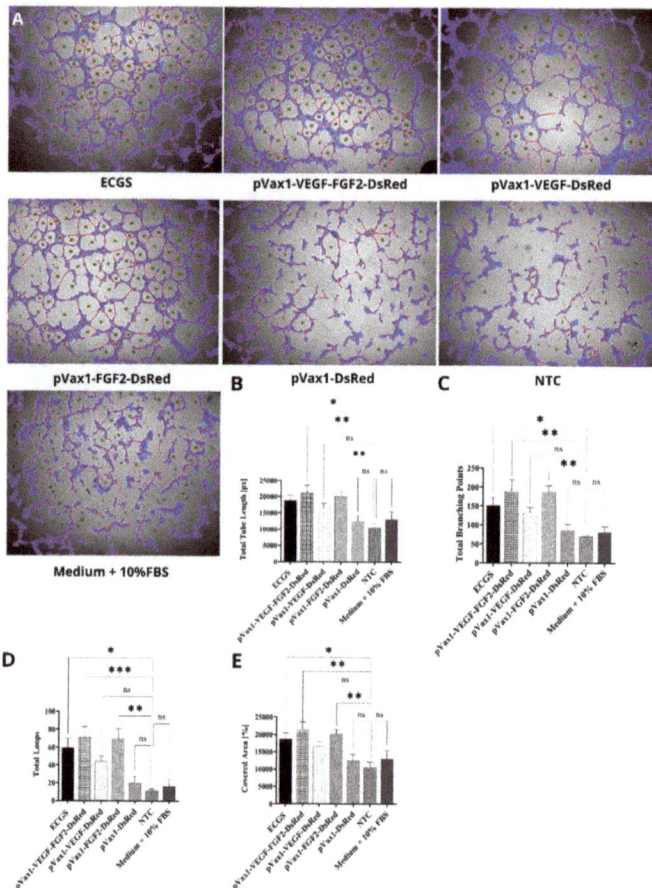

Figure 5. Analysis of tube formation by human umbilical vein endothelial cells (HUVEC). A total of 1×10^4 HUVEC were seeded per well in a 96-well plate. HUVECs were cultivated with conditioned media collected from HEK293T cells transfected with pVax1-VEGF-FGF2-DsRed, pVax1-VEGF-DsRed, pVax1-FGF2-DsRed, pVax1-DsRed, and non-transfected control as well (NTC). ECGS—complete medium containing 10% FBS and Endothelial Cell Growth Supplement (30 µg/mL). Medium+ 10 FBS –medium containing 10% FBS without ECGS. (**A**) Brightfield microscopy image, scale bar 200 µm. (**B**) Length of formed tubes (measured in px), (**C**) Number of branch points formed, (**D**) Number of loops, (**E**) Area of cell coverage. Analysis was carried using Wimasis imaging software package. Data presented as average ± s.e. * indicates statistically significant data relative to control (n = 3; ** $p < 0.01$; *** $p < 0.0001$ ns—non-significant).

4. Discussion

We designed and tested multigene vectors encoding the FGF2, VEGF, and DsRed genes, or combinations of these, combined through the picornoviral 2A-peptide sequences. Our data demonstrated that the expression of mRNA and FGF2 and VEGF proteins in vitro was higher than that observed in the control groups (cells modified with the DsRed plasmid and non-modified cells).

The selection of an appropriate vector system is believed to be one of the essential aspects of developing gene therapy drugs. The vector pVax1 is a non-immunogenic optimized expression system. The content of eukaryotic DNA sequences is critically reduced, thus minimizing the vector's chromosomal integration into the host cell genome. Besides this, pVax1 has been approved by the American Food and Drug Administration (FDA) and is currently used widely to develop DNA vaccines [64]. Considering the world's current situation due to the global spread of severe acute respiratory syndrome 2 (SARS-CoV-2), DNA vaccine development remains an urgent issue [65]. In particular, multicistronic recombinant constructs could be used for the simultaneous equimolar expression of several immunogenic proteins of differing pathogens.

Gene co-expression systems make it feasible to increase the induction efficiency of therapeutic angiogenesis due to the simultaneous delivery of several proangiogenic factors. Application of 2A-peptides may become a strategy employed to achieve stable gene co-expression [66]. This approach is attractive in the expression systems' design when encoding combinations of therapeutic molecules in the same transcriptional unit and provides a large packaging capacity [67]. In addition, it has been tested in a wide range of eukaryotic cells [68,69]. High transgene expression has been confirmed, as has good cleavage of synthesized recombinant proteins [50,68], and the absence of immune responses to system components has also been verified [68]. The application of multicistronic expression systems will therefore simplify the development procedures needed for polygenic constructs to achieve the simultaneous delivery of several therapeutic genes to a particular cell [70,71]. In the current study, HEK293T cells were used as a model system to characterize recombinant plasmids and evaluate the effect of over-expression of VEGF and/or FGF2 on the secretion profile of genetically modified cells. The possibility of successful modulation of the secretion profile of HEK293 by the action of various external factors has been demonstrated previously. In particular, co-cultivation of HEK293 with mesenchymal stem cells that expressed lipocalin 2 resulted in an increased expression of growth factors HGF, IGF-1, and FGF2 by HEK293 cells [72]. Confirmed changes in the secretion of HEK293 IL-2, IL-4, IL-6, IL-8, IL-10, GM-CSF, IFN-γ, TNF-α due to the influence of bovine serum albumin have also been published [73].

In our study, multiplex analysis of soluble factors in the supernatants and cell lysates of HEK293T revealed augmentation of several cytokines, chemokines, and growth factors in transfected cells. However, the differences found, except for VEGF and FGF2, were not statistically significant. Therefore, we suggest that for a deeper understanding of the functioning and effects of VEGF and FGF2 overexpression on the state of modified cells, it is necessary to expand the range of analytes investigated, as well as to select cells that have a pronounced autocrine and paracrine potential relating to the production of the recombinant factors used. In our opinion, mesenchymal stem cells from various origins could serve as appropriate candidates. In particular, we have previously demonstrated that genetic modification and overexpression of proangiogenic factors by cells can modulate the secretory profile of stem cells from human adipose tissue [74]. Shanshan Jin et al., previously reported that overexpression of FGF2 by human gingival mesenchymal stem cells enhanced their secretion of VEGF and TNF-β [75]. Similar results were obtained by Yukita et al., where recombinant FGF2 increased the expression of glial neurotrophic growth factor (GDNF) by dental follicle cells [76]. We assume that such adaptations of the secretome to overexpress angiogenic factors might further increase the transplanted cells' therapeutic potential. The current assay has shown a high correlation between the various techniques used to verify the created structures' functionality. Using an in vitro model of angiogenesis, we have shown that the conditioned medium collected from genetically modified cells caused a stimulating effect on capillary formation by endothelial cells. The presented data are consistent with our earlier obtained results studying two-cassette plasmid vectors providing independent expression of two growth factors [43]. The results indicate that, in the studied model, FGF2 more effectively affects the formation of capillary-like structures by human endothelial cells as compared to VEGF. The slight effect of secreted VEGF on the formation of vascular-like structures in the present study is likely to be due to the short exposure period. When using recombinant VEGF or VEGF expressing plasmid constructs, several studies have demonstrated that significant induction of angiogenesis is only observed 20–30 days after therapeutic exposure [77,78]. At the same time, significant differences were not observed between the pVax1-VEGF-FGF2-DsRed and pVax1-FGF2 groups in the present study. We assume that the critical contribution to the formation of vascular-like structures in vitro is mediated by FGF2 expression. These results are consistent with previous reports showing that FGF2 induced the highest blood vessels density in a mouse cornea model [79]. Cartland et al. have previously indicated that FGF2 is more effective at stimulating angiogenesis in vitro and in vivo than VEGF and TRAIL [80]. This phenomenon may be because VEGF and FGF2 act on a wide range of receptors and, accordingly, activate various signaling cascades and stages of angiogenesis [79–81].

It is worth emphasizing that pro-angiogenic factors are active even in picomolar concentrations and, as a consequence, a slight local increase in their concentration is sufficient to achieve a therapeutic effect. Moreover, in different living species, presumably, since trophic factors are evolutionarily conserved molecules, the same factors can activate similar biological effects. In this regard, it is therefore no coincidence that human molecules, such as growth factors, might be active in various model organisms. Moreover, codon optimization is expected to preserve the biological potential of the synthesized molecules [82]. Simultaneously, alternative data are accumulating, and indicating the negative effect of codon optimization on the translation and structure of the synthesized protein [83], which introduces one more variable that must be taken into account when creating effective, optimized gene therapy systems. Our results show that recombinant constructs expressing different genes are putatively implementing discrete patterns of angiogenesis. Their efficacy for therapeutic use in the induction of angiogenesis should be tested using in vivo models.

5. Conclusions

Our work has constructed and tested, in vitro, a multicistronic system that ensures simultaneous efficient delivery of several therapeutic growth factor genes into cells. Data on the functionality of the synthesized recombinant proteins as the part of the multicistronic construct have also been obtained. We have demonstrated that the proangiogenic factors synthesized in the secretome of genetically modified cells exhibit stimulating effects on the formation of capillary-like structures by HUVEC in vitro. This approach can be used to develop and test gene therapy protocols for various human diseases that require the simultaneous expression of several transgenes to stimulate therapeutic angiogenesis and other regenerative processes.

Author Contributions: Conceptualization, I.I.S., V.V.S. and A.A.R.; methodology, A.P.K. and A.A.R.; investigation, D.Z.G., E.E.G., G.E.S., A.F.M., M.N.Z.; validation, I.I.S. and D.Z.G.; writing—original draft preparation, D.Z.G. and I.I.S.; writing—review and editing, I.I.S. and C.S.R.; supervision, A.A.R. and A.P.K.; funding acquisition, A.A.R. and I.I.S. All authors have read and agreed to the published version of the manuscript.

Funding: This research was partially supported by the Russian Foundation for Basic Research grant No 18-44-160029 and by a subsidy allocated to Kazan Federal University for the state assignment in the sphere of scientific activities (project 0671-2020-0058).

Institutional Review Board Statement: Not applicable.

Informed Consent Statement: Not applicable.

Data Availability Statement: The data presented in this study are available on request from the corresponding author. The data are not publicly available due to privacy.

Acknowledgments: This work is part of Kazan Federal University Strategic Academic Leadership Program.

Conflicts of Interest: The authors declare no conflict of interest.

References

1. The Top 10 Causes of Death. 2020. Available online: www.who.int/news-room/fact-sheets/detail/the-top-10-causes-of-death (accessed on 23 April 2021).
2. Gianni-Barrera, R.; Di Maggio, N.; Melly, L.; Burger, M.G.; Mujagic, E.; Gürke, L.; Schaefer, D.J.; Banfi, A. Therapeutic vascularization in regenerative medicine. *Stem Cells Transl. Med.* **2020**, *9*, 433–444. [CrossRef] [PubMed]
3. Bian, X.; Ma, K.; Zhang, C.; Fu, X. Therapeutic angiogenesis using stem cell-derived extracellular vesicles: An emerging approach for treatment of ischemic diseases. *Stem Cell Res. Ther.* **2019**, *10*, 158. [CrossRef] [PubMed]
4. Makarevich, P.I.; Parfyonova, Y.V. Therapeutic Angiogenesis: Foundations and Practical Application. In *Physiologic and Pathologic Angiogenesis: Signaling Mechanisms and Targeted Therapy*; Simionescu, D., Simionescu, A., Eds.; InTech: Rijeka, Croatia, 2017; ISBN 978-953-51-3023-9.
5. Ferrara, N.; Carver-Moore, K.; Chen, H.; Dowd, M.; Lu, L.; O'Shea, K.S.; Powell-Braxton, L.; Hillan, K.J.; Moore, M.W. Heterozygous embryonic lethality induced by targeted inactivation of the VEGF gene. *Nat. Cell Biol.* **1996**, *380*, 439–442. [CrossRef] [PubMed]
6. Giacca, M.; Zacchigna, S. VEGF gene therapy: Therapeutic angiogenesis in the clinic and beyond. *Gene Ther.* **2012**, *19*, 622–629. [CrossRef]
7. Uccelli, A.; Wolff, T.; Valente, P.; Di Maggio, N.; Pellegrino, M.; Gürke, L.; Banfi, A.; Gianni-Barrera, R. Vascular endothelial growth factor biology for regenerative angiogenesis. *Swiss Med. Wkly.* **2019**, *149*, 20011. [CrossRef]
8. Sanada, F.; Taniyama, Y.; Muratsu, J.; Otsu, R.; Shimizu, H.; Rakugi, H.; Morishita, R. Gene-Therapeutic Strategies Targeting Angiogenesis in Peripheral Artery Disease. *Medicines* **2018**, *5*, 31. [CrossRef]
9. Kim, J.; Mirando, A.C.; Popel, A.; Green, J.J. Gene delivery nanoparticles to modulate angiogenesis. *Adv. Drug Deliv. Rev.* **2017**, *119*, 20–43. [CrossRef]
10. Jazwa, A.; Florczyk, U.; Grochot-Przeczek, A.; Krist, B.; Loboda, A.; Jozkowicz, A.; Dulak, J. Limb ischemia and vessel regeneration: Is there a role for VEGF? *Vasc. Pharmacol.* **2016**, *86*, 18–30. [CrossRef]
11. Gerber, H.-P.; McMurtrey, A.; Kowalski, J.; Yan, M.; Keyt, B.A.; Dixit, V.; Ferrara, N. Vascular Endothelial Growth Factor Regulates Endothelial Cell Survival through the Phosphatidylinositol 3′-Kinase/Akt Signal Transduction Pathway. *J. Biol. Chem.* **1998**, *273*, 30336–30343. [CrossRef]
12. Wu, J.-B.; Tang, Y.-L.; Liang, X.-H. Targeting VEGF pathway to normalize the vasculature: An emerging insight in cancer therapy. *OncoTargets Ther.* **2018**, *11*, 6901–6909. [CrossRef]
13. Gerber, H.-P.; Dixit, V.; Ferrara, N. Vascular Endothelial Growth Factor Induces Expression of the Antiapoptotic Proteins Bcl-2 and A1 in Vascular Endothelial Cells. *J. Biol. Chem.* **1998**, *273*, 13313–13316. [CrossRef]
14. Carmeliet, P.; Ferreira, V.; Breier, G.; Pollefeyt, S.; Kieckens, L.; Gertsenstein, M.; Fahrig, M.; Vandenhoeck, A.; Harpal, K.; Eberhardt, C.; et al. Abnormal blood vessel development and lethality in embryos lacking a single VEGF allele. *Nat. Cell Biol.* **1996**, *380*, 435–439. [CrossRef]
15. Riccardi, E.; Napolitano, E.; Platella, C.; Musumeci, D.; Melone, M.A.B.; Montesarchio, D. Anti-VEGF DNA-based aptamers in cancer therapeutics and diagnostics. *Med. Res. Rev.* **2021**, *41*, 464–506. [CrossRef]
16. Gan, L.-M.; Lagerström-Fermér, M.; Carlsson, L.G.; Arfvidsson, C.; Egnell, A.-C.; Rudvik, A.; Kjaer, M.; Collén, A.; Thompson, J.D.; Joyal, J.; et al. Intradermal delivery of modified mRNA encoding VEGF-A in patients with type 2 diabetes. *Nat. Commun.* **2019**, *10*, 871. [CrossRef]
17. Demidova, O.A.; Bokeria, L.A.; Bokeria, O.L.; Arakelyan, V.S.; Deev, R.V. Neovasculgen" in the treatment of patients with chronic ischemia of the lower limbs, clinical study. Byulleten' NTSSSKH im. A.N. Bakuleva RAMN. *Serdechno Sosud. Zabol.* **2017**, *18*, 210.
18. Shvalb, P.; Gavrilenko, A.; Kalinin, R.; Chervyakov, Y.; Voronov, D.; Staroverov, I.; Gryaznov, S.; Mzhavanadze, N.; Nersesyan, E.; Kiselev, S.; et al. Efficacy and safety of application Neovasculgen in the complex treatment patients with chronic lower limb ischemia (IIb-III phase of clinical trials). *Cell. Transplant. Tissue Eng.* **2011**, *6*, 76–83.
19. Kattoor, A.J.; Mathur, P.; Mehta, J.L. Trials of Angiogenesis Therapy in Patients with Ischemic Heart Disease. In *Biochemical Basis and Therapeutic Implications of Angiogenesis*; Springer Science and Business Media LLC: Berlin/Heidelberg, Germany, 2017; pp. 393–421.
20. Ribatti, D.; Presta, M. The role of fibroblast growth factor-2 in the vascularization of the chick embryo chorioallantoic membrane. *J. Cell. Mol. Med.* **2002**, *6*, 439–446. [CrossRef]
21. Trafermin—Kaken Pharmaceutical. 2001. Available online: https://adisinsight.springer.com/drugs/800009962 (accessed on 23 April 2021).
22. Nie, K.; Li, P.; Zeng, X.; Sun, G.; Jin, W.; Wei, Z.; Wang, B.; Qi, J.; Wang, Y.; Wang, D. Clinical observation of basic fibroblast growth factor combined with topical oxygen therapy in enhancing burn wound healing. *Chin. J. Rep. Rec. Surg.* **2010**, *24*, 643–646. (In Chinese)
23. Walicke, P.A. Basic and acidic fibroblast growth factors have trophic effects on neurons from multiple CNS regions. *J. Neurosci.* **1988**, *8*, 2618–2627. [CrossRef]

24. Del Corral, R.D.; Morales, A.V. The Multiple Roles of FGF Signaling in the Developing Spinal Cord. *Front. Cell Dev. Biol.* **2017**, *5*, 58. [CrossRef]
25. Bikfalvi, A.; Klein, S.; Pintucci, G.; Rifkin, D.B. Biological Roles of Fibroblast Growth Factor-2. *Endocr. Rev.* **1997**, *18*, 26–45. [CrossRef] [PubMed]
26. Kano, M.R.; Morishita, Y.; Iwata, C.; Iwasaka, S.; Watabe, T.; Ouchi, Y.; Miyazono, K.; Miyazawa, K. VEGF-A and FGF-2 synergistically promote neoangiogenesis through enhancement of endogenous PDGF-B–PDGFRβ signaling. *J. Cell Sci.* **2005**, *118*, 3759–3768. [CrossRef] [PubMed]
27. Lee, J.-S.; Kim, J.-M.; Kim, K.L.; Jang, H.-S.; Shin, I.-S.; Jeon, E.-S.; Suh, W.; Byun, J.; Kim, D.-K. Combined administration of naked DNA vectors encoding VEGF and bFGF enhances tissue perfusion and arteriogenesis in ischemic hindlimb. *Biochem. Biophys. Res. Commun.* **2007**, *360*, 752–758. [CrossRef] [PubMed]
28. Spanholtz, T.A.; Theodorou, P.; Holzbach, T.; Wutzler, S.; Giunta, R.E.; Machens, H.-G. Vascular Endothelial Growth Factor (VEGF165) Plus Basic Fibroblast Growth Factor (bFGF) Producing Cells induce a Mature and Stable Vascular Network—a Future Therapy for Ischemically Challenged Tissue. *J. Surg. Res.* **2011**, *171*, 329–338. [CrossRef]
29. Tille, J.C.; Wood, J.; Mandriota, S.J.; Schnell, C.; Ferrari, S.; Mestan, J.; Zhu, Z.; Witte, L.; Pepper, M.S. Vascular endothelial growth factor (VEGF) receptor-2 antagonists inhibit VEGF- and basic fibroblast growth factor-induced angiogenesis in vivo and in vitro. *J. Pharmacol. Exp. Ther.* **2001**, *299*, 1073–1085.
30. Bouïs, D.; Kusumanto, Y.; Meijer, C.; Mulder, N.H.; Hospers, G.A. A review on pro- and anti-angiogenic factors as targets of clinical intervention. *Pharmacol. Res.* **2006**, *53*, 89–103. [CrossRef]
31. Fujita, M.; Ishihara, M.; Simizu, M.; Obara, K.; Ishizuka, T.; Saito, Y.; Yura, H.; Morimoto, Y.; Takase, B.; Matsui, T.; et al. Vascularization in vivo caused by the controlled release of fibroblast growth factor-2 from an injectable chitosan/non-anticoagulant heparin hydrogel. *Biomaterials* **2004**, *25*, 699–706. [CrossRef]
32. Cross, M.J.; Claesson-Welsh, L. FGF and VEGF function in angiogenesis: Signalling pathways, biological responses and therapeutic inhibition. *Trends Pharmacol. Sci.* **2001**, *22*, 201–207. [CrossRef]
33. Carano, R.A.; Filvaroff, E.H. Angiogenesis and bone repair. *Drug Discov. Today* **2003**, *8*, 980–989. [CrossRef]
34. Boilly, B.; Vercoutter-Edouart, A.-S.; Hondermarck, H.; Nurcombe, V.; Le Bourhis, X. FGF signals for cell proliferation and migration through different pathways. *Cytokine Growth Factor Rev.* **2000**, *11*, 295–302. [CrossRef]
35. Martino, M.M.; Ebrkic, S.; Ebovo, E.; Eburger, M.; Schaefer, D.J.; Ewolff, T.; Gärke, L.; Briquez, P.S.; Larsson, H.M.; Barrera, R.E.; et al. Extracellular Matrix and Growth Factor Engineering for Controlled Angiogenesis in Regenerative Medicine. *Front. Bioeng. Biotechnol.* **2015**, *3*, 45. [CrossRef]
36. Springer, M.L.; Chen, A.S.; Kraft, P.E.; Bednarski, M.; Blau, H.M. VEGF Gene Delivery to Muscle. *Mol. Cell* **1998**, *2*, 549–558. [CrossRef]
37. Lukashev, A.N.; Zamyatnin, A.A. Viral vectors for gene therapy: Current state and clinical perspectives. *Biochemistry* **2016**, *81*, 700–708. [CrossRef]
38. Merten, O.-W.; Gaillet, B. Viral vectors for gene therapy and gene modification approaches. *Biochem. Eng. J.* **2016**, *108*, 98–115. [CrossRef]
39. Hardee, C.L.; Arévalo-Soliz, L.M.; Hornstein, B.D.; Zechiedrich, L. Advances in non-viral DNA vectors for gene therapy. *Genes* **2017**, *8*, 65. [CrossRef]
40. Giacca, M.; Zacchigna, S. Virus-mediated gene delivery for human gene therapy. *J. Control. Release* **2012**, *161*, 377–388. [CrossRef]
41. Lundstrom, K. Gene Therapy Today and Tomorrow. *Diseases* **2019**, *7*, 37. [CrossRef]
42. Shaimardanova, A.A.; Chulpanova, D.S.; Kitaeva, K.V.; Abdrakhmanova, I.I.; Chernov, V.M.; Rutland, C.S.; Rizvanov, A.A.; Solovyeva, V.V. Production and Application of Multicistronic Constructs for Various Human Disease Therapies. *Pharmaceutics* **2019**, *11*, 580. [CrossRef]
43. Solovyeva, V.V.; Chulpanova, D.S.; Tazetdinova, L.G.; Salafutdinov, I.I.; Bozo, I.Y.; Isaev, A.; Deev, R.V.; Rizvanov, A.A. In Vitro Angiogenic Properties of Plasmid DNA Encoding SDF-1α and VEGF165 Genes. *Appl. Biochem. Biotechnol.* **2019**, *190*, 773–788. [CrossRef]
44. Salafutdinov, I.I.; Gazizov, I.M.; Gatina, D.K.; Mullin, R.I.; Bogov, A.A.; Islamov, R.R.; Kiassov, A.P.; Masgutov, R.F.; Rizvanov, A.A. Influence of Recombinant Codon-Optimized Plasmid DNA Encoding VEGF and FGF2 on Co-Induction of Angiogenesis. *Cells* **2021**, *10*, 432. [CrossRef]
45. Yu, X.; Zhan, X.; D'Costa, J.; Tanavde, V.M.; Ye, Z.; Peng, T.; Malehorn, M.T.; Yang, X.; Civin, C.I.; Cheng, L. Lentiviral vectors with two independent internal promoters transfer high-level expression of multiple transgenes to human hematopoietic stem-progenitor cells. *Mol. Ther.* **2003**, *7*, 827–838. [CrossRef]
46. Berger, A.; Maire, S.; Gaillard, M.-C.; Sahel, J.-A.; Hantraye, P.; Bemelmans, A.-P. mRNAtrans-splicing in gene therapy for genetic diseases. *Wiley Interdiscip. Rev. RNA* **2016**, *7*, 487–498. [CrossRef] [PubMed]
47. Li, M.; Wang, Y.; Liu, M.; Lan, X. Multimodality reporter gene imaging: Construction strategies and application. *Theranostics* **2018**, *8*, 2954–2973. [CrossRef] [PubMed]
48. Lee, S.; Kim, J.-A.; Kim, H.-D.; Chung, S.; Kim, K.; Choe, H.K. Real-Time Temporal Dynamics of Bicistronic Expression Mediated by Internal Ribosome Entry Site and 2A Cleaving Sequence. *Mol. Cells* **2019**, *42*, 418–425. [CrossRef]

49. Hadpech, S.; Jinathep, W.; Saoin, S.; Thongkum, W.; Chupradit, K.; Yasamut, U.; Moonmuang, S.; Tayapiwatana, C. Impairment of a membrane-targeting protein translated from a downstream gene of a "self-cleaving" T2A peptide conjunction. *Protein Expr. Purif.* **2018**, *150*, 17–25. [CrossRef]
50. Al-Allaf, F.A.; Abduljaleel, Z.; Athar, M.; Taher, M.M.; Khan, W.; Mehmet, H.; Colakogullari, M.; Apostolidou, S.; Bigger, B.; Waddington, S.; et al. Modifying inter-cistronic sequence significantly enhances IRES dependent second gene expression in bicistronic vector: Construction of optimised cassette for gene therapy of familial hypercholesterolemia. *Non Coding RNA Res.* **2019**, *4*, 1–14. [CrossRef]
51. Kim, J.H.; Lee, S.-R.; Li, L.-H.; Park, H.-J.; Park, J.-H.; Lee, K.Y.; Kim, M.-K.; Shin, B.A.; Choi, S.-Y. High Cleavage Efficiency of a 2A Peptide Derived from Porcine Teschovirus-1 in Human Cell Lines, Zebrafish and Mice. *PLoS ONE* **2011**, *6*, e18556. [CrossRef]
52. Lee, K.; Kim, S.Y.; Seo, Y.; Kwon, H.; Kwon, Y.J.; Lee, H. Multicistronic IVT mRNA for simultaneous expression of multiple fluorescent proteins. *J. Ind. Eng. Chem.* **2019**, *80*, 770–777. [CrossRef]
53. Mizuguchi, H.; Xu, Z.; Ishii-Watabe, A.; Uchida, E.; Hayakawa, T. IRES-Dependent Second Gene Expression Is Significantly Lower Than Cap-Dependent First Gene Expression in a Bicistronic Vector. *Mol. Ther.* **2000**, *1*, 376–382. [CrossRef]
54. Minskaia, E.; Nicholson, J.; Ryan, M.D. Optimisation of the foot-and-mouth disease virus 2A co-expression system for biomedical applications. *BMC Biotechnol.* **2013**, *13*, 67. [CrossRef]
55. Doronina, V.A.; Wu, C.; De Felipe, P.; Sachs, M.; Ryan, M.D.; Brown, J.D. Site-Specific Release of Nascent Chains from Ribosomes at a Sense Codon. *Mol. Cell. Biol.* **2008**, *28*, 4227–4239. [CrossRef]
56. Donnelly, M.L.L.; Luke, G.; Mehrotra, A.; Li, X.; Hughes, L.E.; Gani, D.; Ryan, M.D. Analysis of the aphthovirus 2A/2B polyprotein 'cleavage' mechanism indicates not a proteolytic reaction, but a novel translational effect: A putative ribosomal skip. *J. Gen. Virol.* **2001**, *82*, 1013–1025. [CrossRef]
57. De Felipe, P.; Luke, G.A.; Hughes, L.E.; Gani, D.; Halpin, C.; Ryan, M.D. E unum pluribus: Multiple proteins from a self-processing polyprotein. *Trends Biotechnol.* **2006**, *24*, 68–75. [CrossRef]
58. Szymczak, A.L.; Workman, C.J.; Wang, Y.; Vignali, K.M.; Dilioglou, S.; Vanin, E.F.; Vignali, D.A.A. Correction of multi-gene deficiency in vivo using a single 'self-cleaving' 2A peptide–based retroviral vector. *Nat. Biotechnol.* **2004**, *22*, 589–594. [CrossRef]
59. Thomas, G. Furin at the cutting edge: From protein traffic to embryogenesis and disease. *Nat. Rev. Mol. Cell Biol.* **2002**, *3*, 753–766. [CrossRef]
60. Rothwell, D.G.; Crossley, R.; Bridgeman, J.S.; Sheard, V.; Zhang, Y.; Sharp, T.V.; Hawkins, R.E.; Gilham, D.E.; McKay, T.R. Functional Expression of Secreted Proteins from a Bicistronic Retroviral Cassette Based on Foot-and-Mouth Disease Virus 2A Can Be Position Dependent. *Hum. Gene Ther.* **2010**, *21*, 1631–1637. [CrossRef]
61. Fisicaro, N.; Londrigan, S.L.; Brady, J.L.; Salvaris, E.; Nottle, M.B.; O'Connell, P.J.; Robson, S.C.; D'Apice, A.J.F.; Lew, A.M.; Cowan, P.J. Versatile co-expression of graft-protective proteins using 2A-linked cassettes. *Xenotransplantation* **2011**, *18*, 121–130. [CrossRef]
62. Yang, Y.-P.; Li, Y.-H.; Zhang, A.-H.; Bi, L.; Fan, M.-W. Good Manufacturing Practices production and analysis of a DNA vaccine against dental caries. *Acta Pharmacol. Sin.* **2009**, *30*, 1513–1521. [CrossRef]
63. Garanina, E.E.; Mukhamedshina, Y.O.; Salafutdinov, I.I.; Kiyasov, A.P.; Lima, L.M.; Reis, H.J.; Palotás, A.; Islamov, R.R.; Rizvanov, A.A. Construction of recombinant adenovirus containing picorna-viral 2A-peptide sequence for the co-expression of neuro-protective growth factors in human umbilical cord blood cells. *Spinal Cord* **2015**, *54*, 423–430. [CrossRef]
64. Xu, Y.; Zhang, N.-Z.; Tan, Q.-D.; Chen, J.; Lu, J.; Xu, Q.-M.; Zhu, X.-Q. Evaluation of immuno-efficacy of a novel DNA vaccine encoding Toxoplasma gondiirhoptry protein 38 (TgROP38) against chronic toxoplasmosis in a murine model. *BMC Infect. Dis.* **2014**, *14*, 525. [CrossRef]
65. Smith, T.R.F.; Patel, A.; Ramos, S.; Elwood, D.; Zhu, X.; Yan, J.; Gary, E.N.; Walker, S.N.; Schultheis, K.; Purwar, M.; et al. Immunogenicity of a DNA vaccine candidate for COVID. *Nat. Commun.* **2020**, *11*, 2601. [CrossRef] [PubMed]
66. Liu, Z.; Chen, O.; Wall, J.B.J.; Zheng, M.; Zhou, Y.; Wang, L.; Vaseghi, H.R.; Qian, L.; Liu, J. Systematic comparison of 2A peptides for cloning multi-genes in a polycistronic vector. *Sci. Rep.* **2017**, *7*, 2193. [CrossRef] [PubMed]
67. Luke, G.A.; Ryan, M.D. Therapeutic applications of the 'NPGP' family of viral 2As. *Rev. Med. Virol.* **2018**, *28*, e2001. [CrossRef] [PubMed]
68. Daniels, R.W.; Rossano, A.; MacLeod, G.T.; Ganetzky, B. Expression of Multiple Transgenes from a Single Construct Using Viral 2A Peptides in Drosophila. *PLoS ONE* **2014**, *9*, e100637. [CrossRef]
69. Wang, Y.; Wang, F.; Xu, S.; Wang, R.; Chen, W.; Hou, K.; Tian, C.; Wang, F.; Zhao, P.; Xia, Q. Optimization of a 2A self-cleaving peptide-based multigene expression system for efficient expression of upstream and downstream genes in silkworm. *Mol. Genet. Genom.* **2019**, *294*, 849–859. [CrossRef]
70. Geisse, S.; Fux, C. Chapter 15 Recombinant Protein Production by Transient Gene Transfer into Mammalian Cells. In *Methods in Enzymology*; Elsevier BV: Amsterdam, The Netherlands, 2009; Volume 463, pp. 223–238.
71. Vink, T.; Oudshoorn-Dickmann, M.; Roza, M.; Reitsma, J.-J.; de Jong, R.N. A simple, robust and highly efficient transient expression system for producing antibodies. *Methods* **2014**, *65*, 5–10. [CrossRef]
72. Halabian, R.; Roudkenar, M.H.; Jahanian-Najafabadi, A.; Hosseini, K.M.; Tehrani, H.A. Co-culture of bone marrow-derived mesenchymal stem cells overexpressing lipocalin 2 with HK-2 and HEK293 cells protects the kidney cells against cisplatin-induced injury. *Cell Biol. Int.* **2014**, *39*, 152–163. [CrossRef]
73. Serban, A.I.; Stanca, L.; Geicu, O.I.; Dinischiotu, A. AGEs-Induced IL-6 Synthesis Precedes RAGE Up-Regulation in HEK 293 Cells: An Alternative Inflammatory Mechanism? *Int. J. Mol. Sci.* **2015**, *16*, 20100–20117. [CrossRef]

74. Solovyeva, V.; Salafutdinov, I.; Tazetdinova, L.; Khaiboullina, S.; Masgutov, R.; Rizvanov, A. Genetic modification of adipose derived stem cells with recombinant plasmid DNA pBud-VEGF-FGF2 results in increased of IL-8 and MCP-1 secretion. *J. Pure Appl. Microbiol.* **2014**, *8*, 523–528.
75. Jin, S.; Yang, C.; Huang, J.; Liu, L.; Zhang, Y.; Li, S.; Zhang, L.; Sun, Q.; Yang, P. Conditioned medium derived from FGF-2-modified GMSCs enhances migration and angiogenesis of human umbilical vein endothelial cells. *Stem Cell Res. Ther.* **2020**, *11*, 68. [CrossRef]
76. Yukita, A.; Hara, M.; Hosoya, A.; Nakamura, H. Relationship between localization of proteoglycans and induction of neurotrophic factors in mouse dental pulp. *J. Oral Biosci.* **2017**, *59*, 31–37. [CrossRef]
77. Bauters, C.; Asahara, T.; Zheng, L.P.; Takeshita, S.; Bunting, S.; Ferrara, N.; Symes, J.F.; Isner, J.M. Site-specific therapeutic angiogenesis after systemic administration of vascular endothelial growth factor. *J. Vasc. Surg.* **1995**, *21*, 314–325. [CrossRef]
78. Takeshita, S.; Weir, L.; Chen, D.; Zheng, L.P.; Riessen, R.; Bauters, C.; Symes, J.F.; Ferrara, N.; Isner, J.M. Therapeutic Angiogenesis Following Arterial Gene Transfer of Vascular Endothelial Growth Factor in a Rabbit Model of Hindlimb Ischemia. *Biochem. Biophys. Res. Commun.* **1996**, *227*, 628–635. [CrossRef]
79. Cao, R.; Eriksson, A.; Kubo, H.; Alitalo, K.; Cao, Y.; Thyberg, J. Comparative Evaluation of FGF-2–, VEGF-A–, and VEGF-C–Induced Angiogenesis, Lymphangiogenesis, Vascular Fenestrations, and Permeability. *Circ. Res.* **2004**, *94*, 664–670. [CrossRef]
80. Cartland, S.P.; Genner, S.W.; Zahoor, A.; Kavurma, M.M. Comparative Evaluation of TRAIL, FGF-2 and VEGF-A-Induced Angiogenesis In Vitro and In Vivo. *Int. J. Mol. Sci.* **2016**, *17*, 2025. [CrossRef]
81. Song, M.; Finley, S.D. ERK and Akt exhibit distinct signaling responses following stimulation by pro-angiogenic factors. *Cell Commun. Signal.* **2020**, *18*, 114. [CrossRef]
82. Lanza, A.M.; Curran, K.A.; Rey, L.G.; Alper, H.S. A condition-specific codon optimization approach for improved heterologous gene expression in Saccharomyces cerevisiae. *BMC Syst. Biol.* **2014**, *8*, 33. [CrossRef]
83. Alexaki, A.; Hettiarachchi, G.K.; Athey, J.C.; Katneni, U.; Simhadri, V.; Hamasaki-Katagiri, N.; Nanavaty, P.; Lin, B.; Takeda, K.; Freedberg, D.; et al. Effects of codon optimization on coagulation factor IX translation and structure: Implications for protein and gene therapies. *Sci. Rep.* **2019**, *9*, 15449. [CrossRef]

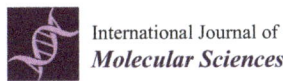

Article

Assessment of Microvessel Permeability in Murine Atherosclerotic Vein Grafts Using Two-Photon Intravital Microscopy

Fabiana Baganha [1,2], Laila Ritsma [3], Paul H. A. Quax [1,2] and Margreet R. de Vries [1,2,]*

1. Department of Surgery, Leiden University Medical Center, 2333 ZA Leiden, The Netherlands; F.Baganha_Carreiras@lumc.nl (F.B.); P.H.A.Quax@lumc.nl (P.H.A.Q.)
2. Einthoven Laboratory for Experimental Vascular Medicine, Leiden University Medical Center, 2333 ZA Leiden, The Netherlands
3. Department of Cell and Chemical Biology, Leiden University Medical Center, 2333 ZC Leiden, The Netherlands; L.M.A.Ritsma@lumc.nl
* Correspondence: M.R.de_Vries@lumc.nl; Tel.: +31-71-526-5147

Received: 6 November 2020; Accepted: 1 December 2020; Published: 3 December 2020

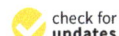

Abstract: Plaque angiogenesis and plaque hemorrhage are major players in the destabilization and rupture of atherosclerotic lesions. As these are dynamic processes, imaging of plaque angiogenesis, especially the integrity or leakiness of angiogenic vessels, can be an extremely useful tool in the studies on atherosclerosis pathophysiology. Visualizing plaque microvessels in 3D would enable us to study the architecture and permeability of adventitial and intimal plaque microvessels in advanced atherosclerotic lesions. We hypothesized that a comparison of the vascular permeability between healthy continuous and fenestrated as well as diseased leaky microvessels, would allow us to evaluate plaque microvessel leakiness. We developed and validated a two photon intravital microscopy (2P-IVM) method to assess the leakiness of plaque microvessels in murine atherosclerosis-prone ApoE3*Leiden vein grafts based on the quantification of fluorescent-dextrans extravasation in real-time. We describe a novel 2P-IVM set up to study vessels in the neck region of living mice. We show that microvessels in vein graft lesions are in their pathological state more permeable in comparison with healthy continuous and fenestrated microvessels. This 2P-IVM method is a promising approach to assess plaque angiogenesis and leakiness. Moreover, this method is an important advancement to validate therapeutic angiogenic interventions in preclinical atherosclerosis models.

Keywords: angiogenesis; vessel maturity; vessel permeability; hemorrhage; atherosclerosis; two-photon intravital microscopy

1. Introduction

Plaque angiogenesis and plaque hemorrhage are major players in the destabilization and rupture of atherosclerotic lesions [1]. Plaque microvessels increase in numbers via angiogenesis during vulnerable stages of the disease, and microvessels density has been associated with the onset of rupture and clinical manifestations [2,3]. Plaque angiogenesis arises from reduced oxygen availability in the plaque, caused by lesion growth and presence of metabolic active inflammatory cells. Triggered by hypoxia, endothelial cells proliferate and migrate from the vasa vasorum to form microvessels to overcome the oxygen demand in the lesion [1]. However, these plaque microvessels are characterized by poor pericyte coverage, lack of cell junctions, and are highly susceptible to leakage of erythrocytes, leucocytes, and plasma lipids, together described as intraplaque hemorrhage [4,5].

Healthy microvessels are present in most organs and tissues, have a well-organized architecture, act as a protection barrier, and provide nutrients and oxygen by passive diffusion to their surroundings.

The type of endothelial lining determines the permeability of the vessel. While in continuous microvessels (abundantly found in the ear skin) the endothelial cell lining is uninterrupted, fenestrated microvessels (found in secreting glands) have more pores to increase molecular diffusion of molecules (up to 66 kDa) without compromising their barrier function [6,7]. Contrarily, microvessels in atherosclerotic lesions in their pathological and immature state are thought to have a compromised barrier function and are as such more permeable [4,8–11].

To date, clinical available imaging techniques to study plaque angiogenesis and subsequent intraplaque hemorrhage, such as PET [12], CT [13], and MRI [14], do not have sufficient spatial resolution to visualize cellular events or image the detailed microvessels network in small size animal models. Two-photon intravital microscopy (2P-IVM), due to its high resolution, can overcome these limitations, allowing detailed 3D reconstructions of plaque angiogenesis and real-time evaluation of target dynamic processes, such as in vivo hemorrhage [7,15,16].

We hypothesized that permeability of healthy continuous and fenestrated microvessels in living mice can be compared to plaque microvessel permeability to assess pathological leakiness. Permeability can be evaluated by quantification of extravasation of 40 kDa-size dextrans [7,17]. It should leak from all vessels [7,17], but is expected to leak more from fenestrated vessels than continuous, and more from pathological vessels than healthy vessels. Moreover, it, is known that capillaries with poor pericytes coverage in context of inflammation can be permeable to large dextrans up to 2000 kDa [17]. Therefore, we also hypothesized that evaluation of 2000 kDa dextran extravasation in the same experimental setting, might be relevant to further assess the pathological permeability.

In this study, we set up an advanced 2P-IVM method to visualize atherosclerotic vein graft (VG) lesions in the neck region of living anesthetized mice. (Figure 1B). With this technique the architecture of adventitial and intimal plaque microvessels in advanced atherosclerotic VG lesions can be visualized (Figure 1C). This model was chosen since in mice, vasa vasorum angiogenesis only occurs at a very old age and most spontaneous atherosclerotic lesions in mice do not show intraplaque angiogenesis [11]. We previously showed that hypercholesterolemic ApoE3*Leiden VG lesions, due to their lesion size and state of hypoxia, present with vasa vasorum derived neovascularization, [8] with the unique characteristic of leaky intimal microvessels and intraplaque hemorrhage [9]. Furthermore, we report a 2P-IVM method to assess vessel permeability by quantification of 40 kDa and 2000 kDa-labeled dextrans extravasation in healthy microvessels and plaque microvessels in real-time (Figure 1D,E). We show that plaque microvessels are pathological more permeable in comparison with healthy continuous and fenestrated microvessels, which advocates for their destabilizing role in plaque rupture.

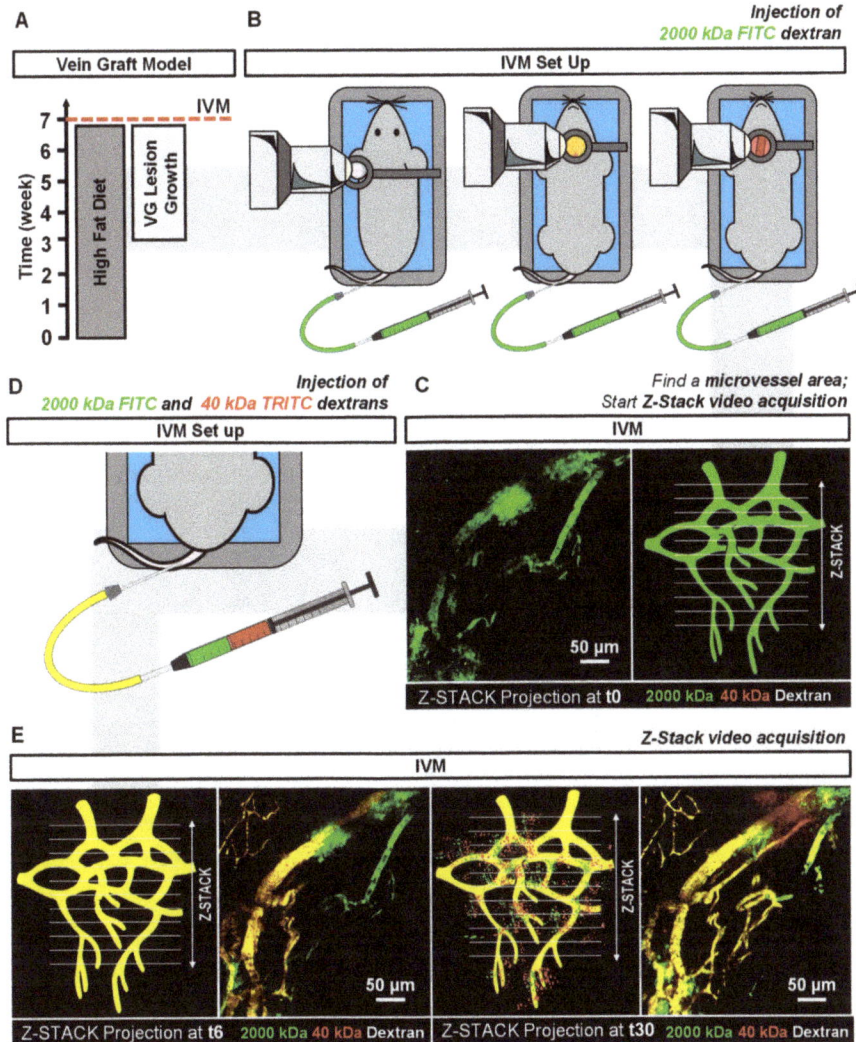

Figure 1. 2P-IVM pipeline to image plaque angiogenesis in advance atherosclerotic lesions and to assess dextrans extravasation in continuous, fenestrated and plaque microvessels. (**A**) After 3 weeks of hypercholesteremic diet, ApoE3*Leiden mice (n = 12) undergo VG surgery. Four weeks later, (**B**) mice are prepared for IVM and plaque microvessels in the VG lesions, continuous microvessels in ear skin, fenestrated microvessels in parotid glands are imaged by injection of 2000 kDa-FITC dextran intravenously. (**C**) Areas of interest are evaluated by time-lapse Z-stack acquisition over 20 min. (**D**,**E**) Injection of 40 kDa-TRITC 2000 kDa-FITC dextran solution is used to assess vessel permeability by quantification of FICT and TRITC fluorescence extravascular intensities in Z-stack projections.

2. Results

*2.1. Detection of Plaque Angiogenesis in ApoE3*Leiden Mice Vein Graft Lesions*

Plaque angiogenesis was detected by 2P-IVM in advanced atherosclerotic lesions of the ApoE3*Leiden mice VG model by injection of the plasma tracer 2000 kDa-FITC dextran as depicted in Figure 1B,C. Here, we imaged for the first time the VG in the neck using high resolution intravital microscopy. We designed a circular metal frame was designed with a coverslip on top connected to a pole by a stalk (Figure 1B,C). The frame could be fixed to the pole at varying heights by a screw. The thin stalk enabled us to image the vessels at high resolution without putting too much pressure on the sternum/chest region or throat.

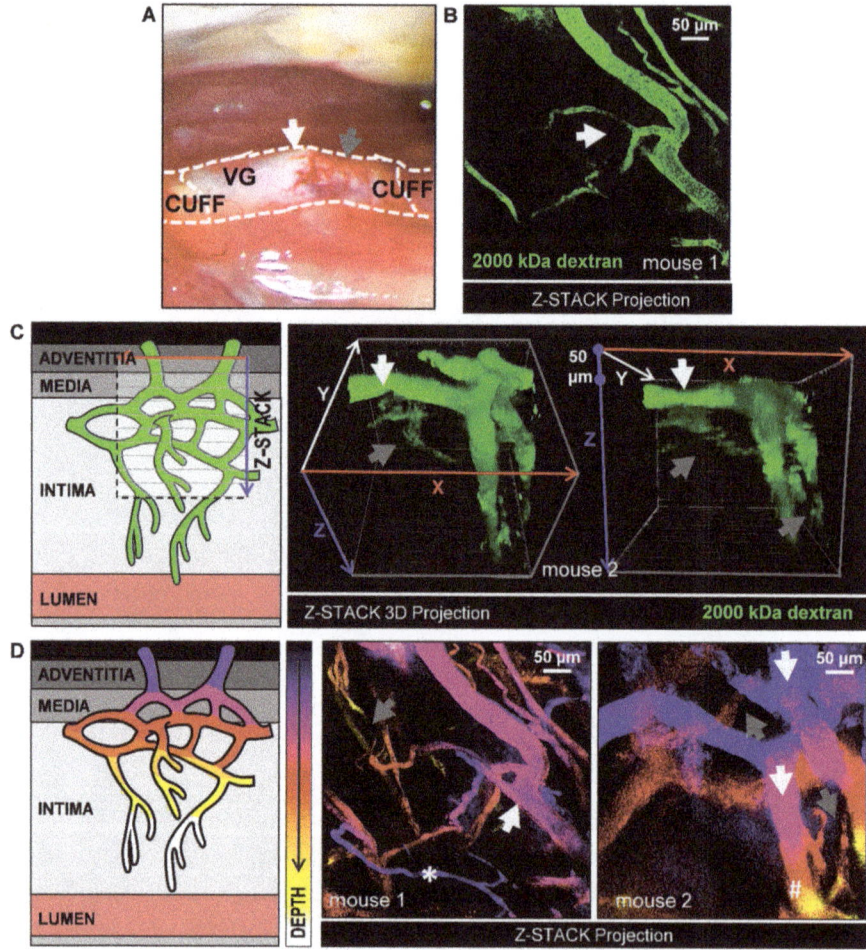

Figure 2. Detection of plaque angiogenesis by 2P-IVM by injection of the plasma tracer 2000 kDa-FITC dextran in atherosclerotic lesions in ApoE3*Leiden mice VGs. (**A**) 28 days after surgery, areas of interest (white arrows: white thick regions, grey arrows: red thin regions) were imaged to study the architecture of plaque microvessels. (**B**) Z-stack projection of plaque microvessels (white arrows: branching). See also Video 1 (total Z-depth of 111 μm, 2 μm step); (**C**) Illustration of Z-stack acquisition in VG lesions and representative Z-stack 3D projections of adventitial (white arrows) and intimal microvessels (grey arrows) from one mouse at two different angles. See also video 2 for 360 view. Note that the large adventitial microvessels are also extending in Z because they are curved around the vein. (**D**) Z-stack projections from two mice with a Z-depth color code filter (white arrows: Adventitial microvessels; grey arrows: Intimal microvessels). Due to the curved nature of the vein: (*) Intimal microvessel is discriminated from adventitial microvessel based on its size, despite being located in a top Z layer; (#) Adventitial microvessel is discriminated from an intimal microvessel based on its size, despite being located in a deeper Z layer.

Thick white fatty atherosclerotic regions were observed along the conduit (Figure 2A). Compared to red thin lesion regions, these white regions show a prominent presence of microvessels. Therefore, white fatty thick spots were chosen to image the architecture of plaque angiogenesis (Figure 2B). FITC signal was homogenously distributed within the intravascular space of the microvessels with no signs of blood flow obstructions. Branching features, characteristic of immature or angiogenic vessels [18] were also observed (Figure 2B and Video 1). In video 1, a 111-μm deep z-stack projection of the image of Figure 2B is shown. This video offers an in depth view of the plaque microvessels throughout the adventitia, media, and intima.

Using 3D stack projections, vasa vasorum angiogenesis is observed throughout the lesion depth (Figure 2C and Video 2). Vasa vasorum angiogenesis expands towards hypoxic plaque areas, (intima) and these intimal microvessels were observed to be narrower than most preexisting adventitial vessels. Bigger adventitial microvessels were usually detected at 50–100 μm depth and narrower intimal microvessel structures, from >100 μm. Accordingly, size and depth were required to discriminate adventitial microvessels from intimal microvessels.

To easily visualize this in a single image, Z depth color coding was used (Figure 2D). As an example of the different variations seen in mice, two examples are given (mouse 1 and mouse 2). Here, vessels which are located deep in Z (in the intimal layer) are differently colored from vessels located high in Z (adventitial layer). Adventitial microvessels are shown in a blue to purple color gradient (Figure 2D, grey arrows) while intimal microvessels are shown in a red to yellow color gradient (Figure 2D, white arrows).

Due to the curved nature of the vein graft, some microvessels not match the color-code (* and #). Indeed, a thin vessel (*) is excluded as an adventitial microvessel based on its caliber, despite being located in a top Z layer. In addition, a thick microvessel (#) is partially located in the deeper Z layers. As can be appreciated in the 3D rendering (Figure 2C), the thick vessel is curved around the vein graft, and therefore extending into the deeper Z layer, and should be excluded as an intimal microvessel. As shown by the represented examples, vessel depth, microvessel caliber, and 3D rendering have to be considered to distinguish adventitial and intimal microvessels.

2.2. Evaluation of Dextran in Microvessels

To determine the amplitude and speed at which dextrans become visible in the various microvessels, we first injected mice with 2000 kDa-FITC to detect the microvessels and assess a region of interest, and then injected mice with a mixture of 2000 kDa-FITC and 40 kDa-TRITC dextran during timelapse imaging. We plotted the relative fluorescence intensity (RFI, normalized to t6) of 2000 kDa-FITC and 40 kDa-TRITC dextran over time for continuous (Figure 3A), fenestrated (Figure 3B), and plaque microvessels (Figure 3C).

Residual 2000 kDa-FITC fluorescence from the first injection ($t \leq 5$) was observed in all groups (Figure 3A–C). As shown in Figure 2D, residual FITC RFI at t5 is similar between the groups (Figure 3D).

As expected, after injection of 2000 kDa-FICT and 40 kDa-TRITC dextrans at t5, intravascular FITC RFI increases significantly until t6 in all groups, as demonstrated in Figure 3D (continuous microvessels: $p < 0.0001$, fenestrated microvessels: $p = 0.0007$, plaque microvessels: $p = 0.0106$). TRITC RFI increased even more than FITC RFI, as depicted in Figure 3E, most likely due to the residual FITC from the first injection (continuous microvessels: $p < 0.0001$, fenestrated microvessels: $p < 0.0001$, plaque microvessels: $p < 0.0001$).

During the next 24 image recordings, intravascular FITC and TRITC signal remained stable (~1) in all groups (Figure 3A–C). As shown in Figure 3D,E, FITC and TRITC RFI between t6 and t30 did not differ between continuous, fenestrated and plaque microvessels. Representative sequences of FITC and TRITC fluorescence intensities in continuous, fenestrated and plaque microvessels, observed in real-time, at t5 and t6, are shown in Figure 3F.

Thus, tail vein-injected dextrans appear quickly and with the same dynamics in the various microvessels, and remain so in similar concentration throughout the course of imaging.

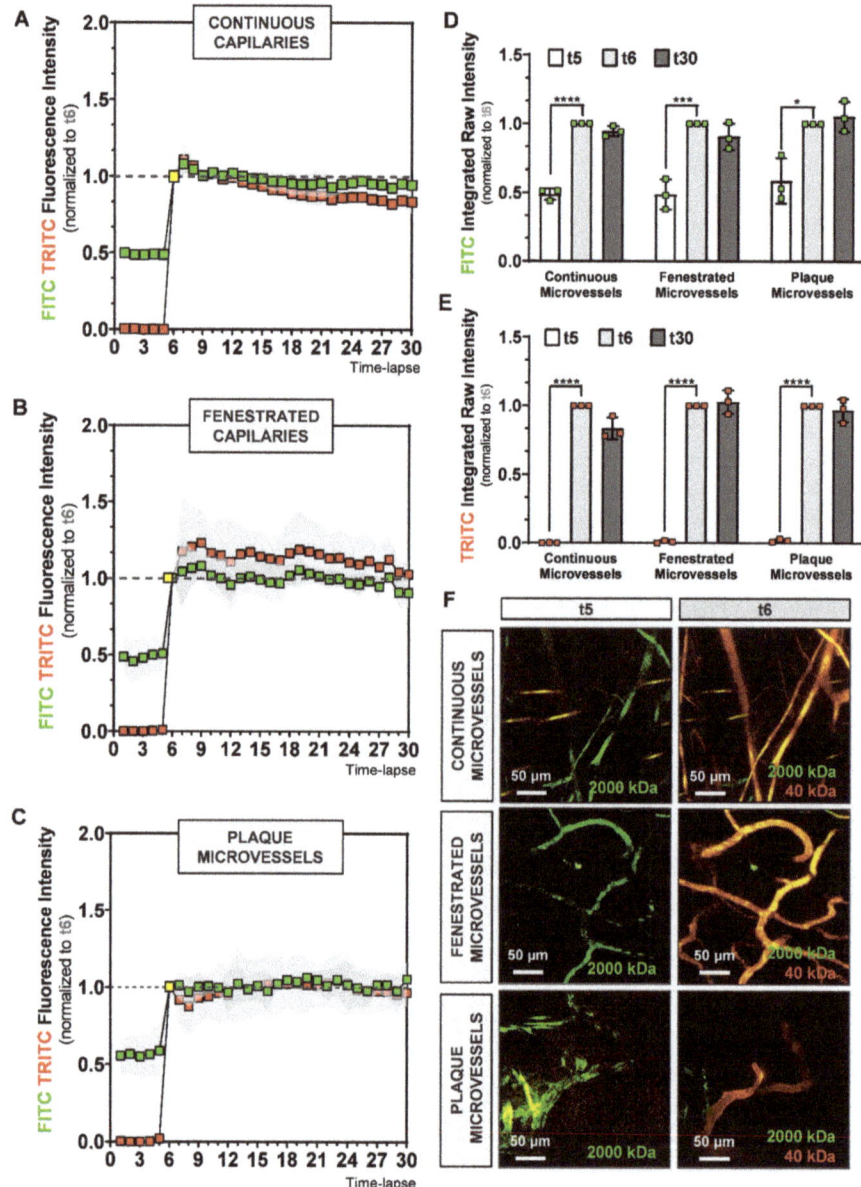

Figure 3. Evaluation of time-lapse imaging of 2000 kDa-FITC and 40 kDa-TRITC RFI inside the microvessel structures of (**A**) continuous, (**B**) fenestrated and (**C**) plaque microvessels. (**D,E**) Quantification of FITC and TRITC intravascular RFI at time-lapse 5, 6 and 30. (**F**) Representative max-projection of FITC and TRITC signal in continuous, fenestrated and plaque microvessels at t5 and t6. Data presented as mean ± SD. * $p \leq 0.05$, *** $p \leq 0.001$, **** $p \leq 0.0001$ by 1-way-ANOVA.

2.3. Evaluation of Dextran Extravasation into the Extravascular Space

Next, we determined if it was possible to visualize dextran extravasation from the vasculature. In the same time-lapse movies as used for Figure 3, we measured the extravascular RFI (normalized to t6) for 2000 kDa-FITC and 40 kDa-TRITC dextran for continuous (Figure 4A), fenestrated (Figure 4B), and plaque (Figure 4C) microvessels.

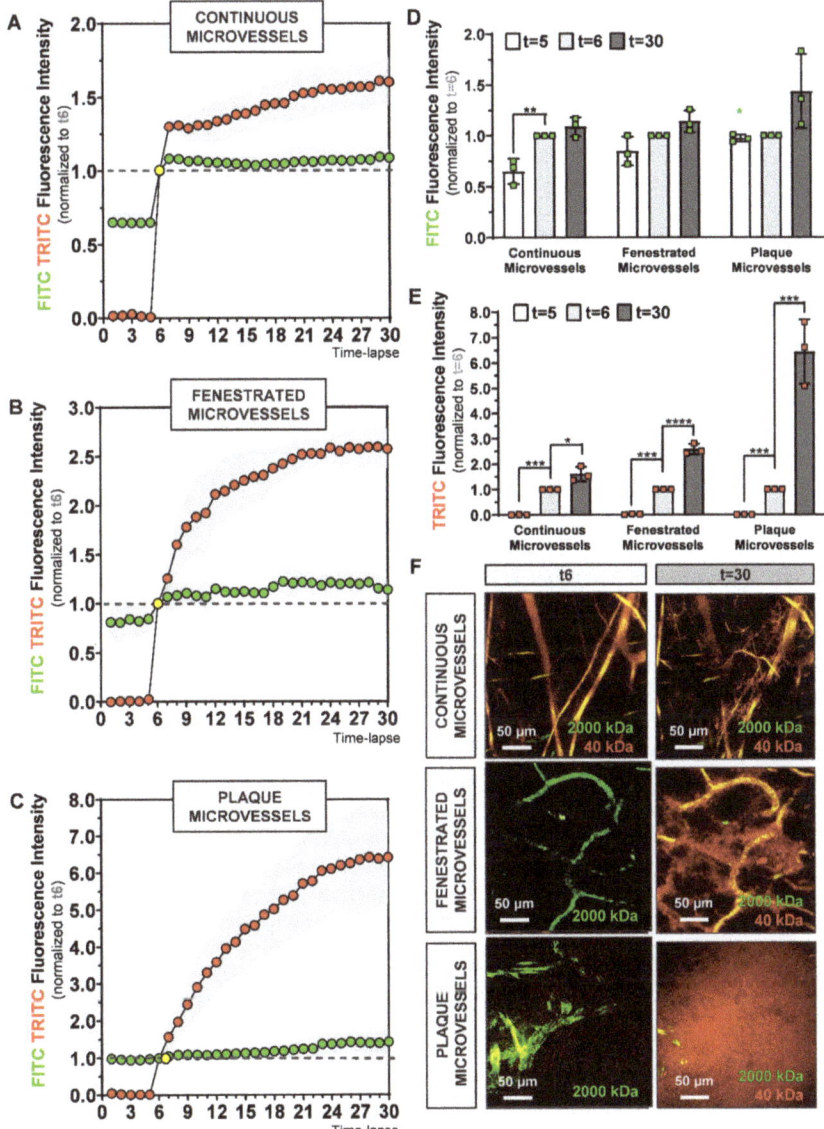

Figure 4. Evaluation of time-lapse imaging of 2000 kDa-FITC and 40 kDa-TRITC RFI outside the microvessel structures of (**A**) continuous, (**B**) fenestrated and (**C**) plaque microvessels. (**D,E**) Quantification of FITC and TRITC extravascular RFI at time-lapse 5, 6 and 30. (**F**) Representative max-projection of FITC and TRITC signal in continuous, fenestrated and plaque microvessels at t6 and t30. Data presented as mean ± SD. * $p \leq 0.05$, ** $p \leq 0.001$, *** $p \leq 0.001$, **** $p \leq 0.0001$ by 1-way-ANOVA; Green star (* $p \leq 0.05$): FITC RFI at t5 between continuous and plaque microvessels.

Residual fluorescence from the 2000 kDa-FITC first injection ($t \leq 5$) was detected in all groups in the extravascular space as shown in Figure 4A–C. FITC RFI at t5 is different between continuous and plaque microvessels groups (0.652 ± 0.14 vs. 0.973 ± 0.14, $p = 0.0274$, Figure 4D, green star).

After injection of 2000 kDa-FICT and 40 kDa-TRITC dextrans at t5, TRITC extravascular RFI increases significantly between t5 and t6 in all groups, as shown in Figure 3E ($p < 0.001$). However, FITC extravascular RFI (Figure 3D) varies between the groups. While it significantly increases between t5 and t6 in continuous microvessels ($p = 0.0274$), no differences are observed between t5 and t6 (~1) in plaque microvessels (Figure 4C,D).

In the next 24 image recordings, TRITC extravascular RFI increases in all microvessels, as shown in Figure 4A–C. In contrast, FITC extravascular RFI between t6 and t30 does not differ in continuous and fenestrated microvessels, (Figure 3D). However, in plaque microvessels, a trend towards an increase in FITC extravascular RFI is detected at t30 compared to t6, ($p = 0.0827$, Figure 4D).

Importantly, the mean TRITC extravascular RFI at t30 is 1.63 ± 0.29, 63% higher in comparison to t6 ($p = 0.01$) in the continuous microvessels group (Figure 4E). In fenestrated microvessels, TRITC RFI mean at t30 is 2.58 ± 0.21, 158% higher compared to t6 ($p < 0.0001$, Figure 4E). In plaque microvessels, TRITC mean intensity is 6.64 ± 1.27, 564% higher compared to t6 ($p = 0.0003$, Figure 4E). Representative sequences of FITC and TRITC signal in continuous, fenestrated and plaque microvessels, observed in real-time at t0, t6 and t30 are shown in Figure 4F.

Overall, 40 kDa dextran extravasates more than 2000 kDa dextran. 40 kDa dextran continues to extravasate over time, whereas 2000 kDa dextran shows an initial peak in extravasation and then stops.

2.4. Comparison Dextrans Extravasation in Continuous, Fenestrated and Plaque Microvessels

To better understand 2000 kDa and 40 kDa dextran extravasation differences between continuous, fenestrated and plaque microvessels, we compared FITC or TRITC fluorescence intensities outside the vessel structures (Figure 5).

FITC extravascular fluorescence intensities show small and non-significant increases over time in all groups as depicted in Figure 5A. Extravasation of 2000 kDa-FITC dextran is comparable between the groups at t18, t24, and t30 as demonstrated in Figure 5B.

The 40 kDa dextran profile displays, strong changes in TRITC extravascular RFI between the groups, which increases in time (Figure 5C). After t6, TRITC intensity increases differently between groups. While in continuous microvessels, TRITC signal increases, reaching a stable value of 1.30 ± 0.10, at t8, in the fenestrated microvessels group, TRITC signal at t8 is already 1.60 ± 0.23 and stabilizes at t18 (2.38 ± 0.19). In plaque microvessels, TRITC RFI raises continuously, with 1.98 ± 0.53 at t8 and 5.03 ± 1.13 at t18. As shown in Figure 5D, extravasation of 40 kDa TRITC-dextran in the plaque microvessels was 3.4-fold higher ($p = 0.0016$) in comparison to continuous microvessels, and 1.8-fold higher ($p = 0.0072$) in comparison to fenestrated capillaries at t18.

At the end of the observation period (t30), TRITC RFI was 1.60 ± 0.29 in continuous microvessels, 2.58 ± 0.11 in fenestrated microvessels and 6.42 ± 1.27 in plaque microvessels ($n = 3$). Extravasation of 40 kDa TRITC-dextran in plaque microvessels was four-fold higher ($p = 0.0006$) compared to continuous microvessels and 2.5-fold higher ($p = 0.0020$) compared to fenestrated capillaries. Thus, continuous, fenestrated, and plaque microvessels are all permeable to 40 kDa size-dextrans but follow different and vessel specific extravasation curves. Importantly, plaque microvessels show the largest permeability.

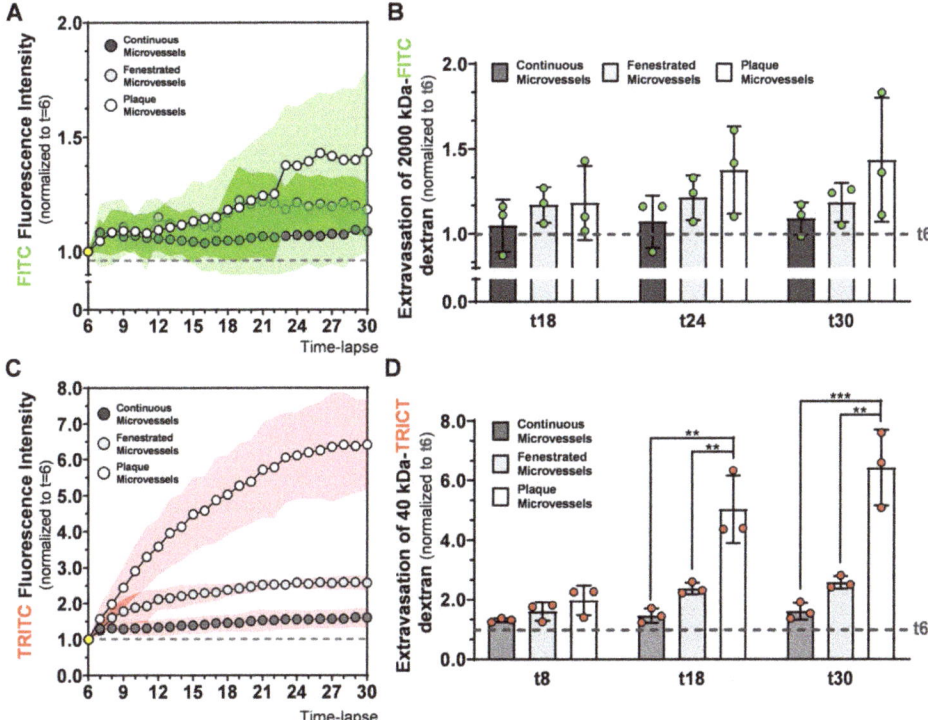

Figure 5. Evaluation of 2000 kDa-FITC and 40 kDa-TRITC dextrans extravasation in continuous, fenestrated and plaque microvessels. Time dependent evolution of (**A**) FITC and (**C**) TRITC extravascular RFI between groups. Comparison of (**B**) 2000 kDa and (**D**) 40 kDa extravasation at different timepoint between groups. Data presented as mean ± SD (SD is expressed as a green (**A**) or red (**C**) cloud). ** $p \leq 0.001$, *** $p \leq 0.001$, by 1-way-ANOVA.

3. Discussion

In this study, we used 2P-IVM to visualize adventitial and intimal plaque microvessels in advanced atherosclerotic lesions in ApoE3*Leiden VGs. In this model, a non-diseased caval vein from a donor mouse is used as an interposition in the carotid artery of a hypercholesterolemic ApoE3*Leiden mouse, within 28 day an atherosclerotic lesion forms with adventitial and intimal plaque microvessels with various forms of maturity [8,9]. We report a 2P-IVM method to evaluate plaque microvessels leakiness in vivo, by comparing the extravasation of 40 kDa dextran in healthy, continuous, and fenestrated, as well as diseased, plaque microvessels. We demonstrated in real-time, that microvessels in advanced atherosclerotic lesions in VGs are pathologically permeable.

By injecting 2000 kDa-FITC dextrans, we were able to observe in vivo microvessels networks throughout the adventitia, media and extending into the intimal layer of the VG lesion. Larger vessels were detected in the adventitia layer, while more narrow vessel structures were detected further deep in the plaque. We here confirm in vivo the abundant presence of intimal microvessels in advance atherosclerotic lesions in the ApoE3*Leiden VG model that was previously shown with histology [8,9]. This is a rare feature seldomly seen in other atherosclerotic mouse models [19,20]. These microvessel networks are characterized by typical vessel features of ongoing angiogenesis, as observed by the irregular microvessel architecture with accentuated turns and branching. Moreover, using 3D and color-depth Z-Stack projections, we demonstrate how vasa vasorum angiogenesis evolves throughout the lesion including the intima.

Fenestrated microvessels (observed in salivary glands) are more permeable than continuous microvessels (located in the ears) due to their increased number of pores, which drives faster molecule diffusion [6,7]. Accordingly, we observed that continuous and fenestrated microvessels follow different 40 kDa dextran extravasation signatures. While in continuous microvessels, extravasation of 40 kDa dextran reached a stable value rapidly in the observation period, extravasation of the 40 kDa dextran in fenestrated microvessels took more time and was more extensive.

Healthy microvessels have a well-organized architecture that acts as a protection barrier but which does let molecules such as nutrients cross. Plaque microvessels, in contrast, have a disorganized structure with a lack of proper pericyte coverage, diminished VE-cadherins junctions, heterogeneous basement membrane and show an unbalance in angiopoietin 1 and 2 expression [9]. This unbalanced architecture leads to dysfunctionality as shown by their co-localization with extravasated erythrocytes and inflammatory cells, in part explained by the increased expression of VCAM-1 and ICAM-1, as previously described by histological analysis [8,9]. By comparing 40 kDa extravasation patterns in healthy microvessels with the plaque microvessels, we demonstrate in real-time, that microvessels in advanced atherosclerotic lesions are pathological permeable. Their 40 kDa-FITC extravasation curves of the plaque microvessels were clearly different and at the end of the observation period, extravascular 40 kDa dextran was four-fold higher compared to continuous microvessels and 2.5-fold higher compared to fenestrated microvessels. This increased permeability can contribute to the extravasation of erythrocytes and leukocytes which drive plaque instability [4].

In the 2000 kDa dextran extravasation patterns in continuous, fenestrated, and plaque microvessels FITC extravascular RFI between t6 and t30 showed a trend towards an increase in the plaque microvessels. FITC extravascular RFI at t30 was similar between the groups. The reason why we were not able to detect different FITC extravascular RFI at t30 might be related to the immature nature of the plaque microvessels. Recent studies have shown that microvessels with an immature structure drive macromolecules accumulation by the enhanced permeability and retention (EPR) effect [21,22].

In this study, we used two injections of 2000 kDa dextran with the same fluorescent dye (FITC), with the first to visualize blood flow and the second to quantify vessel permeability. After the second injection, FITC intravascular RFI increased significantly between t5 and t6, in all groups. However, FITC extravascular RFI between t5 and t6, only increased significantly in continuous microvessels and did not differ in plaque microvessels. Moreover, when we compared FITC extravascular residual fluorescence (from the first injection) at t5 between groups, it was significantly higher in plaque microvessels compared to continuous microvessels.

Therefore, it is possible that 2000 kDa dextran (from the first injection) accumulates in the extravascular space of plaque microvessels due to the EPR effect, thereby decreasing signal differences during quantification of 2000 kDa extravasation in the second injection. In future approaches that aim to quantify extravasation patterns of macromolecules (such as 2000 kDa dextrans) other methods (e.g., dextrans with differently colored dyes) to detect blood flow should be considered.

Nevertheless, this 2P-IVM imaging methodology allows direct imaging of adventitial and intimal microvessels but also the quantification of the permeability of the microvessels by 40 kDa extravasation in a more realistic test environment compared to post-mortem tissue. Moreover, this technique could be easily adapted to further investigated the dynamics of intraplaque angiogenesis and intraplaque hemorrhage. By injecting fluorescent-labelled cells (such as erythrocytes or inflammatory cells), their extravasation, transmigration, and interaction with the endothelium could easily be monitored and quantified in vivo. Therefore, this 2P-IVM method is a promising approach to validate therapeutic angiogenic interventions targeting advance atherosclerosis in preclinical models in real-time.

4. Materials and Methods

4.1. Animals

All experiments were carried out with approval of the Animal Welfare Committee of the Leiden Medical University Center (28 March 2018; approval number 116002106645-18-096) and in compliance the Directive 2010/63/EU of the European Parliament. Male ApoE3*Leiden mice ($n = 12$), 10–16 weeks old, were fed with a high-cholesterol inducing diet (2.5% cholesterol and 0.05% cholate w/w, AB diets, Woerden, The Netherlands) during all the experiment. Mice were housed under standard laboratory conditions and received food and water ad libitum.

4.2. Vein Graft Surgery

VG surgery consists of the interposition of the caval vein from a donor mouse in the carotid artery of a recipient mouse, as described before [8]. In brief, the recipient mouse was fixed in a supine position, and an incision was made in the neck. The parotid glands were put aside exposing the right carotid artery. Next, the carotid artery was ligated and cut in middle, a cuff was placed at both ends of the arterial segments. Subsequently, the ends were everted over the cuffs and ligated. The vena cava was harvested from the donor mouse and positioned between the carotid artery by sleeving it over the cuffs and tightened with 8/0 sutures. Pulsatile flow through the venous conduit confirms a successful procedure. Finally, the parotid gland is put back in position and the skin is sutured. Within 28 days after the surgery, the VG lesions develop from a few cell layers at the start of the engraftment, to a massive thickened vessel wall [23].

Mice were anesthetized (intraperitoneally) with 5 mg/kg of midazolam (Roche Diagnostics, Basel, Switzerland), 0.5 mg/kg of dexmedetomidine (Orion Corporation, Espoo, Finland) and 0.05 mg/kg of fentanyl (Janssen Pharmaceutical, Beerse, Belgium). After the surgery, the anesthesia was antagonized with 2.5 mg/kg of atipamezole (Orion Corporation,) and 0.5 mg/kg of flumazenil (0.5 mg/kg, Fresenius Kabi, Bad Homburg vor der Höhe, Germany). Then, 0.1 mg/kg of buprenorphine (MSD Animal Health, Boxmeer, The Netherlands) was given for pain relief.

4.3. Two-Photon Intravital Microscopy

Four weeks after the surgery (Figure 1A), mice ($n = 12$) were anesthetized and prepared for intravital imaging on a Zeiss LSM 710 NLO upright multiphoton microscope equipped with a Mai Tai Deep See multiphoton laser (690–1040 nm).

Neck and ear regions were shaved, and a catheter was placed in the tail vein for intravenous injections. To image fenestrated microvessels (in the parotid glands) and plaque microvessels (in the VGs), mice were placed in a supine position on an inset located under the microscope (Figure 1B). Parotid glands were extracorporated, and VGs were carefully exposed from the surrounding connective tissue. To image continuous microvessels (in the ear skin), mice were placed in prone position on the inset (Figure 1B). In both positions, temperature was controlled and breathing was monitored. On top of the target tissue, a metal frame was placed. This metal frame was specially designed to allow the use of a water immersion objective (W Plan Apochromat 20×/1.0 DIC M27 75 mm objective) in the different tissues of the mouse body (Figure 1B).

To select areas of interest in the different microvessels types (continuous, fenestrated and plaque), mice were injected with 50 µL of 100 mg/mL FITC-conjugated 2000 kDa dextran (a blood tracer), via the vein catheter (Figure 1B). These areas were imaged by cycles of time-lapse Z-stacks (40 s each) over 20 min by multiphoton excitation at 488 nm (FITC) and 555 nm (TRITC). Emission was collected by two LSM PMTs at 500–558 nm (FITC) and 578–700 nm (TRITC). At the 5th frame of the time-lapse (t5) a mixture of 100 µL of a 100 mg/mL 40 kDa Dextran-TRITC (42874, Sigma-Aldrich, Zwijndrecht, The Netherlands) and 2000 kDa Dextran-FITC (FD2000S, Sigma-Aldrich, Zwijndrecht, The Netherlands) solution was injected to assess vessel permeability in real-time in all the groups (Figure 1C).

To study plaque angiogenesis in particular, a separate group of three mice was used to study the architecture of intimal and adventitial microvessels. Then, 50–150 µm depth Z-stacks were acquired by multiphoton excitation at 488 nm, after injection of 50 µL 100 mg/mL FITC-conjugated 2000 kDa dextran, via the tail vein catheter. Directly after imaging, all mice were euthanized by exsanguination.

4.4. Data Analysis

4.4.1. Quantification of FITC and TRITC Fluorescence Integrated Density Inside and Outside the Vessel Structures

To quantify FITC and TRITC fluorescence integrated density inside and outside the vessel structures, we converted 2P-IVM time-lapse acquisition files in maximal intensity Z-stack projections (RBG). Based on the literature, 2000 kDa-size dextrans are less prone to extravasate in microvascular structures due to their big size [17]. Therefore, we used the FITC channel to apply a tight automatic threshold and define vessel structures surface, denominated as Vessel Mask. Vessel Mask comprises all pixels inside the vessel value as 1 (defined by the automatic threshold) and all the pixels outside the vessel value as 0, at all the timelapses. The Outside Mask was created via inversion. Both Vessel Mask and Outside Mask were then multiplied by the FITC and TRITC channel, generating four additional files: FITC pixels inside the vessel, FITC pixels outside the vessel, TRITC pixels inside the vessel, TRITC pixels outside the vessel.

For the all the six files, relative fluorescence intensity (RFI) was calculated by RawIntegrated density function. Since the area between intravascular and extravascular space are different between mice and organs, FITC and TRITC integrated densities were divided by the number of pixels of theVessel Mask or Outside Mask. Subsequently, FITC and TRITC fluorescence integrated densities reflect all the pixel intensities inside or outside the vessel structures. Since 40 kD and 2000 kDa dextran injection was detected intravitally at the 6th frame of the time-lapse (t6), FITC and TRITC fluorescence integrated intensities, intra and extravascular, were normalized to t6 values, and plotted in XY graphs.

4.4.2. Video Processing of FITC and TRITC Fluorescence Time-Lapse Series Acquired by 2P-IVM

To evaluate 40 kDa and 2000 kDa dextran extravasation patterns, we generated video time-lapse series of maximal FITC and TRITC fluorescence Z-stack projections. 2000 kDa dextran is visualized in the green channel and 40 kDa dextran is visualized in the red channel.

Plaque microvessels in advanced atherosclerotic VG lesions were processed by maximal FITC fluorescence Z-stack projections. Moreover, we generated 3D stack projections using Imaris 3D rendering software (Imaris, Zurich, Switzerland). In both renderings 2000 kDa-FITC dextran is visualized in the green channel.

To distinguish between adventitial and intimal microvessels, we used the temporal color-coding plugin in ImageJ FIJI that used a color LUT based on Z-depth and projects this in a maximum projection image.

4.5. Statistical Analysis

Results are shown as mean ± standard deviation error (SD). One-way ANOVA was used to compare differences between groups. Differences were considered significant when $p* \leq 0.05$, $p** \leq 0.01$, $p*** \leq 0.001$ or $p**** \leq 0.001$.

Author Contributions: Conception and design of the work: F.B. and L.R.; Animal surgeries and data acquisition: F.B., L.R. and M.R.d.V.; Data analysis: F.B. and L.R.; The first draft of the manuscript was written by F.B., and revised by M.R.d.V., P.H.A.Q. and L.R. Supervision: M.R.d.V. and P.H.A.Q. All authors have read and agreed to the published version of the manuscript.

Funding: This work was supported by a grant from the European Union, MSCA joint doctoral project MoGlyNet [675527]. It was also supported by a Veni grant (016.176.081, NOW), a gisela thier grant (LUMC) and a Leids Universiteits Fonds grant (CWB 7204) awarded to LR.

Conflicts of Interest: The authors declare no conflict of interest.

Abbreviations

2P-IVM Two-photon intravital microscopy
RFI   Relative fluorescence intensity

References

1. Parma, L.; Baganha, F.; Quax, P.H.A.; De Vries, M.R. Plaque angiogenesis and intraplaque hemorrhage in atherosclerosis. *Eur. J. Pharmacol.* **2017**, *816*, 107–115. [CrossRef]
2. Sluimer, J.C.; Daemen, M.J. Novel concepts in atherogenesis: Angiogenesis and hypoxia in atherosclerosis. *J. Pathol.* **2009**, *218*, 7–29. [CrossRef] [PubMed]
3. Kalucka, J.; Bierhansl, L.; Wielockx, B.; Carmeliet, P.; Eelen, G. Interaction of endothelial cells with macrophages—Linking molecular and metabolic signaling. *Pflügers Arch. Eur. J. Physiol.* **2017**, *469*, 473–483. [CrossRef]
4. De Vries, M.R.; Quax, P.H. Plaque angiogenesis and its relation to inflammation and atherosclerotic plaque destabilization. *Curr. Opin. Lipidol.* **2016**, *27*, 499–506. [CrossRef]
5. Pérez-Medina, C.; Binderup, T.; Lobatto, M.E.; Tang, J.; Calcagno, C.; Giesen, L.; Wessel, C.H.; Witjes, J.; Ishino, S.; Baxter, S.; et al. In Vivo PET Imaging of HDL in Multiple Atherosclerosis Models. *JACC Cardiovasc. Imaging* **2016**, *9*, 950–961. [CrossRef] [PubMed]
6. Stan, R.V.; Tse, D.; Deharvengt, S.J.; Smits, N.C.; Xu, Y.; Luciano, M.R.; McGarry, C.L.; Buitendijk, M.; Nemani, K.V.; Elgueta, R.; et al. The Diaphragms of Fenestrated Endothelia: Gatekeepers of Vascular Permeability and Blood Composition. *Dev. Cell* **2012**, *23*, 1203–1218. [CrossRef]
7. Ono, S.; Egawa, G.; Kabashima, K. Regulation of blood vascular permeability in the skin. *Inflamm. Regen.* **2017**, *37*, 1–8. [CrossRef]
8. De Vries, M.R.; Niessen, H.W.M.; Löwik, C.W.G.M.; Hamming, J.F.; Jukema, J.W.; Quax, P.H.A. Plaque Rupture Complications in Murine Atherosclerotic Vein Grafts Can Be Prevented by TIMP-1 Overexpression. *PLoS ONE* **2012**, *7*, e47134. [CrossRef]
9. De Vries, M.R.; Parma, L.; Peters, H.A.B.; Schepers, A.; Hamming, J.F.; Jukema, J.W.; Goumans, M.-J.; Guo, L.; Finn, A.V.; Virmani, R.; et al. Blockade of vascular endothelial growth factor receptor 2 inhibits intraplaque haemorrhage by normalization of plaque neovessels. *J. Intern. Med.* **2019**, *285*, 59–74. [CrossRef] [PubMed]
10. Marsch, E.; Theelen, T.L.; Demandt, J.A.; Jeurissen, M.; Van Gink, M.; Verjans, R.; Janssen, A.; Cleutjens, J.P.; Meex, S.J.R.; Donners, M.M.; et al. Reversal of Hypoxia in Murine Atherosclerosis Prevents Necrotic Core Expansion by Enhancing Efferocytosis. *Arter. Thromb. Vasc. Biol.* **2014**, *34*, 2545–2553. [CrossRef]
11. Rademakers, T.; Douma, K.; Hackeng, T.M.; Post, M.J.; Sluimer, J.C.; Daemen, M.J.; Biessen, E.A.; Heeneman, S.; Van Zandvoort, M. Plaque-Associated Vasa Vasorum in Aged Apolipoprotein E–Deficient Mice Exhibit Proatherogenic Functional Features In Vivo. *Arter. Thromb. Vasc. Biol.* **2013**, *33*, 249–256. [CrossRef] [PubMed]
12. Alie, N.; Eldib, M.; Fayad, Z.A.; Mani, V. Inflammation, Atherosclerosis, and Coronary Artery Disease: PET/CT for the Evaluation of Atherosclerosis and Inflammation. *Clin. Med. Insights Cardiol.* **2014**, *8*, 13–21. [CrossRef] [PubMed]
13. Tsujita, K.; Kaikita, K.; Araki, S.; Yamada, T.; Nagamatsu, S.; Yamanaga, K.; Sakamoto, K.; Kojima, S.; Hokimoto, S.; Ogawa, H. In Vivo optical coherence tomography visualization of intraplaque neovascularization at the site of coronary vasospasm: A case report. *BMC Cardiovasc. Disord.* **2016**, *16*, 1–4. [CrossRef] [PubMed]
14. Neeman, M. Perspectives: MRI of angiogenesis. *J. Magn. Reson.* **2018**, *292*, 99–105. [CrossRef]
15. Taqueti, V.R.; Jaffer, F.A. High-resolution molecular imaging via intravital microscopy: Illuminating vascular biology in vivo. *Integr. Biol.* **2013**, *5*, 278–290. [CrossRef]
16. Ritsma, L.; Ponsioen, B.; Van Rheenen, J. Intravital imaging of cell signaling in mice. *IntraVital* **2012**, *1*, 2–10. [CrossRef]
17. Egawa, G.; Nakamizo, S.; Natsuaki, Y.; Doi, H.; Miyachi, Y.; Kabashima, K. Intravital analysis of vascular permeability in mice using two-photon microscopy. *Sci. Rep.* **2013**, *3*, srep01932. [CrossRef]

18. Rattigan, S. Faculty Opinions recommendation of In vivo imaging shows abnormal function of vascular endothelial growth factor-induced vasculature. *Hum. Gene Ther.* **2007**, *515*–524. [CrossRef]
19. Eriksson, E.E. Intravital Microscopy on Atherosclerosis in Apolipoprotein E–Deficient Mice Establishes Microvessels as Major Entry Pathways for Leukocytes to Advanced Lesions. *Circulation* **2011**, *124*, 2129–2138. [CrossRef]
20. Perrotta, P.; Pintelon, I.; De Vries, M.R.; Quax, P.H.; Timmermans, J.-P.; De Meyer, G.R.; Martinet, W. Three-Dimensional Imaging of Intraplaque Neovascularization in a Mouse Model of Advanced Atherosclerosis. *J. Vasc. Res.* **2020**, *57*, 348–354. [CrossRef]
21. Debefve, E.; Cheng, C.; Schaefer, S.; Yan, H.; Ballini, J.-P.; Bergh, H.V.D.; Lehr, H.-A.; Ruffieux, C.; Ris, H.-B.; Krueger, T. Photodynamic therapy induces selective extravasation of macromolecules: Insights using intravital microscopy. *J. Photochem. Photobiol. B* **2010**, *98*, 69–76. [CrossRef] [PubMed]
22. Maeda, H.; Wu, J.; Sawa, T.; Matsumura, Y.; Hori, K. Tumor vascular permeability and the EPR effect in macromolecular therapeutics: A review. *J. Control. Release* **2000**, *65*, 271–284. [CrossRef]
23. Lardenoye, J.H.; de Vries, M.R.; Lowik, C.W.; Xu, Q.; Dhore, C.R.; Cleutjens, J.P.; van Hinsbergh, V.W.; van Bockel, J.H.; Quax, P.H. Accelerated Atherosclerosis and Calcification in Vein Grafts: A Study in Apoe*3 Leiden Transgenic Mice. *Circ. Res.* **2002**, *7*, 577–584. [CrossRef] [PubMed]

Publisher's Note: MDPI stays neutral with regard to jurisdictional claims in published maps and institutional affiliations.

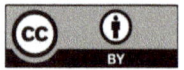

© 2020 by the authors. Licensee MDPI, Basel, Switzerland. This article is an open access article distributed under the terms and conditions of the Creative Commons Attribution (CC BY) license (http://creativecommons.org/licenses/by/4.0/).

MDPI
St. Alban-Anlage 66
4052 Basel
Switzerland
Tel. +41 61 683 77 34
Fax +41 61 302 89 18
www.mdpi.com

International Journal of Molecular Sciences Editorial Office
E-mail: ijms@mdpi.com
www.mdpi.com/journal/ijms

www.ingramcontent.com/pod-product-compliance
Lightning Source LLC
LaVergne TN
LVHW070413100526
838202LV00014B/1451